# Men'sHealth®

# TOTAL
# FITNESS
# GUIDE
# 2008

# Men'sHealth.
# TOTAL FITNESS GUIDE 2008

RODALE

© 2008 by Rodale Inc.

All rights reserved. No part of this publication may be reproduced or transmitted in any form or by any means, electronic or mechanical, including photocopying, recording, or any other information storage and retrieval system, without the written permission of the publisher.

*Men's Health* is a registered trademark of Rodale Inc.

Printed in the United States of America

Rodale Inc. makes every effort to use acid-free ∞, recycled paper ♻.

ISBN 13: 978–1–59586–697–5

ISBN 10: 1–59486–697–X

Book design by Susan Eugster

2   4   6   8   10   9   7   5   3      hardcover

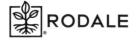

**RODALE**

WE **INSPIRE** AND **ENABLE** PEOPLE TO IMPROVE
THEIR LIVES AND THE WORLD AROUND THEM

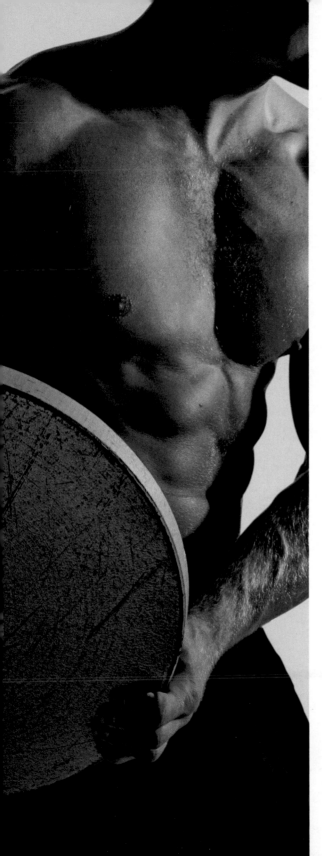

# Contents

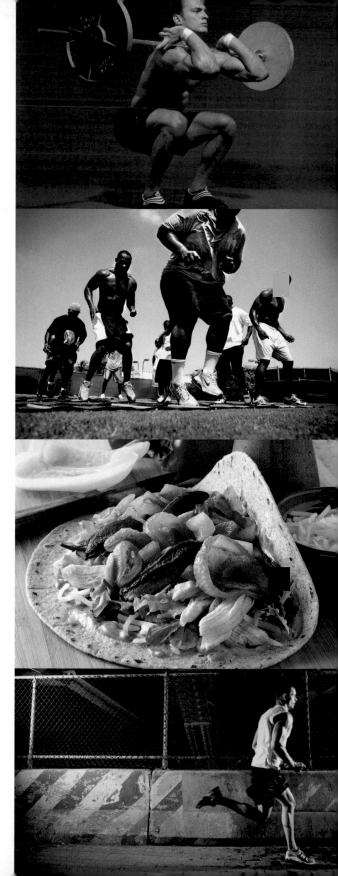

# Introduction

**W**ant to change your life? There's no better way than to change your body.

But don't make an idle promise to yourself. Each year, 40 percent of guys tell themselves, "I'm going to get back in shape"—five or more times! And then they do little to change. It's a safe bet that if you keep on doing what you're doing, you're going to keep on getting what you're getting.

You can change all that with the book you're holding in your hands. It's the ultimate guide to your fitness. We interviewed dozens of experts to put together this collection of the best fitness advice out there.

Perhaps the first thing you need to do is drop some pounds. That's why we begin the book with the Lose Weight section. Our simple plan will show you how to drop 30 pounds of your deadweight in just 3 months. Next, you'll learn why losing your gut is critical for getting glances on the beach but also for adding years to your life and life to your years. And we have the belly-busting workout to help you get there in less than 30 minutes, three times a week. Then, use our total-body workout to get leaner than ever. To fuel all of this activity, you need to eat right. So we offer a plan to shop once and eat all week. You'll enjoy 10 simple-to-make

meals that build muscle, fight fat, save time, and cost half as much as eating out.

Because we don't know anyone who has time to spare, the second section of the book, Get Fit, aims at getting you fit—fast. First, you'll rebuild your entire body with our three-step plan. Then, following the examples of five of the world's best athletes, you'll unleash your faster, stronger self to become a force to be reckoned with. Plus, you'll get a glimpse inside the NFL's secret training camp to steal their best muscle, speed, and agility workouts.

In the third part of the book, Muscle Up, we tackle the topic of building more muscle. You'll experience the greatest workout known to man using the power of Olympic weight lifting. With our four-step lifting plan, you'll transform your workout—and your body. Is poor posture ruining your workout? You didn't know it could? In this section, you'll learn how to get it straight and build a better body. And to improve that ultimate measure of a man, the bench press, you'll learn from a master how to press twice as much as you do now—in less than 60 days.

Part Four helps you tackle and improve troublesome parts. Spot Train offers advice on building your abs, back, chest, arms, shoulders, and more. First, we offer the greatest abs workout ever: Chisel them in just 24 minutes a day. Then, build a bigger, stronger back with our workout that delivers the ultimate upper body. Next, sculpt a powerful chest. After that, you can add 2 inches to your arms in just 24 minutes a workout. Finally, build the rock-solid shoulders you want—in the time that you have. And more.

Take it outdoors with our fifth section, Run Fast. Here you'll read the story of one runner's quest to discover what really matters as he runs across the Sahara. You'll learn how to train for and run your first race—no doubt slimming down, beating stress, and rewarding yourself with a huge dose of satisfaction in the process. Next, you'll find a troubleshooter's guide to the hazards of the road and learn how to stay safe from SUVs, dogs, knee pain, blisters, and lightning. You'll shore up your weak links by focusing on five things that wreck your form and learning the running rehab to fix them. Then, you'll change your leg workout with the best exercise you're not doing—the single-leg squat.

In the last part of this book, Have Fun, we talk about all things sports. One of the top trainers in college sports offers advice on how to build a bigger, stronger, faster body. Is skiing or snowboarding your thing? Learn how to build some muscle in order to shred the slopes this winter. To shrink your golf handicap, start working out like the pros. You'll unleash your golfing power and add 30 yards to your drive. Then, because nothing knocks a guy onto the bench faster than a bum knee, we discuss how to get a handle on knee problems and get back in the game.

This book is filled with information and advice to help you make hundreds of positive changes. Sometimes change can be scary. Sometimes change can be hard. But in this case—when you're talking about your health, your body, your life—change is good.

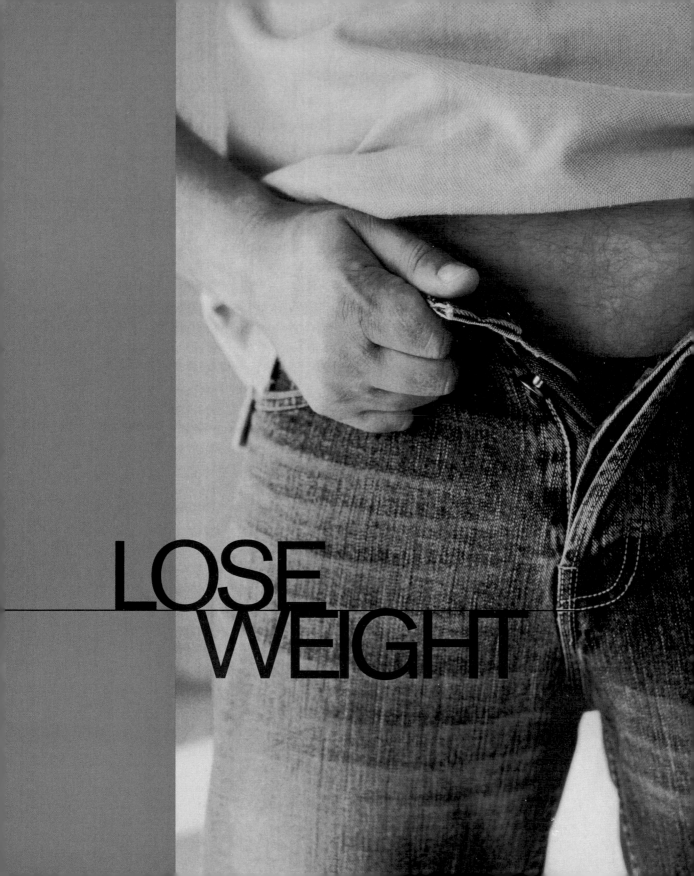

LOSE
WEIGHT

Each year, 59 million Americans resolve to lose weight. That's one in five of us. Unfortunately, since one in three of us is overweight and another one in three is obese, that's probably not enough. If you don't find yourself in the third of Americans at their ideal weight, at least you have a lot of company.

And you've come to the right place. In the pages that follow, you'll pick up hundreds of tips and tricks from experts on losing weight. First, our simple action plan will show you how to lose 30 pounds in just 3 months. Next, you'll learn why losing your gut is not only imperative for getting appreciative glances on the beach but also for adding years to your life. And we have the belly-busting workout to help you get there in less than 30 minutes, three times a week. Then, our total-body workout will leave you leaner than ever. To fuel all of this, we offer a plan to shop once and eat right all week. You'll enjoy 10 simple-to-make meals that fight fat, build muscle, save time, and cost less than $50.

Losing weight probably won't be easy. But it's a change that will have an enormous impact on your looks and on your life.

ESSENTIAL READING

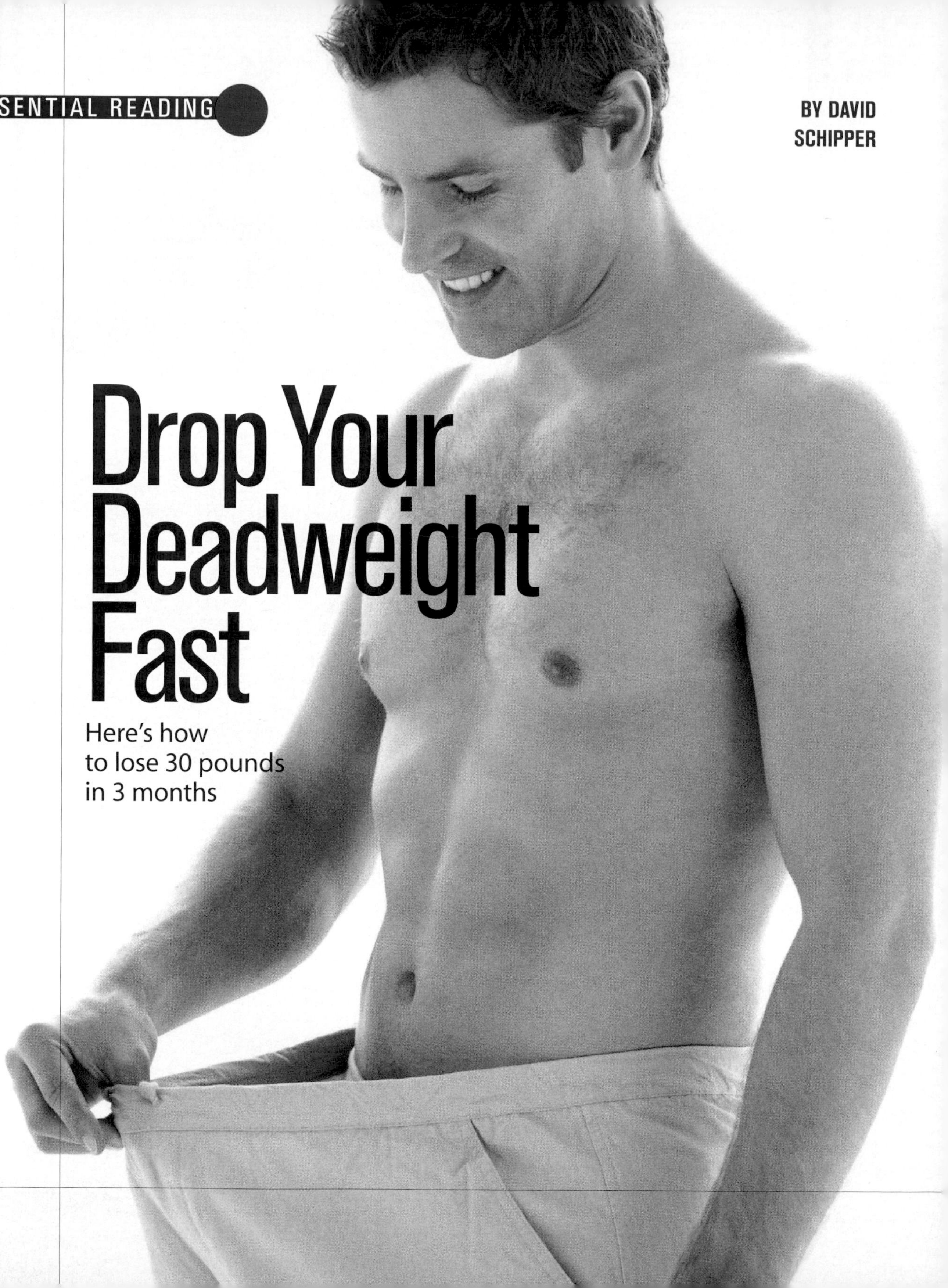

BY DAVID SCHIPPER

# Drop Your Deadweight Fast

Here's how to lose 30 pounds in 3 months

**T**hree months before my wedding, I had a realization: I didn't want to be a fat groom. After all, a cummerbund can only help so much.

And besides, what kind of man would marry a beautiful woman knowing he's going to die young?

That's not hyperbole. My 5'9" frame tipped the scales at 231 pounds, easily qualifying me as obese—a designation that advanced my biological age of 26 by 2 decades, according to a UCLA study.

More disturbing, a blood test showed that I was on the verge of diabetes, despite having no obvious symptoms (other than a bulging belly). For the first time, being fat felt irresponsible.

But dramatic change doesn't take as long as you might think. In 12 weeks, I lost 33 pounds and whittled 5 inches off my waist— just in time for our big day. And, even better, my latest blood work came back nearly normal. How'd I do it? Keep reading.

## The Tipping Point

Like most overweight men, I wasn't proud of carrying around all that extra flab— especially since I'm an editor at *Men's Health*. But it wasn't until I literally feared for my life that I became fully committed to change. That day arrived when I met with Keith Berkowitz, MD, medical director of the Center for Balanced Health in New York City. His specialty: turning the obese thin.

When I showed up at his office, Dr. Berkowitz first analyzed a blood test I'd had done in preparation for our meeting. My

triglycerides (a measure of the fat circulating in my bloodstream) were more than double what's considered normal. I was also insulin resistant. That means my body had to produce 10 times the amount of insulin—a

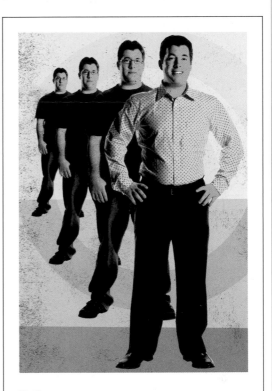

**Before**
Weight: 231 pounds
Waist: 42 inches
Blood pressure: 125/80
Triglycerides: 328
Resting heart rate: 84

**After**
Weight: 198 pounds
Waist: 37 inches
Blood pressure: 116/70
Triglycerides: 161
Resting heart rate: 72

## A Day on the Diet

You don't have to starve yourself to lose weight fast. Here's a snapshot of what I consumed in a typical day. (Not shown: the total amount of water I drank.) Because each meal was packed with protein and fat, I never felt hungry, even though my overall calorie intake was far lower than before I started the plan.

### 7 a.m.: Breakfast
    3 scrambled eggs
    Large bowl of cantaloupe
    8 ounces green tea

### Noon: Lunch
    Large salad of lettuce, cucumbers, and green peppers, topped with 6 ounces tuna mixed with mayonnaise
    16 ounces water

### 3 p.m.: Snack
    Quarter-pound hamburger, no bun
    2 ounces string cheese
    Diet soda

### 6:30 p.m.: Dinner
    8 ounces salmon fillet
    2 servings steamed broccoli
    Bowl of cucumbers
    16 ounces water

hormone that signals your body to store fat—normally secreted by a healthy guy my age. Both of these measurements are key predictors of future heart disease. Can you say "instant motivation"?

Chances are, if you're overweight, your blood work may look similar. Research shows that heavier men have higher choles-terol, triglycerides, and blood pressure than their leaner counterparts. And, according to Dr. Berkowitz, almost half of the population is insulin resistant. The most telling physical sign: abdominal fat. Still need a kick in the pants? Ask your physician for a complete blood profile; fear is a great motivator.

## The Action Plan

Much to my horror, Dr. Berkowitz recommended a "controlled-carbohydrate diet." That doesn't mean cutting out carbohydrates altogether. Rather, you restrict the types that significantly raise your blood sugar and thus your insulin levels, such as those found in soda, candy, and foods made with flour, which happen to be the carbs I like the most. And, surprisingly, my don't-eat list even included whole grains at first. The reason? Although healthy for men with normal insulin function, whole grains still raise insulin levels. For me, that made them a food to avoid until I lost weight and saw improvements in my blood work, at which time I could add them back slowly in the form of high-fiber crackers or flaxseed bread. (See "Your Flex Plan" on page 7.)

The upshot is that this plan limited my carbs to those found in vegetables and fruit, which was a drastic change from my regular carbohydrate-laden diet. It meant I had to give up Entenmann's night. (I'll leave the menu to your imagination.) So I wasn't sure I could stick with it.

Enter Valerie Berkowitz. While Keith

# Super Substitutions

I consider myself a sandwich connoisseur. So when I started this diet, I was concerned about eliminating bread, along with crunchy snack foods like chips. But my 3-month stint wasn't hard time. In fact, I enjoyed it. And these foods are the reason.

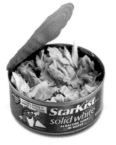

**Baked cheese:** It crunches like chips. Place slices of your favorite cheese on a baking sheet, pop them in an oven preheated to 350°F, and bake for 5 to 6 minutes, or until light brown, then let them cool.

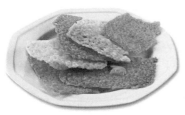

**Tuna:** I used it for small meals and as a substitute for salad dressing. A salad topping

of tuna mixed with mayonnaise is a great alternative to bottled dressing, which is low in protein or lacks it altogether.

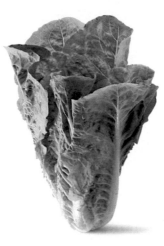

**Romaine lettuce:** You can jam everything from turkey to whitefish salad—which I buy at the deli counter—into one leaf, roll it up, and eat. Does it taste like a real sandwich? No. It might taste better.

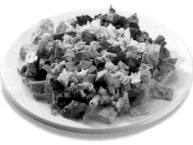

**A big salad:** Load it with ham, turkey, and chicken, and

it'll have more meat in it than most sandwiches—and, of course, far more vegetables. Try dressing it with blue cheese or oil and vinegar, both of which are carb-free.

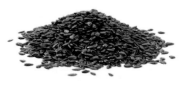

**Flaxseed:** It's not only healthy, it's a great pseudo-breading. Sprinkle 2 teaspoons over a cooked piece of salmon or chicken breast for added flavor and texture.

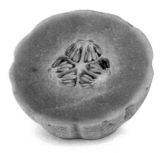

**Melons:** Cantaloupe and honeydew provide slow-digesting carbs that help assuage the craving for bread. Plus, the sweetness of a fresh scoop seems like dessert after you've cut out candy and baked goods.

## The Gut-Busting Workout

Finish off the flab with this full-body fat-burning routine from Michael Mejia, CSCS, author of *The Better Body Blueprint*. It's designed to speed your results and improve your fitness, while protecting your hard-earned muscle—all in just 3 days a week.

### How to Do It

**Warmup:** Before each workout, warm up with 5 minutes of light aerobic exercise or calisthenics.

**Weight training:** Do the weight workout that follows 3 days a week, resting at least a day after each session. Perform the exercises as a circuit, completing one set of 10 to 12 repetitions of each movement before resting for 60 seconds. Then repeat the entire sequence once or twice, for a total of two or three circuits. Every other workout, reverse the order in which you do the exercises. So in one session, you'll start with the overhead squat, and the next you'll begin with the pushup.

1. Overhead squat
2. Pushup-position row
3. Lying hip extension
4. Lat pulldown
5. Russian twist
6. Pushup

**Cardio:** After each weight-training session, finish up with 12 to 15 minutes of aerobic exercise—running, cycling, rowing—using an intensity that you judge to be a 7 or 8 on a 10-point scale.

Berkowitz served as general manager of my diet, his wife, Valerie—a registered dietitian and director of nutrition at the Center for Balanced Health—took the job of head coach. She helped me create an eating plan that was user-friendly and required no calorie counting. Basically, my instructions were to eat only when hungry and to the point of fullness, incorporating the five simple rules that follow. I could eat as much meat and vegetables as I wanted, and I was allowed 3 to 5 ounces of cheese and two servings daily of low-glycemic fruits—berries, melons, peaches, plums, apples, oranges, and kiwifruit.

I was also advised to drink 80 ounces of water daily. Use these guidelines, and you, too, can lose 30 pounds in 3 months.

## 1. Cut Out Fast-Digesting Carbs

For the most part, these are foods that are made with sugar or are high in starch, such as bread, pasta, any other flour-based food, potatoes, and rice. Because they all contain high amounts of glucose, they raise blood sugar quickly. "This is the trigger that signals your body to release a flood of insulin," says Valerie. Eliminate these foods, and insulin levels stay near rock bottom, which simultaneously improves your health and speeds fat loss. In fact, when University of Connecticut researchers analyzed why low-carb dieters were so successful, they calculated that 70 percent of their weight loss stemmed from low insulin levels. (One note: Because milk has a significant number of carbohydrates, it was also off-limits until my blood profile showed I was healthier.)

## 2. Eat More Vegetables

This may be the ultimate diet cliché, but there's no question it works. In fact, a study of more than 2,000 low-carb dieters found that, on average, the biggest losers were consuming four servings of nonstarchy vegetables a day. That's virtually any vegetable of your choice other than potatoes (white, sweet, or fried), carrots, and corn. "Eating more produce increases the amount of fiber in your diet, which helps keep you full," says Valerie. For an even greater fiber boost, I added a daily glass of Metamucil (the sugar-free version). If you've never taken Metamucil, its effectiveness in reducing your appetite is nothing short of amazing.

## 3. Have Protein at Every Meal

This is especially important at breakfast and with snacks, when guys are most likely to skimp on this muscle-building nutrient. (Thanks a lot, cereal.) Case in point: University of Illinois scientists report that, on average, people consume 65 percent of their protein after 6 p.m. More important, the researchers found that to optimally preserve your muscle as you lose weight, you need to take in protein at each meal throughout the day. "Besides nourishing your muscles, the added protein will help keep you from overeating," says Valerie. The best sources are beef, chicken, fish, dairy, and eggs.

## 4. Don't Be Afraid of Natural Fat

That's right, the kind that's found in a piece of meat, an omelet, an avocado, olives, or olive oil–based dressing. Because fat alone doesn't raise your insulin levels, it has little to do with making you fat, contrary to popular opinion, says Valerie. High amounts of carbs coupled with high amounts of fat are the real culprits, she explains, because

## Your Flex Plan

After 6 weeks, you can add a limited amount of whole grains back into your diet. The key is to monitor your weight to ensure that the grains don't slow fat loss. To start, trade one serving of fruit for any of these items.

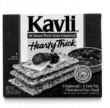

**Two Kavli Hearty Thick crispbread:** These nutty Norwegian slices with 7.5 grams carbs each can be found online at www.germandeli.com.

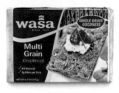

**Two Wasa crackers:** Packed with whole grains and fiber, these Swedish flat crackers are sold in your supermarket's organic or deli section and at www.amazon.com.

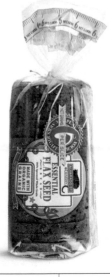

**Two slices of Alvarado Street Essential Flax Seed Bread:** Each slice contains just 7.5 grams of carbohydrates, about 60 percent of the amount in regular bread. Find it at www.alvaradostreetbakery.com.

they stimulate the release of insulin, causing your body to store fat instead of burn it. But what about heart health? In a review of 13 studies published in the *Journal of Nutrition*, researchers determined that low-carbohydrate diets—all of which provided at least 50 percent of daily calories from fat—were more effective at reducing heart-disease risk than traditional low-fat diets.

### 5. Forget about Processed Foods

Prediet, I lived on lunchmeat. But Valerie nixed these packaged meats quickly because most contain added salt (affecting weight and blood pressure) and sugar, as well as nitrates, which are associated with an increased risk of cancer. Instead, I ate ground beef and ground turkey. (Both take only a few minutes to cook at night and taste great cold the following day.) I did slip up, though. On my 15th day on the program, I discovered Terra vegetable chips. "A delicious potpourri of exotic vegetables," the bag says. Sounded healthy to me, so I crunched on them hard during long days at work. A week later, when I told Valerie about my new favorite addiction, a sharp scolding followed. I'd been suckered by the word *vegetable*. These chips are made from starchy root vegetables, so their carbohydrate count is similar to that of potato chips, and they're loaded with salt. The scale reflected my mistake. If you follow only one rule, make it this: If it comes in a box or a bag, skip it. I guarantee you'll have success.

BY CASSANDRA FORSYTHE AND ADAM CAMPBELL

# Nutrition Fiction

Read beyond the marketing hype and
avoid the dirty-dozen "health" foods

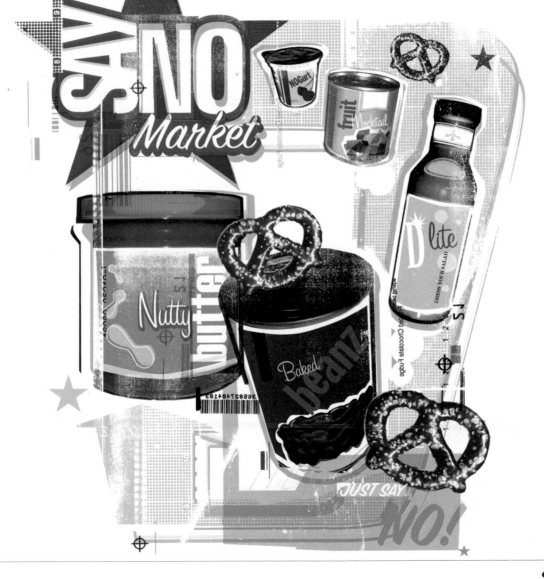

**T**ake a moment and consider this logic: 1. Fat-free foods are healthy. 2. Skittles are fat-free. 3. Therefore, Skittles are healthy. Make sense? Of course not. But it's exactly the type of reasoning that food manufacturers want you to use.

You see, in our example, we started with a false premise. That's because the term "fat-free" is often code for "high-sugar"—an attribute that makes a product the opposite of healthy. Case in point: Johns Hopkins University researchers recently determined that high blood sugar is an independent risk factor for heart disease. So high-glycemic foods—those such as sugars and starches that raise your blood sugar dramatically—are inherently unhealthy. (See Skittles, above.)

Unfortunately, faulty food logic is far less obvious when you're shopping outside the candy aisle. Why? Because making healthy choices isn't as simple as knowing that beans are packed with fiber, or that fruits are loaded with disease-fighting antioxidants. After all, manufacturers often add ingredients, such as sugar, that can instantly turn a good snack bad. As a result, many of the products that you think are wholesome are anything but. And that's why we've created

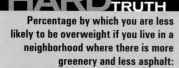

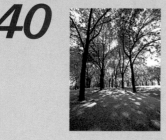

our list of the dirty dozen: 12 "healthy" foods that you can—and should—live without.

## Yogurt with Fruit at the Bottom

**The upside:** Yogurt and fruit are two of the healthiest foods known to man.

**The downside:** Corn syrup is not. But that's exactly what's used to make these products super sweet. For example, a cup of Colombo blueberry yogurt contains 36 grams of sugar, only about half of which is found naturally in the yogurt and fruit. The rest comes in the form of "added" sugar—or what we prefer to call "unnecessary."

**The healthy alternative:** Opt for Dannon Light 'n Fit Carb & Sugar Control Yogurt, which has 90 percent less sugar than regular yogurt.

## Baked Beans

**The upside:** Beans are packed with fiber, which helps keep you full and slows the absorption of sugar into your bloodstream.

**The downside:** The baked kind are typically covered in a sauce made with brown and white sugars. And because the fiber is located inside the bean, it doesn't have a chance to interfere with the speed at which the sugary glaze is digested. Consider that 1 cup of baked beans contains 24 grams of sugar: That's about the same amount in 8 ounces of regular soda.

**The healthy alternative:** Red kidney beans, packed in water. You get the nutritional benefits of legumes, but without the extra sugar. They don't even need to be heated: Just open the can, rinse thoroughly, and serve. Try splashing some hot sauce on top for a spicy variation.

## California Roll

**The upside:** The seaweed it's wrapped in contains essential nutrients, such as iodine, selenium, calcium, and omega-3 fats.

**The downside:** It's basically a Japanese sugar cube. That's because its two other major components are white rice and imitation crab, both of which are packed with fast-digesting carbohydrates and almost no protein.

**The healthy alternative:** Real sushi made with tuna or salmon. These varieties have fewer bad carbohydrates, while providing a hefty helping of high-quality protein. Better yet, skip the rice, too, by ordering sashimi.

## Granola Bars

**The upside:** Granola is made with whole oats, a nutritious food that's high in fiber.

**The downside:** The oats are basically glued together with ingredients such as high-fructose corn syrup, honey, and barley malt—all of which quickly raise blood sugar.

**The healthy alternative:** Grab a low-sugar meal replacement bar that contains no more than 5 grams of net carbs—those are the ones that affect blood sugar—and at least 15 grams of protein. We like Myoplex Carb Sense.

## Pasta Salad

**The upside:** Most pasta-salad recipes include a variety of fresh vegetables.

## The Cheater's Diet

Don't count out Atkins just yet: Cutting back on carbs may help you burn more fat during exercise. In a recent study, Australian researchers fed trained cyclists a low-carbohydrate diet for 5 out of 6 days. On another occasion, the cyclists followed a high-carbohydrate diet for all 6 days. When the cyclists exercised on day 7, the scientists found they burned 45 percent more fat after their low-carbohydrate week of eating. Credit the boost in fat burning to an improved ability of the muscles to extract energy from fat stores on a low-carb diet, says Jeff Volek, PhD, RD, an exercise-and-diet researcher at the University of Connecticut. The bottom line: If you're exercising regularly and eating a low-carbohydrate diet, give yourself license to "cheat" once a week; you'll keep burning fat and may be more likely to stick with your diet. Surprising health news, too: A new review in the *Journal of Nutrition* found that since 2003, all 13 studies comparing low-carbohydrate and low-fat diets reported that low-carb eating was superior to the low-fat approach in reducing heart-disease risk factors.

**The downside:** The main ingredient is white-flour pasta, a close relative of white bread.

**The healthy alternative:** Egg salad has no impact on blood sugar, and a University of Connecticut review reports that there is no connection between egg consumption and heart disease.

## English Muffins

**The upside:** One English muffin—two halves—has half as many calories as two slices of bread. So it's better for a breakfast sandwich.

**The downside:** Most English muffins not only raise blood sugar significantly but are nearly devoid of fiber, protein, and vitamins. This makes them a great example of a food that provides only empty calories.

**The healthy alternative:** One hundred percent whole-wheat English muffins are a decent start, but we like the kind made from sprouted grains, which contain no flour and are packed with nutrients. For instance, Food for Life sprouted-grain English muffins have twice as much fiber and 30 percent more protein compared with the typical 100 percent whole-wheat version. (For stores, check www.foodforlife.com.)

## Croutons

**The upside:** They're so small they contribute very few calories to your overall meal, yet they add a satisfying crunch.

**The downside:** Most croutons are made with the same refined flour that's used in white bread, a food with a higher glycemic index than sugar.

**The healthy alternative:** Sliced roasted almonds. They're crunchy, sugar-free, and high in monounsaturated fats, the same type of healthy fats found in olive oil. In fact, Harvard University researchers estimate that substituting nuts for an equivalent amount

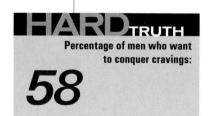

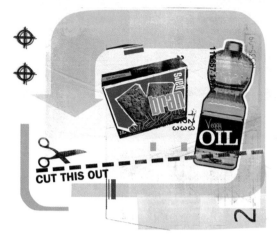

CUT THIS OUT

of carbohydrates results in a 30 percent reduction in heart-disease risk.

## Fat-Free Salad Dressing

**The upside:** Cutting out the fat reduces the calories that a dressing contains.

**The downside:** Sugar is added to provide flavor. But perhaps more important is that the removal of fat reduces your body's ability to absorb many of the vitamins found in a salad's vegetables. Ohio State University researchers discovered that people who ate a salad dressing that contained fat absorbed 15 times more beta-carotene and five times more lutein—both powerful antioxidants—than when they downed a salad topped with fat-free dressing.

**The healthy alternative:** Choose a full-fat dressing that's made with either olive oil or canola oil and has less than 2 grams of carbs per serving.

## Fruit Cocktail

**The upside:** The main ingredient is fruit.

**The downside:** If you don't read the label closely, you may choose a brand that's packed in heavy syrup. For instance, a $1/2$-cup serving of syrupy fruit cocktail contains 23 grams of added sugar.

**The healthy alternative:** Look for fruit cocktail canned in "100 percent juice," not syrup.

## Reduced-Fat Peanut Butter

**The upside:** Even the reduced-fat versions pack a substantial quantity of heart-healthy monounsaturated fat.

**The downside:** Many commercial brands are sweetened with "icing sugar"—the same finely ground sugar used to decorate cupcakes. In fact, each tablespoon of Skippy contains a half teaspoon of the sweet stuff. Reduced-fat versions are the worst of all, because they contain less healthy fat and even more icing sugar.

**The healthy alternative:** An all-natural, full-fat peanut butter—such as Crazy Richard's or Teddy's—that contains no added sugar.

## Pretzels

**The upside:** One ounce has just 110 calories.

**The downside:** These twisted low-fat snacks have one of the highest glycemic indexes of any food. In fact, they rank above ice cream and jelly beans in their ability to raise blood sugar.

**The healthy alternative:** Cheese crisps—baked pieces of cheese that crunch like chips.

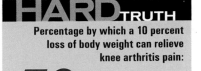

**HARD**TRUTH

Percentage by which a 10 percent loss of body weight can relieve knee arthritis pain:

**50**

## Corn Oil

**The upside:** It contains omega-6 fatty acids—unsaturated fats that don't raise cholesterol.

**The downside:** Corn oil has 60 times more omega-6s than omega-3s, the type of healthy fats found in fish, walnuts, and flaxseed. Studies suggest that a high intake of omega-6 fats relative to omega-3 fats increases inflammation, which boosts your risk of cancer, arthritis, and obesity.

**The healthy alternative:** Olive or canola oils, which have a far better ratio of omega-6s to omega-3s.

BY JOHN BERARDI, PhD, CSCS

# The Metabolism Advantage Exercise Plan

Incinerate 500 to 1,000 daily
calories with these moves

When Alex first came to me, he was carrying 180 pounds on his 5'6" frame. He had been chubby since childhood and had gained more weight during and after college.

He ran 2 miles a day and ate almost nothing, yet he couldn't get his weight to budge. At 30 percent fat, the 23 year old was officially considered obese. I put Alex on the exercise program you'll find in this chapter. In just 8 weeks, he dropped 19 pounds of fat and gained 12 pounds of lean mass, lowering his body fat to 20 percent. He accomplished all of this while eating 500 to 700 *additional* daily calories. Here's how Alex burned off his blubber—and how you will do the same.

>> **During exercise:** The Metabolism Advantage exercise plan includes three 60-minute strength-training sessions and three 30-minute cardio sessions each week. This amount of exercise will burn roughly 300 to 600 calories per day during your workouts.

>> **After exercise:** Because of the intensity of the Metabolism Advantage workouts, your body will continue to burn calories at a higher rate after you leave the gym. After your weight-training sessions, for example, your muscles will restock fuel and repair proteins for roughly 12 to 24 hours, elevating your metabolism by anywhere from 5 to 10 percent. Finally, research shows that intense weightlifting and cardio boosts the calories your body burns to digest food at your next meal by as much as 73 percent. All told, you can

expect to burn an additional 100 to 200 calories per day due to this afterburn.

>> **All day long:** Your weight-training sessions will build larger, stronger muscle fibers that must gobble up more calories to maintain themselves. All the organs in your body burn calories both to conduct their daily functions and to renew themselves. Your muscles are no exception. The more muscle you have, the faster your metabolism runs. On the Metabolism Advantage plan, you can expect to increase your resting metabolism by 7 percent or more. As long as you stick with the program, this boost is permanent, allowing you to burn up to 100 to 200 additional calories per day.

The Metabolism Advantage exercise plan will boost calorie burning by 500 to 1,000 calories daily during your workouts, after your workouts, and all day long.

No matter how much you currently exercise—ranging from not at all to hours a day—the Metabolism Advantage exercise plan can take you from a sluggish metabolism to a speedy one. The program will help reverse the age-related drop in metabolism caused by either inactivity or the wrong types of activity. Indeed, you can exercise—even exercise a lot—and still have a slow metabolism. In order to speed up things, you must do the right types and right amounts of exercise.

## Metabolism-Boosting Exercise

The prevalence of best-selling diet books that promise fantastic results in just 8 minutes a day or less has led me to this conclusion: Many people want results, but they don't want to put in the time needed to get those results. I won't sugarcoat things for you. To speed up your metabolism in a permanent way, you have to spend some serious time in the gym. According to piles and piles of well-conducted scientific studies, you must do the following in order to boost metabolism and shed fat.

**Exercise for at least 5 hours a week.** Research from the University of Wyoming clearly demonstrates that it takes at least 5 hours a week to see real body composition results. In this survey of more than 1,000 people, researchers concluded that people who work out for less than 5 hours a week tend to be unhappy with the way they look and feel. On the other hand, people who work out for more than 5 hours a week tend to be happy with the way they look and feel. According to scientifically based U.S. government guidelines, you must exercise for 30 minutes a day to improve your health and 60 minutes a day to burn fat. In research conducted on weight gainers and maintainers, maintainers spent 80 minutes or more per day exercising, whereas gainers spent 20 minutes or less.

Because of that research and more, the Metabolism Advantage exercise plan includes six weekly workouts that add up to roughly 5 hours of exercise a week. Now if you're doing no exercise at the moment, that may seem like a heck of a lot of time. Let's put things in perspective. When you con-sider that the average North American watches about 28 hours of television per week (that's right, 28), finding 5 hours to exercise shouldn't seem so problematic. Just turn off *COPS*, Spike TV's James Bond-a-thon, or the current race on Speedvision, put on your sneaks, and get to the gym!

I don't want to hear any grumbling about your demanding job or busy home life. No matter what your current schedule, you can succeed on this program. How do I know? I've seen all types of people of all ages, from 30-year-old professionals to 60-year-old empty nesters, fit these workouts into their lives. To date, I have not met a client who was too busy to make this program work. Finding time to exercise is a mindset. Do you want to lose fat, gain muscle, and boost your metabolism 24 hours a day? Then commit yourself to this program, put your workouts on the calendar, and make them nonnegotiable.

**Make every workout count.** To maximize your afterburn and your resting metabolic rate (RMR), you'll focus on intense strengthening and cardio workouts. In the weight room, at least once a week, you'll lift weights that are heavy enough to completely fatigue your muscles within 5 to 7 repetitions. This high-resistance, low-repetition method will target the maximum number of muscle fibers in each workout. The more muscle fibers you fatigue *during* your workout, the more your body must repair *after* your workout, maximizing your afterburn. The same is true of cardio. The Metabolism

Advantage cardio plan prescribes interval training. In these high-intensity workouts, you'll alternate between surges of fast-paced cardio, which boost your heart rate above 90 percent of your maximum, and a slower recovery pace. Studies show that this type of intense cardio revs up your metabolism not only during your workout but also for many hours afterward.

**Give your body time to recover.** To build a faster metabolism, you must build bigger muscles. To build bigger muscles, you must apply the principles of the stress-recovery cycle. You stress your muscles during your weight-training and cardio workouts, then you rest them, giving them time to recover. During this recovery phase, your muscles restock their fuel stores, repair microtrauma, and replace protein. If you stress and stress and stress your muscles and provide no recovery time, you hinder your results and may even end up overtrained, a condition that may even *slow* your metabolism. So, no matter how gung-ho you are, resist the urge to earn extra credit by sneaking in extra workouts!

During the first 8 weeks of the main Metabolism Advantage plan, you'll take off 1 day each week, giving your body the downtime it needs to repair itself. (In subsequent weeks or in alternate plans, you may take off an additional day.) Through upper-body, lower-body, and total-body sessions, you'll also strength train each major muscle group just twice a week. This provides the stimulus your muscles need to grow as well as the rest they need to repair themselves. You must always give your muscles the rest they need.

**Change your program every 4 weeks.** No matter how intense your workouts, if you do the same type of exercises week after week, your body may adapt to those exercises, and your results may plateau. As with any other stressor (exercise is a stressor, you know—a good one, but a stressor nonetheless), the body adapts to all demands placed upon it. Therefore, to prevent it from adapting too well to the program (thereby leaving you stalled out and making no further progress), the Metabolism Advantage plan changes every 4 weeks.

During weeks 1 through 4, you'll repeatedly complete three strength-training workouts: one for the upper body, one for the lower body, and one total-body session. During this time, you'll adapt to these movements. As you gain strength, you'll lift heavier weights. By week 4, however, these workouts will become as familiar to you as your morning commute. So, to maximize afterburn, you'll challenge your muscles— and mind—with a completely new set of moves. For the same reason, your cardio workouts will change as well.

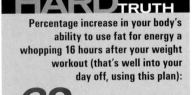

**HARD TRUTH**

Percentage increase in your body's ability to use fat for energy a whopping 16 hours after your weight workout (that's well into your day off, using this plan):

**62**

**Be flexible.** In the following pages, you'll find one way to execute the Metabolism Advantage exercise plan. I'd be oversimplifying things, however, if I told you it was the only way. As long as you follow the principles of the plan—by completing intense workouts, giving your body time to recover, and changing your program every 4 weeks—you can easily customize it to your personal goals and lifestyle and still reap the results. In fact, doing so will increase your success. When you design a program that fits your lifestyle, you increase your odds of sticking with it!

## Metabolism Advantage Strength Training

Whether you're young or old, strength training is critical to your metabolism and overall well-being. Even if you're in your nineties, regular strength training can triple your strength.

If you do only cardio and no strength training, you can expect to lose strength, gain fat, struggle with lower-back pain, and eventually become more reliant on others for physical tasks. Balance the right types of cardio workouts with the right type of strength training, however, and you can expect to build and preserve muscle as you age and remain lean, strong, and injury-free.

When you lift weights, you challenge your muscles to do something they are unaccustomed to doing. Lifting damages muscle fibers, creating areas of dead and dying tissue. Your immune system then sends in specialized cells called leukocytes and macrophages to break down both the damaged tissue and some healthy tissue.

Although this sounds like a bad thing, it's not. Once the leukocytes and macrophages finish their demolition duty, more immune cells rush in. These create new, thicker, stronger proteins to replace the proteins that the leukocytes and macrophages just destroyed and hauled away.

Think of your immune cells as construction workers who have been hired to repair a hurricane-ravaged house. They tear off the roof and other damaged structures and then nail on new shingles and other materials, creating a stronger house able to withstand higher-force winds. During their demolition and construction work, these workers burn a lot of calories.

It's the same with your immune cells. During the 24 hours after your workout, these busy cells elevate your metabolism by 5 to 10 percent. The bigger you are, the more muscle you damage during a workout, giving you an even greater afterburn.

These bigger, stronger muscle fibers increase your metabolism 24 hours a day. All tissues in your body—including your muscles—go through a regular program of turnover. You may be familiar with skin turnover, for example. Every day, old skin flakes off, and new skin forms underneath it. Every organ in your body goes through this process, which gobbles up a great number of calories. You can't do much to speed up the turnover rates of most of your organs, but you *can* increase the turnover rate of your muscles. The more muscle you have, the more muscle cells your body must continually recycle. As I've mentioned, 1 extra pound of muscle burns up to 50 extra calories a day. Add 5 pounds of tight, lean muscle, and you'll boost your body's energy needs by 250 calories per day.

For optimal results, you'll do the following on the Metabolism Advantage plan.

**Mix high-intensity with moderate-intensity lifting.** You've probably heard at least three theories about how much weight and how many repetitions you should complete when weightlifting. Guys who are after big muscle will tell you to do heavy weights and low reps. Some exercise physiologists recommend the standard 10 to 12 reps. And some personal trainers tell women to do 15 or more reps to tone rather than bulk. Who's right? As it turns out, no one.

To boost your metabolism to the max, you need to perform a combination of high-intensity, low-repetition training and moderate-intensity, moderate-weight training. This varied approach will ensure that you target all of your muscle fibers, boosting your afterburn and overall metabolism.

Typical strength-training plans that tell you to lift a weight 8, 10, or 15 times target predominantly type I and IIa fibers. When you weight train, these fibers attempt to shoulder the load. Type IIb fibers, a third type, are difficult to target, but seeking them out is well worth the effort. If you work only your type I and type IIa fibers, you leave roughly a third of your muscle fibers untrained. This reduces your burn during and after your workout and prevents you from maximizing your RMR.

To work and break down type IIb fibers, you need to lift a weight that's heavy enough to fatigue the muscle you are working in 5 to 7 reps. (Some programs targeting IIb fibers recommend working in the 1-to-3-rep range as well.) That's why, during two of your weekly weight workouts on the main Metabolism Advantage program, you'll try to reach muscle failure within 5 to 7 repetitions. In other words, you will choose a weight that you can lift no more than seven times. If you tried to bang out another rep, you wouldn't be able to lift the bar. This type of weightlifting will help to target all of your muscle fibers.

So if low-rep, high-intensity lifting trains all of your muscle fibers, why not lift this way all the time?

This type of lifting is very stressful to your nervous system. Do it more than twice a week, and you raise your risk of burnout and injury to joints and other supporting structures. Also, mixing up your weights and reps provides variety in your program, which helps stimulate muscle growth. That's why one of your weekly workouts calls for 8 to 10 reps rather than 5 to 7.

**Do compound movements instead of isolation movements.** Roughly 80 percent of the weightlifting moves you'll find in the pages that follow consist of compound movements. In contrast to isolation exercises, such as preacher curls that zero in on the biceps muscles, compound movements target more than one muscle at a time by working more than one joint at a time. This increases your calorie burn during your workout because you're using more muscles at once. It also makes each workout more efficient.

There are various types of compound-movement exercises. Some of them, such as the bench press, require multiple muscles to complete one movement. To press the bar away from your chest, you must use your deltoids (shoulders), pectorals (chest), lats (back), triceps (upper arms), and rotator cuff (small muscles around the shoulder joint). Other exercises work the entire body in multiple movements. For example, in the push press, you work your legs as you squat, your core as you extend to standing, and your shoulders as you hoist the bar overhead. Finally, for some of the exercises, you'll use a Swiss ball to put you off-balance. This forces you to work your core—and many other muscles—to remain balanced.

**Use a balanced approach.** When left to their own devices, most people do the exercises they like and avoid the ones they hate. The result: They make their already strong muscles stronger and their weaker muscles even weaker! The Metabolism Advantage plan will help you work all of the muscle groups in your body equally. In addition to helping to build muscle throughout your body—creating more overall muscle and boosting your metabolism—this balanced approach helps prevent injuries due to muscle imbalances. It also improves your posture. And hey, it creates a more symmetrical appearance.

**Recover after every set.** On the Metabolism Advantage program, your muscles will need roughly 1 to 1$^1$/$_2$ minutes to rest between sets.

**Lift fast.** To recruit the maximum number of muscle fibers, lift as quickly as you can, but lower the weight fairly slowly, to a count of three. Because you'll lift heavy weights, *fast* is obviously a relative term here, so just put everything you have behind each lift. I want you to focus all of your mental energy on the lift, not on counting, so work with a partner to egg you on during the lifting phase of the movement and encourage you to slow things down during the lowering phase.

## The Workouts

In the following pages, you'll find two lower-body, two upper-body, and two total-body strength-training workouts. To find the right weight for you, take a list of all of the exercises in the program to the gym and, exercise by exercise, experiment with different weights until you find the right weight to fatigue your muscles in either five reps (for the upper- and lower-body workouts) or eight reps (for the total-body workout). This means, seriously, that if someone held a gun to your head, you couldn't do another rep beyond the five or eight that you just completed—not even to save your life.

Warm up before each workout with 5 minutes of light cardio, and cool down afterward with another 5 minutes of light cardio.

## LOWER BODY

### BARBELL SQUAT

**Quads, Glutes, Hamstrings**

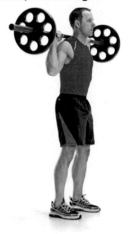

Position a barbell along the backs of your shoulders, holding the bar with an overhand grip.

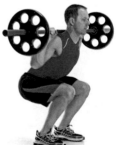

With your body weight equally distributed between your heels and forefeet, bend your knees, lowering your torso until your thighs are parallel to the floor. Keep your head forward, your back straight, and your feet flat on the floor.

Extend your knees and hips and rise until your legs are straight. Complete two sets of five to seven reps.

### OVERHEAD BARBELL SQUAT

**Quads, Core Muscles**

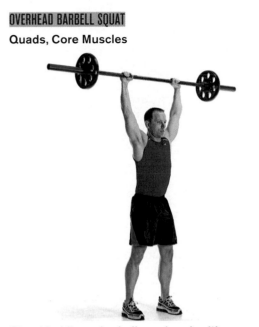

Stand holding a barbell overhead, with your arms extended.

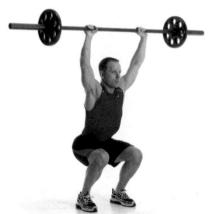

With your body weight equally distributed between your heels and forefeet, bend your knees, lowering your torso until your thighs are parallel to the floor. Keep your head forward, your back straight, and your feet flat on the floor.

Extend your knees and hips and rise until your legs are straight. Complete two sets of five to seven reps.

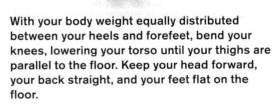

## BARBELL DEADLIFT

Glutes, Hamstrings, Lower Back

## DUMBBELL WALKING LUNGE

Glutes, Hamstrings, Quads

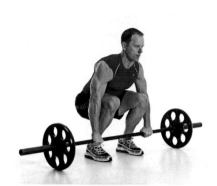

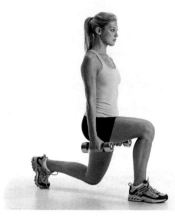

Place a barbell on the floor and stand with your feet hip-width apart under the center of the bar. Bend your knees, squat down, and grasp the bar with an overhand grip, with your hands shoulder-width or slightly farther apart.

Hold a pair of dumbbells at your sides. Lunge forward with your right leg, landing on your heel and then your forefoot. Lower your body by bending your knees until they both form right angles and the knee of your left leg is almost in contact with the floor.

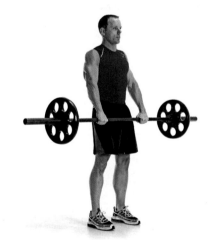

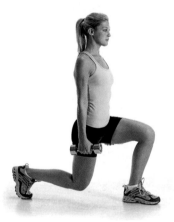

Keeping your arms and back straight, extend your knees and hips as you lift the bar and stand. As you lift, keep the bar close to your body. Pull your shoulders back at the top of the lift. Complete three sets of five to seven reps.

Step forward with your left leg, landing on your heel and then your forefoot.

Continue lunging forward until you've completed five to seven repetitions on each side. Complete two sets.

## SINGLE-LEG SWISS BALL LEG CURL
Hamstrings, Glutes

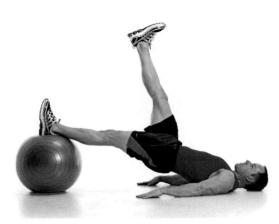

Lie on your back with your heels and lower calves on a Swiss ball. Lift your hips until your body forms an incline. Lift your right leg into the air, balancing your body weight with just your left leg against the ball.

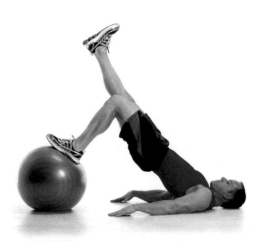

Bend your left knee and pull the ball toward you.

Pause for a second, then slowly reverse the sequence. Complete five to seven reps, then repeat with the other leg. Complete two sets per leg.

## STEPUP
Glutes, Quads, Hamstrings

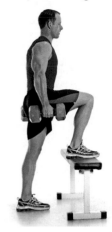

Holding dumbbells at your sides, stand in front of a weight bench or step that's at least 12 inches high. Place your right foot on top of the bench or step.

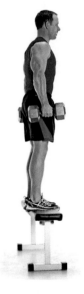

Press into your right foot and extend your right leg as you lift your body over the bench or step. Place your left foot on the bench or step.

Then step down onto the floor with your right foot. Keeping your torso upright, continue alternating sides until you've stepped up five to seven times on each side. Complete two sets.

## UPPER BODY

### BENT-OVER BARBELL ROW

Upper and Lower Back, Biceps

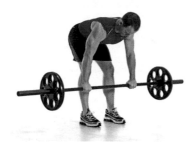

Bend your knees slightly and bend forward with your back straight. Grasp a barbell with an overhand grip, with your hands slightly more than shoulder-width apart.

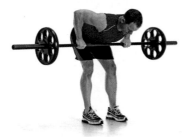

Bend your elbows, bringing them toward the ceiling as you pull the bar toward your midsection.

Then extend your arms to the starting position, allowing your shoulders to stretch forward slightly. Complete two sets of five to seven reps.

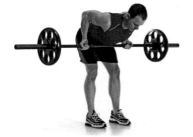

Next, change your hand position so your palms are facing upward in an underhand grip and complete one more set of five to seven reps.

### FLAT BARBELL BENCH PRESS

Chest, Shoulders, Triceps

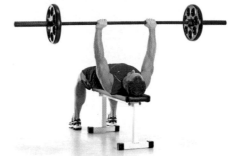

Lie on a flat bench and position your body so the barbell on the supports is above your face. Grasp the bar with your hands shoulder-width apart. Keep your feet flat on the floor as you lift the weight off the supports and hold the bar above your chest.

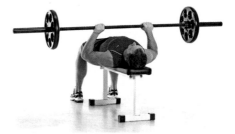

Bend your elbows to the sides as you lower the bar toward your upper chest, stopping when your elbows are in line with your torso. Pause at the bottom for a second, then press back up. Complete five to seven reps.

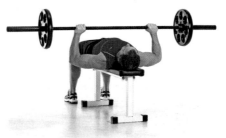

After one set, change your hand position to a wide grip—more than shoulder-width apart—and complete one more set of five to seven reps.

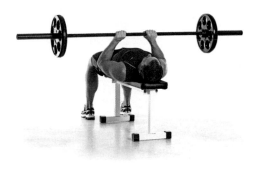

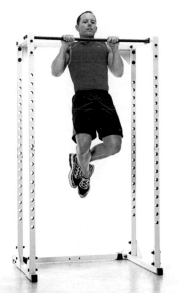

Next, do the press with a narrow grip—less than shoulder-width apart—and complete one more set of five to seven reps.

## PULLUP

Upper Back, Biceps, Brachialis

Pull yourself up until your chin clears the bar.

Lower and repeat, completing five to seven reps.

**Note:** If you can't pull up your entire body weight, do assisted pullups, either with a partner pushing against your lower back or on a pull-up machine that supports some—but not all—of your body weight.

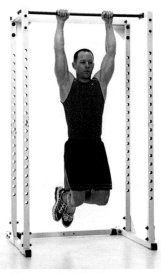

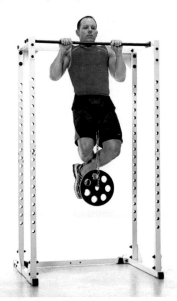

Hang from an overhead bar with an overhand grip, with your hands shoulder-width apart.

If you can easily do five to seven reps, either wear a weighted belt or hold a dumbbell between your ankles. Complete two sets.

## BARBELL OVERHEAD PRESS
Shoulders, Trapezius, Triceps

## SINGLE-ARM BARBELL BICEPS CURL
Biceps

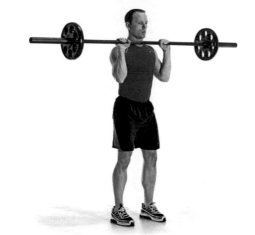

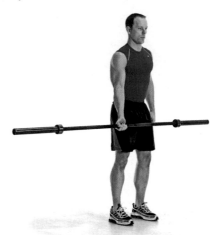

Take a barbell off the supports of a squat rack and hold it at collarbone level with an overhand grip, with your hands shoulder-width apart.

Grasp either a long or short barbell (depending on your strength) with your right hand, holding the center of the bar in an underhand grip.

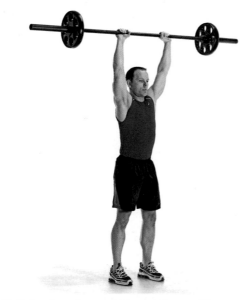

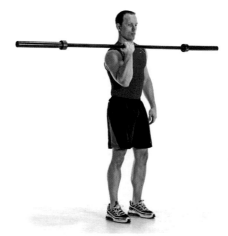

Walk back a step or two and then, with your knees slightly bent, press the bar overhead until your arms are straight. Lower the bar to chin level and repeat. Complete two sets of five to seven reps.

Keeping your right elbow close to your side, raise the bar until your right forearm is vertical. Then lower it until your arm is fully extended. Complete five to seven reps, then repeat with your left arm. Complete two sets for each arm.

## DIP

**Triceps, Chest**

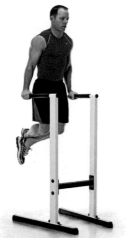

## PUSHUP ON SWISS BALL

**Chest**

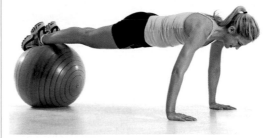

Kneel with your belly on a Swiss ball. Roll forward until you are in a plank position, with your hands on the floor under your chest and your feet on the ball.

Depending on your strength, you can do this exercise either on a dip bar with or without weight or on a dip/pullup machine that supports some of your weight. If you need added weight, either use a weighted belt or hold a dumbbell between your ankles.

Mount the dip bar or machine with your palms facing in and your arms extended.

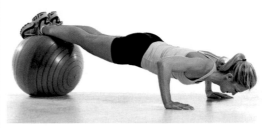

Keeping your back straight, bend your elbows and lower your chest to the floor. Extend your arms to return to the starting position. Complete two sets of 8 to 10 reps.

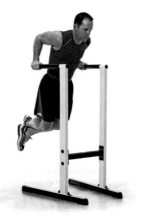

Keeping your elbows close to your body, bend your elbows and lower your torso until your shoulders are slightly stretched. Extend your arms and return to the starting position. Complete two sets of five to seven reps.

## SUITCASE DEADLIFT

Glutes, Hamstrings, Quads, Core Muscles

Grasp a barbell in the center with your right hand and hold it at your right side as if it were a heavy suitcase.

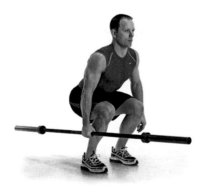

Bend your knees and squat down as if you were trying to place your suitcase on the floor. Keeping your arms and back straight, extend your knees and hips and return to the starting position. Complete three sets of 8 to 10 reps with each arm.

## BARBELL CLEAN

Hips, Shoulders, Legs, Upper Back

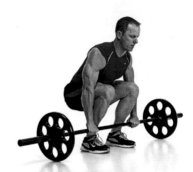

1. Place a barbell on the floor and stand with your feet slightly more than hip-width apart just under the bar. Squat down and grasp the bar with an overhand grip, with your hands slightly more than shoulder-width apart. With your back arched slightly, position your shoulders over the bar.

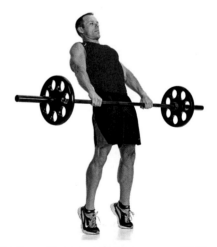

2. Extend your knees and hips as you lift the bar, at first keeping your arms extended.

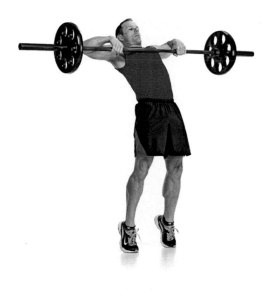

## DUMBBELL OVERHEAD WALKING LUNGE
### Glutes, Quads, Hamstrings, Core Muscles

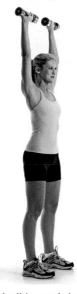

Holding a dumbbell in each hand, stand with your arms extended overhead.

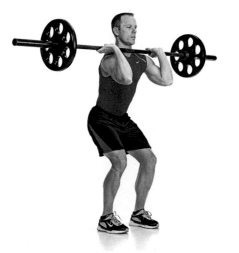

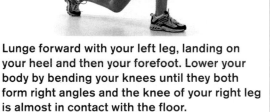

3. Once the bar reaches your knees, vigorously raise your shoulders and pull the barbell up as you flex your elbows to the sides in an upright rowing motion. Keep the bar close to your body the entire time, then catch it at the top position. Lower and repeat. Complete three sets of 8 to 10 reps.

Lunge forward with your left leg, landing on your heel and then your forefoot. Lower your body by bending your knees until they both form right angles and the knee of your right leg is almost in contact with the floor.

Then step forward with your right leg, landing on your heel and then your forefoot. Continue lunging forward until you've completed 8 to 10 repetitions on each side. Complete two sets.

### BRIDGE

Core Muscles

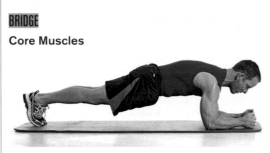

Assume a pushup position, but instead of straightening your arms, rest your weight on your forearms. Suck in your belly button and contract your glutes to flatten the arch in your lower back. Hold for 30 seconds. Complete two sets.

### SIDE BRIDGE

Obliques, Abdominals

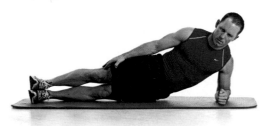

Lie on your left side with your left forearm lined upright beneath your shoulder, perpendicular to your torso.

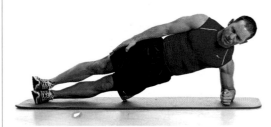

Keeping your body straight, contract your abdominals and obliques as you raise your lower torso, hips, and legs off the floor. In the top position, your body should form a diagonal line from your feet to your head. Hold for 30 seconds.

Then switch sides and repeat. Complete two sets for each side.

## WEEKS 5–8

### LOWER BODY

### BARBELL GOOD MORNING

Hamstrings, Lower Back

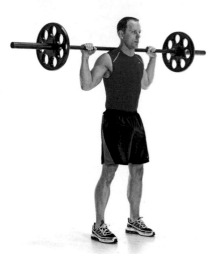

Position a barbell along the backs of your shoulders, grasping it with an underhand grip, with your hands slightly more than shoulder-width apart.

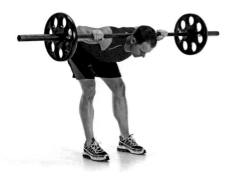

Bend forward from the hips as if you were bowing, but keep your back flat (not rounded). Stop when your torso is parallel to the floor.

Keeping your back and knees extended, return to the starting position. Complete three sets of five to seven reps.

## BARBELL HACK SQUAT

Quads, Glutes, Hamstrings

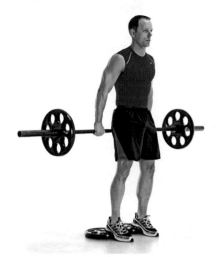

Set a 25-pound weight plate about a foot behind each support of a squat rack. Set a barbell on the rack at about hip level and stand with your back to it, then grasp it behind your back with a shoulder-width, overhand grip. Next, slowly walk backward toward the weight plates until both your heels are elevated on them.

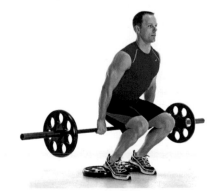

Keeping your back as straight as possible, bend your knees and squat down as far as you can.

When you've reached your lowest point, push your feet into the floor to rise to the starting position. Complete three sets of five to seven reps.

## STIFF-LEG DEADLIFT

Upper and Lower Back, Glutes, Hamstrings

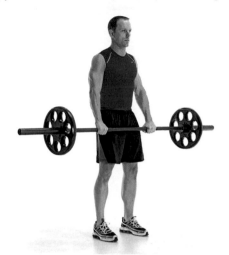

Stand with your feet shoulder-width apart. Hold a barbell at thigh level in an overhand grip, with your hands shoulder-width apart and arms extended.

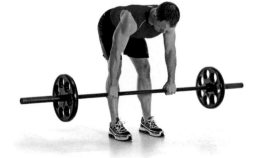

With your knees slightly bent, bend forward from the hips, lowering the bar toward your feet until you feel a mild stretch in your hamstrings.

Then, with your knees bent, lift the bar as you stand upright. Complete two sets of five to seven reps.

## OVERHEAD DUMBBELL SQUAT

Quads, Glutes, Core Muscles

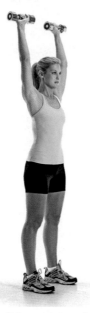

Grasp a dumbbell in each hand and extend your arms overhead.

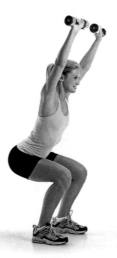

Bend your knees and lower your torso until your thighs are parallel to the floor.

Then extend your knees and hips and stand up. Keep your head forward, your back straight, and your chest high. Complete two sets of five to seven reps.

## LEG PRESS

Quads

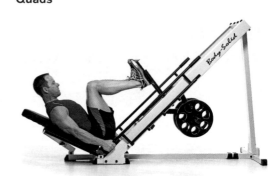

Sit on a leg press machine with your back against the padded support. Place your feet on the platform and grasp the handles at your sides for support.

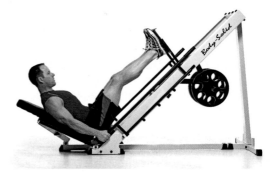

Extend your knees and hips to push the platform away from you.

Bend your knees to return to the starting position. Keep your knees pointed up; don't let them splay outward. Also, don't let your heels rise off the platform. Complete two sets of five to seven reps.

## UPPER BODY

### CHINUP

**Upper Back, Biceps**

You can do chinups wearing a weighted belt or with a dumbbell between your feet, assisted by a partner, or on a chinup machine.

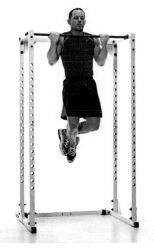

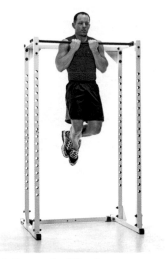

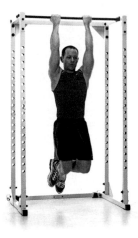

**1. To do a basic chinup, hang from an overhead bar with an underhand grip, with your hands shoulder-width apart.**

**2. Extend your chest and pull yourself up until your chin clears the bar or your chest touches it.**

**Lower and repeat. You can do chinups with a number of different grips and hand positions. For this workout, do the following.**

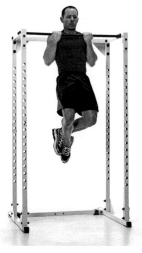

**3. One set of five to seven reps with your hands in an overhand grip (that is, do a pullup as on page 25, with a wide grip) slightly more than shoulder-width apart.**

**4. One set of five to seven reps with your hands slightly less than shoulder-width apart.**

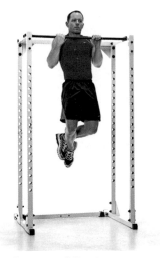

**5. One set of five to seven reps with your right hand in an overhand grip and your left in an underhand grip. Space your hands slightly more than shoulder-width apart.**

**One set of five to seven reps with your left hand in an overhand grip and your right in an underhand grip. Space your hands slightly more than shoulder-width apart.**

## ALTERNATING DUMBBELL INCLINE PRESS

Pectorals, Deltoids, Triceps

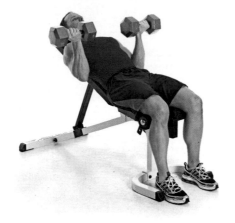

1. Sit on an incline bench holding dumbbells in an underhand grip so they rest on your lower thighs. Bring the weights up to your shoulders and lean back against the bench. Position the dumbbells at the sides of your upper chest, with your elbows below the dumbbells.

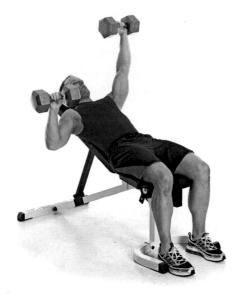

3. Switch to an overhand grip and do two sets of five to seven reps.

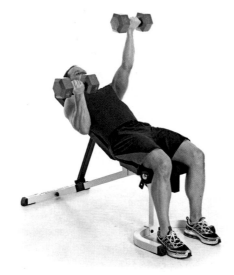

2. Press one dumbbell up until your arm is extended.

Lower the weight to your upper chest and repeat with the other arm. Continue alternating arms until you've completed one set of five to seven reps.

## BARBELL CLEAN

Hips, Shoulders, Legs, Upper Back

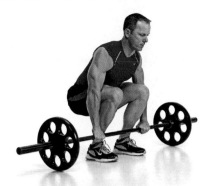

1. Place a barbell on the floor and stand with your feet slightly more than hip-width apart just under the bar. Squat down and grasp the bar with an overhand grip, with your hands slightly more than shoulder-width apart. With your back arched slightly, position your shoulders over the bar.

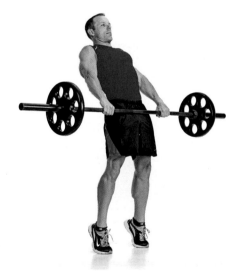

2. Extend your knees and hips as you lift the bar, at first keeping your arms extended.

3. Once the bar reaches your knees, vigorously raise your shoulders and pull the barbell up as you flex your elbows out to the sides in an upright rowing motion. Keep the bar close to your body the entire time, then catch it at the top position. Lower and repeat. Complete two sets of five to seven reps.

## ALTERNATING DUMBBELL SHOULDER PRESS ON SWISS BALL

Deltoids, Triceps

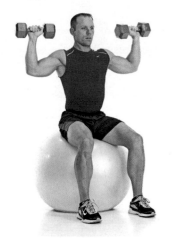

Sit on a Swiss ball with your knees bent and your feet flat on the floor. Hold a dumbbell with an overhand grip next to each shoulder, with your elbows under your wrists.

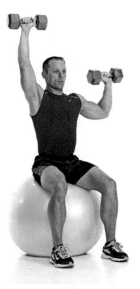

Press one dumbbell up until that arm is extended overhead.

Lower and repeat with the other arm. Complete two sets of five to seven reps with each arm.

## ALTERNATING DUMBBELL CURL ON SWISS BALL

Biceps

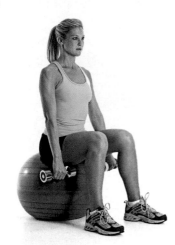

Sit on a Swiss ball with your knees bent and your feet flat on the floor. Hold a dumbbell in an overhand grip at each side, with your arms straight.

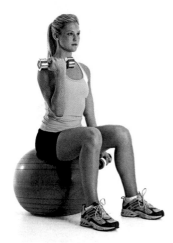

Keeping your elbows close to your sides, raise one dumbbell, rotating your forearm until it is vertical and your palm faces your shoulder.

Lower to the starting position and repeat with the other arm. Continue alternating left and right until you've completed two sets of five to seven reps with each arm.

## CLOSE-GRIP BENCH PRESS
Chest, Shoulders, Triceps

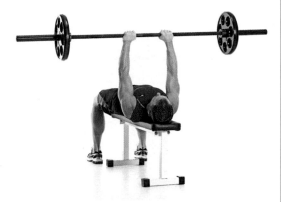

Lie on a flat bench and position your body so the barbell on the supports is above your face. Grasp the bar with your hands less than shoulder-width apart. Keep your feet flat on the floor as you lift the weight off the supports and hold the bar above your chest.

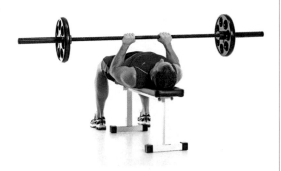

Bend your elbows to the sides as you lower the bar toward your upper chest, stopping when your elbows are in line with your torso.

Pause at the bottom for a second, then press back up. Complete two sets of five to seven reps.

## TOTAL BODY

## SUITCASE DEADLIFT
Glutes, Hamstrings, Quads, Core Muscles

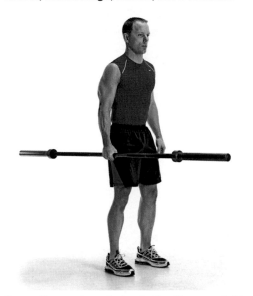

Grasp the center of a barbell with your right hand and hold it at your right side as if it were a heavy suitcase.

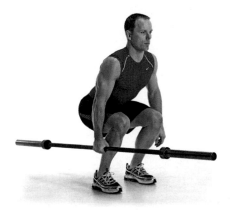

Bend your knees and squat down as if you were trying to place your suitcase on the floor.

Keeping your arms and back straight, extend your knees and hips and return to the starting position. Complete three sets of 8 to 10 reps with each arm.

## DUMBBELL OVERHEAD WALKING LUNGE

Glutes, Quads, Hamstrings, Core Muscles

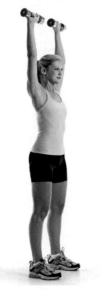

Grasp a dumbbell in each hand and extend your arms overhead.

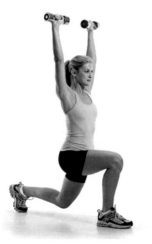

Lunge forward with your left leg, landing on your heel and then your forefoot. Lower your body by bending your knees until they both form right angles and the knee of your right leg is almost in contact with the floor.

Step forward with your right leg, landing on your heel and then your forefoot. Continue lunging forward until you've completed 8 to 10 repetitions on each side. Complete three sets.

## PUSH PRESS

Quads, Deltoids, Triceps

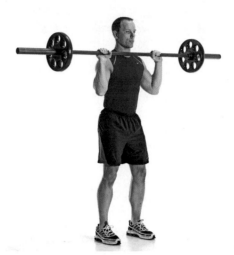

1. Grasp a barbell at chest level with an overhand grip, with your hands slightly more than shoulder-width apart.

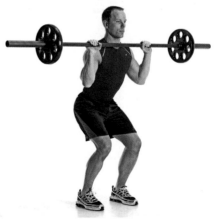

2. Bend your knees and squat down.

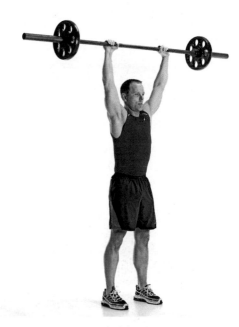

## BENT-OVER BARBELL ROW
### Upper and Lower Back, Biceps

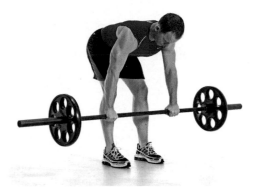

Bend your knees slightly and bend forward with your back straight. Grasp a barbell with an overhand grip, with your hands slightly more than shoulder-width apart.

3. Explosively straighten your legs as you drive the barbell up, vigorously extending your arms overhead in a shoulder press motion.

Lower the barbell to your chest and repeat. Complete three sets of 8 to 10 reps.

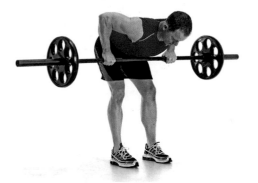

Bend your elbows, bringing them toward the ceiling as you pull the bar toward your midsection.

Extend your arms to the starting position, allowing your shoulders to stretch forward slightly. Complete three sets of 8 to 10 reps.

## BRIDGE
Core Muscles

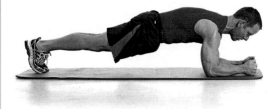

Assume a pushup position, but instead of straightening your arms, rest your weight on your forearms. Suck in your belly button and contract your glutes to flatten the arch in your lower back. Hold for 30 seconds. Complete two sets.

## SIDE BRIDGE
Obliques, Abdominals

Lie on your left side with your left forearm lined upright beneath your shoulder, perpendicular to your torso.

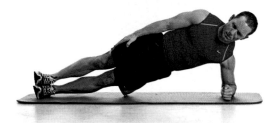

Keeping your body straight, contract your abdominals and obliques as you raise your lower torso, hips, and legs off the floor. In the top position, your body should form a diagonal line from your feet to your head. Hold for 30 seconds.

Then switch sides and repeat. Complete two sets.

## Metabolism Advantage Cardio

Although high-intensity cardiovascular exercise won't give you the same long-term metabolic boost as weight training, it will help you burn more calories in two ways:

1. During your workouts

2. During the 24-hour recovery window after your workouts

The biggest mistake people make? Not pushing themselves hard enough. Forget about that fat-burning zone you may have heard about. According to that theory, your body burns more fat than carbohydrate at low intensities. This is true, but your goal is to burn calories, and during your workout, it doesn't matter where those calories come from. Your muscles stock a type of fuel called glycogen (a type of stored carbohydrate) for ready access during exercise. After a workout, your muscles replace the glycogen they burned during exercise. To enable this process, the body shuts off carbohydrate burning, shuttling dietary carbohydrate to your muscles, where it's converted to glycogen. Your body still needs fuel for energy, so it switches to burning fat. So don't worry about the type of fuel you're burning during your workout. Just burn it!

High-intensity workouts burn more calories during and after exercise than low-intensity workouts. When you run, swim, bike, and do other types of high-intensity cardio, you fatigue and slightly damage your muscles, which must repair and strengthen themselves for subsequent efforts. During this recovery period, your body clears acid and metabolic byproducts from your muscles and replenishes the ATP (adenosine triphosphate, the energy source your muscles use for short bursts of power) and glycogen you burned during exercise. It also changes the makeup of protein in your muscles, replacing damaged muscle protein with new proteins capable of withstanding high-intensity endurance efforts. This process elevates your metabolism slightly for 24 to 48 hours.

How long you maintain your afterburn depends on the intensity of your effort. In one experiment, eight women cycled at either a fairly easy pace or at an extremely intense pace. When they cycled intensely, they not only burned significantly more calories during the 60-minute cycling session but also continued to burn more calories for 24 hours afterward, a metabolism boost equivalent to 150 calories.

In addition to boosting your metabolism, this type of exercise will also extend your life. The Harvard Alumni Health Study, a 4-year study of more than 17,000 men, found that only vigorous—not moderate—exercise reduced risk of death.

## Science Made Simple

**VO$_2$ max:** This scientific term stands for the maximal (max) volume (V) of oxygen (O$_2$) that one can consume during maximal exercise and is a measure of aerobic fitness.

On the Metabolism Advantage cardio plan, you'll complete bursts of intense exercise called intervals. By pushing your pace for a specified period of time and then backing off and recovering, you'll be able to boost your $VO_2$ max. This is a scientific term for the maximal (max) volume (V) of oxygen $(O_2)$ that one can consume during maximal exercise. It's a measure of your aerobic fitness.

To perform this type of interval exercise, select two intensities and alternate between them for the prescribed number of repetitions. On a scale of 0 to 10—with 0 being comatose and 10 being the hardest you could ever work—you should hit an intensity of 9 during your 30-second intervals, 8 during 60-second intervals, and 7 during 90-second intervals. During your recovery period, aim for an intensity of 3.

Experiment to find the right high and low intensities for you. You'll know you've found the right level when you can keep the high- and low-intensity levels constant throughout the duration of the interval session. If you can't do this without excessive fatigue, you need to lower the intensity. You want to feel exhausted by the last few reps, but not sooner.

For example, during a cycling session on a stationary bike, you might cycle for 30 seconds at the bike's preset level 10 and 120

rpm, then decrease your intensity to level 1 and 80 rpm for 90 seconds. For a running interval session on a treadmill, you might run at 12 miles per hour on an incline of 5 percent for 60 seconds and walk for the next 60 seconds at 4 miles per hour on an incline of 0 percent. For rowing intervals, you might row at 40 strokes per minute for 90 seconds of high-intensity rowing, then at 20 strokes per minute for 180 seconds of low-intensity rowing.

Those are just examples of exercise modes and intensity settings. The Metabolism Advantage program doesn't lock you into only these types of exercise. That's right, you can pick whatever type of exercise you like, whether it's cycling, running, rowing, stairclimbing, swimming, or something else. As long as you follow the prescribed intensities and durations, you'll get the benefits you're looking for.

## YOUR INTERVAL WORKOUTS

Here are the interval workouts you'll follow. Choose your favorite form of cardio—such as running, rowing, or cycling—to complete these workouts.

### WORKOUT #1

5-minute low-intensity cardio warmup

Intervals: 30 seconds at high intensity, 90 seconds at low intensity

Weeks 1–4: Perform 7 total intervals

Weeks 5–8: Perform 10 total intervals

5-minute low-intensity cardio cooldown

### WORKOUT #2

5-minute low-intensity cardio warmup

Intervals: 60 seconds at high intensity, 60 seconds at low intensity

Weeks 1–4: Perform 7 total intervals

Weeks 5–8: Perform 10 total intervals

5-minute low-intensity cooldown

### WORKOUT #3

5-minute low-intensity cardio warmup

Intervals: 90 seconds at high intensity, 180 seconds at low intensity

Weeks 1–4: Perform 4 total intervals

Weeks 5–8: Perform 5 total intervals

5-minute low-intensity cooldown

## Your Weekly Schedule

During each week of this plan, your exercise schedule works like this:

**Monday:** Lower-body strengthening workout

**Tuesday:** Interval workout #1

**Wednesday:** Upper-body strengthening workout

**Thursday:** Interval workout #2

**Friday:** Total-body strengthening workout

**Saturday:** Interval workout #3

**Sunday:** Off

Keep in mind that you are not locked into this schedule. You can rearrange the workouts to accommodate your life—just be sure that you get all of them in each week!

## Exercise by the 90 Percent Rule

On the Metabolism Advantage exercise plan, you need not adhere to the program 100 percent of the time. I'm putting you under no pressure to be perfect. Since the difference between 90 percent and 100 percent is negligible, I allow and encourage 10 percent "wiggle room."

So how can you best follow the 90 percent rule when it comes to exercise? Let's do the math. You're going to do an average of six exercise sessions per week. That translates to about 24 exercise sessions per month. Ten percent of that is about 2.4 total workouts. Therefore, in addition to your formal day off each week, you have 2 or 3 more days off (or light days) to play with each month.

If you follow the plan 100 percent of the time, that's great. Keep it up! If you need to skip a workout every now and then, rest assured that you'll still meet your goals as long as you follow the 90 percent rule.

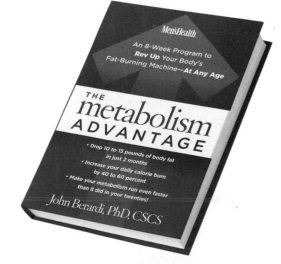

Excerpted from *The Metabolism Advantage* by John Berardi, PhD, CSCS, copyright 2006 by John Berardi. Published by Rodale Inc. Available wherever books are sold.

BY PETER GREENBERG

# Take It on the Road

Hooked on junk food, 50 pounds overweight, and traveling 400,000 miles a year, here's how one man took control of his weight and his life

The last time I weighed what I was supposed to weigh was in 1969. I remember it well.

It was New Year's Eve, and that was the night I gave up smoking.

Three days later, I was in Israel, near Syria, covering a continuing border war. We were in foxholes, and someone had launched mortars toward the Israeli positions. As the explosions came way too close for comfort, the other journalists with me were convinced we were going to die.

Suddenly, a pair of Israeli soldiers appeared behind me and began handing out disgusting French cigarettes. Two of the other journalists, guys who had never smoked, accepted them and lit up. When the soldiers got to me, I tried to decline politely, saying I was "trying to quit." For about 15 seconds, the war seemed to stop while everyone looked at me incredulously, as if to say, "You're trying to quit? We're all about to die anyway. Take the cigarette!"

I didn't. We lived. And I haven't had a cigarette since.

Okay, so much for the good news. From the morning of January 6, 1970, when I returned home, I was on Oreo patrol. Snack food, junk food—you name it, I went for it. And it showed. If it's true that you are what you . . . overeat, then I was the *pie* piper.

I became obsessed with certain "foods." I had an obscene relationship with Diet Pepsi, drinking up to 20 cans a day. I ordered cherry-flavored Swedish Fish candies in bulk. Around my office, you'd always find Peanut M&M's, Snickers bars, and Brach's Root Beer Barrels. By the time I became an executive at Paramount Pictures, I was having boxes of chocolate-chip cookies delivered to the office.

In 1987, I went on a serious diet supervised by a doctor, and I lost 51 pounds.

Then I started traveling for *Good Morning America*. In 7 years, I gained that weight back—and then some. Why? Because I love snacking, and snacks were everywhere. There were potato chips and popcorn in the office, pretzels and peanuts on the plane, chocolates waiting in my hotel room when I arrived. Let's not talk about the minibar. And we haven't even gotten to the social breakfasts, lunches, and dinners that go along with the job.

As the son of a doctor and with my travel schedule, I was religious about getting a checkup every 3 months. And the results, despite my weight, were never cause for alarm. My blood pressure was always a little high, as were my triglycerides and choles-

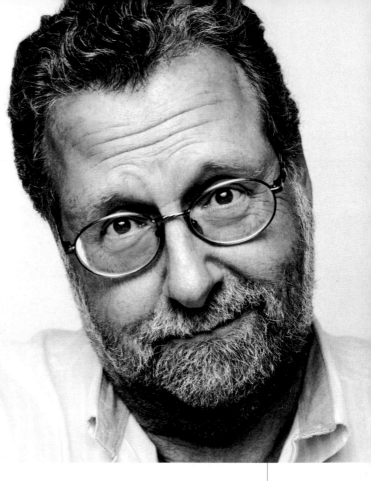

terol, but nothing was out of control. I hadn't smoked in more than 30 years; I hardly drink alcohol and never drink coffee.

Dostoyevsky once wrote that every man lies to himself. Well, I fooled myself into thinking that since I lacked certain vices, my excess weight was an acceptable trade-off for career success.

Then, in March 2005, I went to see my doctor for another checkup. On this visit, the numbers caught up with me. My blood pressure was 145/95, and the cholesterol and triglyceride levels were frightening. Then it was time to stand on the scale. Nothing prepared me for the number that confronted me: 284 pounds!

That was my wakeup call. I knew I had to start taking better care of myself or face serious health problems, but where to begin? That night, I had dinner with Stephen Perrine, the editor-in-chief of *Best Life* magazine. I told him of my disappointing checkup and that I was now motivated to lose weight. "But you travel more than anyone else I know," he said. (As travel editor for NBC's *Today*, I visit 35 countries a year.) "How can you possibly stick to a diet and exercise program?" The problem, as I'm sure most of you can attest, is that travel disrupts discipline and makes it easy to jettison even the most well-intentioned of diets.

Like any good traveler, I needed a road map. First, Perrine made me keep a food diary for a week. And when I was finished with it, it didn't make for pretty reading. Without realizing it, I had become the poster child for the Nabisco-dependency telethon—Chips Ahoy!, Fig Newtons, and the real killers: Wheat Thins. I consumed entire boxes in a single sitting.

## Road Rules for the Traveling Man

**1.** Drink 1 cup of water per hour on the plane. (You may substitute orange juice, tea, seltzer, or tomato juice but not beer, wine, or mixed drinks.)

**2.** Call ahead to your hotel and ask them to have a salad, fruit, yogurt, an omelet, or hard-cooked eggs waiting for you upon arrival.

**3.** Don't get a key for the minibar. Better yet, ask that it be removed from your room. If you stare at that $8 Snickers bar long enough, you're going to eat it.

**4.** Buy an apple or an orange to keep in your room for the morning.

**5.** Work out in the morning before you fly, if possible. Take a walk when you get to your destination if time allows, especially if it is daylight.

**6.** Walk the aisle every 90 minutes during the flight to stretch your legs.

**7.** Buy snacks for the airport and flight—there will be delays. Good choices: Au Bon Pain salads and/ or fruit-yogurt parfait; dried apricots and nuts; Nature Valley Crunchy Granola Bars.

**8.** Don't eat a main meal after 8 p.m.

## The Diet Plan

Seeing my terrible eating habits spelled out in black-and-white was sufficient to convince me to get help. My next stop was a meeting with nutritionist Heidi Skolnik, MS, CDN, a contributor to *Men's Health*. Skolnik is a sports-nutrition consultant to the New York Giants and the School of American Ballet—perfect, I thought, for a defensive-tackle-size guy like me who's light on his feet.

"The key for travelers," Skolnik explained, "is to create structure in an unstructured world. This means looking ahead in the day and anticipating when your three meals and snacks will be—even if you have to eat in a taxi while going across town to a meeting." And in my particular case, Skolnik studied my schedule and determined I was already sabotaging myself. "You schedule your day so tightly, you forget about you in there," she said. Skolnik put me on a 2,200-calorie-a-day diet, which broke down like this:

Protein (25 percent of calories): 137 grams

Fat (24 percent): 59 grams

Carbohydrate (51 percent): 280 grams

She suggested that I never skip breakfast and always eat four to six smaller meals a day, including one or two snacks. Here are some sample menus she created for me.

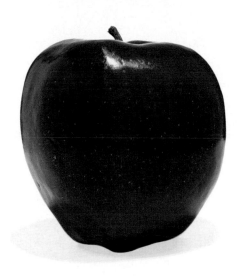

## BREAKFAST

**Option 1:** 2 pancakes with $1^1/_4$ cups berries and 2 pats butter; 2 slices Canadian bacon; 1 cup 1 percent milk

**Option 2:** 2 eggs; English muffin with 2 teaspoons peanut butter; 1 cup 1 percent milk; 1 banana

**Option 3:** 1 cup oatmeal with $^1/_4$ cup dried fruit (like raisins) and 12 almonds or cashews; 2 egg whites with 1 ounce cheese; 1 cup 1 percent milk

## LUNCH

**Option 1:** Tuna salad pita (3 ounces tuna, rinsed and drained; 2 tablespoons low-fat mayonnaise; and $^1/_4$ cup chopped celery in a pita with 2 slices tomato and 1 large romaine lettuce leaf); 1 cup carrot sticks; $^1/_2$ cup canned pineapple; Swedish Fish; 1 cup fat-free, no-added-sugar yogurt

**Option 2:** Turkey sandwich (3 ounces sliced turkey breast on 2 slices whole-wheat bread with 1 slice cheese and 1 teaspoon mustard, 2 slices tomato, and 1 large romaine lettuce leaf); 1 granola bar; salad (1 cup cucumber slices, $^1/_4$ cup

chopped onion, and 2 tablespoons low-fat dressing); 1 medium apple

**Option 3:** 1 cup minestrone soup; 6 Triscuits; 2 tablespoons Parmesan cheese; grilled chicken with $^1/_2$ cup beans over salad; 2 plums

## DINNER

**Option 1:** 5 ounces grilled fish; 1 teaspoon lemon juice; 1 cup brown rice; $^1/_2$ cup cooked spinach; $^1/_2$ cup mushrooms sautéed in 2 teaspoons oil; 1 small whole-wheat roll

**Option 2:** 6-piece shrimp cocktail; $1^1/_3$ cups pasta with $^1/_2$ cup tomato sauce, 5 ounces turkey meatballs, and 2 tablespoons Parmesan cheese; salad ($^1/_4$ cup sliced fresh mushrooms, $^1/_2$ cup spinach, $^1/_4$ cup freshly grated carrots, 1 tablespoon sunflower seeds, 2 tablespoons fat-free dressing)

**Option 3:** 5-ounce steak (New York strip or filet mignon); 1 cup mashed potatoes with 2 tablespoons sour cream; 1 cup mixed vegetables (broccoli, carrots, green beans, and the like) cooked with 1 teaspoon oil; 2 small rolls; mixed green salad; ¾ cup sorbet

## SNACK

**Option 1:** 1 cup fat-free, no-added-sugar yogurt; ¼ cup Grape-Nuts; 12 almonds

**Option 2:** 1 slice whole-wheat bread with 1 tablespoon peanut butter; 1 cup 1 percent milk

**Option 3:** 2 rice cakes with 1 tablespoon peanut butter; 1 banana

My biggest challenges were breakfast and Diet Pepsi. I don't eat breakfast, and some would say I was addicted to Diet Pepsi. That's a definite double negative. So I started eating breakfast and drastically limiting my Diet Pepsi drinking. Within a week, an amazing thing happened: I found myself falling asleep at 8 o'clock each evening. I was actually coming down from the caffeine!

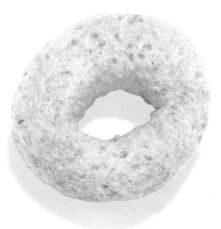

## ON THE ROAD

Okay, the preceding menus might work at home, but what about on the road?

Skolnik became my personal portion teller. She allowed me to have high-fat meat twice a week, but it all came down to portion size. Unless I was a 7' basketball center, a 20-ounce rib eye was lethal and off-limits. At Chinese restaurants, chicken with vegetables was acceptable. Orange chicken (which is fried) was verboten. And since I'm partial to Asian food, Skolnik taught me a trick: Ask for an extra plate, and move a serving from the main platter to the extra plate. This encourages me to eat just one serving, and it also leaves the calorie-laden sauce behind. At Thai restaurants, pad Thai is allowed only if I share the dish.

Airplanes were another hurdle. I fly 400,000 miles a year! The problem with flying is that people turn it into a special event that allows them to break sound nutrition rules, says Susan Bowerman, MS, RD, the assistant director for the UCLA Center for Human Nutrition. To counter that, Bowerman advised me to pack my own food, especially on short flights, because of the high calorie content of the snacks offered by the airlines. What's best? Fresh fruit and raw vegetables, which have the most nutrients and fewest calories per bite, says Bowerman, along with unsalted nuts, dried fruit, protein bars, hard-cooked eggs, sports drinks, yogurt, Cheerios, and dried soups in a cup (you can always get hot water on the plane). Bowerman says that when she flies, she avoids the hot breakfasts—quiches, omelets, French toast, and other calorie-laden dishes—and opts for yogurt or high-fiber cereal. If the airline is offering a sandwich, she removes the cheese and scrapes away any mayonnaise; then, if there is a side salad (since they're usually tiny), she dumps it on the sandwich so she won't be tempted to eat the dressing. All good advice that I try to follow.

## The Fitness Plan

I don't care what anyone else tells you about exercise. If they say they love to do it, they're lying. If they insist it's fun, they are delusional. And if they can't wait to get up in the morning to run to the gym, then they are not to be trusted.

To me, exercise was always nothing more than doing penance for my past sins, and it certainly wasn't my goal. That's why I never looked forward to it; that is, until I met Annette Lang, a certified master trainer and owner of Annette Lang Education Systems (www.annettelang.com) at a gym in midtown Manhattan. Our first session was, to say the least, embarrassing. Annette took my measurements.

Chest: 50¼ inches

Right arm: 15¼ inches

Left arm: 15 inches

Waist: 51 inches

Hips: 48¾ inches

And then it was on to the treadmill, lat pulldowns, leg curls, bridges on a Swiss ball, reverse crunches, straight-arm pulldowns,

and shoulder presses. Impressed? Don't be. I was pathetic. I was breathing hard, and the entire workout lasted 8 minutes. Ugh.

That brief workout gave Lang a solid but sorry picture of what she had to deal with. But she was kind, describing me in her notes as "deconditioned." Then she created a circuit workout for me. "The goal is to do two or three circuits, two to four times a week," she said. We agreed to meet twice a week at the health club at the New York Sheraton on West 53rd Street. Since I would be on the road for the other two workouts, they would be my responsibility.

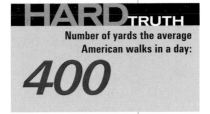

HARD TRUTH

Number of yards the average American walks in a day:

400

At the gym, Lang started me with a lot of machine choices, since many health clubs do not offer free weights. Here's a look at a typical hour-long workout: I start with cardio for 5 to 10 minutes, then move to resistance training with a goal of 15 repetitions for each exercise, but not to the point of muscle failure. Suggestions for substitutions are given below in case you don't have the equipment.

### CIRCUIT 1

Life Fitness elliptical machine: manual level 8, at least 50 rpm, 5 minutes

Straight-arm cable pulldown: 70 pounds (substitute: some kind of pulling exercise; try to get different angles)

Biceps curl into overhead press: 15-pound dumbbells

Cable core rotation: standing; use three weight plates. Hold grips with both hands, arms straight at midsection height; rotate, letting legs move with rotation. (substitute: rotation with dumbbell or medicine ball).

Leg press: 45-pound plates on each side

Deadlift: 15-pound dumbbells

Hip extension: On a slant board

## CIRCUIT 2

Treadmill: manual mode, 7 percent incline, 3 mph, 5 minutes

Lat pulldown: 80 pounds (substitute: pulling exercise)

Leg curl: 40 pounds (substitute: deadlift or bridge)

Leg extension: 60 pounds

Reverse fly machine: 40 pounds (substitute: cable pull with elbows out to sides)

Single-arm cable row: 3 plates, with opposite leg in front (substitute: row with dumbbells or machine)

Pushup: 12 reps on knees

Reverse crunch: 12 reps

Swiss ball bridge: Hold ball to keep stable (substitute: bridge on floor).

Lateral hold: Lie on side propped on elbow with knees bent behind you and body in a straight line with knees; raise hips and hold 8 seconds.

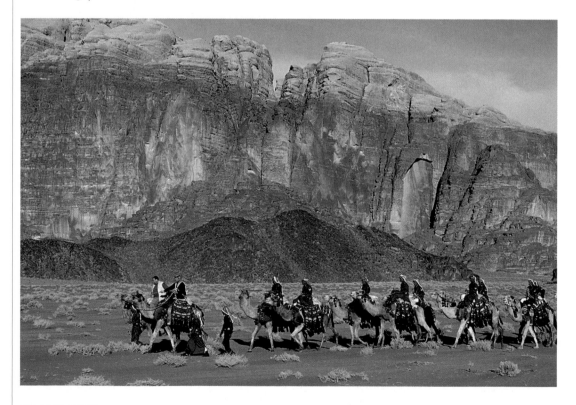

## CIRCUIT 3

Elliptical machine: same as before

Repeat one of the circuits above or do something else, depending on equipment in your facility.

To mix things up, we started visiting Gravity, the health club at Le Parker Meridien in New York City, where executive director Mark Natale introduced me to a weight-training program he calls the Quickie. Designed for speed, it boils a workout down to one set of nine lifts using heavy weight and performed until muscle failure. By combining Lang's cardio circuit with the Quickie, I started dropping 1 to $1^1/_2$ pounds weekly.

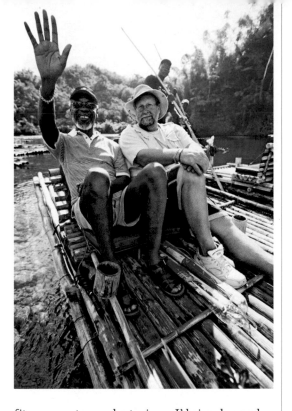

## ON THE ROAD

Let's be honest. You're not going to burn many calories while sitting on an airplane for hours, but one way to reduce stress and make sure you build exercise into your day is to arrive at the airport early and get in some extra laps around the terminal. Due to draconian, people-unfriendly airport design, you're going to walk whether you want to or not. For example, Miami International Airport is great for the long march. Recently, I landed at the new American Airlines Concourse D and had to go through customs and connect to a flight in Concourse C. Total distance covered: 1 mile! And that was while schlepping my luggage.

Luckily, I was able to maintain my fitness regimen on the road because before I flew anywhere, I'd find out if my hotel had a fitness center and a trainer. I'd simply send an e-mail to the hotel detailing my cardio and weight-lifting protocols and arrange for a trainer to meet me the minute I checked in. He would take me immediately to the hotel gym—no detours or diversions. The key to making the traveler's diet work is understanding that we don't change our lifestyle when we change our locations. So instead of checking into my hotel room and immediately logging on to the Internet, I would log in my exercise right away.

That's how I did it over the course of a year in more than 40 cities in Sheratons, Marriotts, and Hiltons; individual hotels like the Broadmoor in Colorado Springs and the Atlantic in Fort Lauderdale, Florida; and even on the Celebrity cruise ship *Summit*.

Each hotel gym was different, of course, but I was able to adapt much if not all of

Lang's training regimen to every location. More often than not, both the trainer and I had to improvise when the equipment wasn't similar. But the important thing is it worked! Four months into the workout regimen, I had lost almost 22 pounds. It was beginning to show. Friends and co-workers were starting to give me compliments, and that positive reinforcement was and continues to be great motivation for me.

While I hadn't changed all my bad patterns—I still was not eating proper breakfasts—I did do something I thought I'd never do: I kicked the Diet Pepsi habit. I

went from 22 cans a day (I never actually finished one) down to four, then two, and then . . . none.

And I replaced the Diet Pepsi with water. I began with the equation of drinking: Divide your weight in pounds by two, and drink that many ounces of water every day. Since I had started at 284 pounds, I had to drink about 140 ounces (more than a gallon) of water daily. By the end of the summer, I was down to 261 pounds and 130 ounces of water. It became an effective tool of my weight-loss program.

In the meantime, the workouts in New York continued to increase in frequency and intensity.

## SAMPLE CIRCUIT

Elliptical machine: 6 minutes, level 14

Flat chest press: 25-pound dumbbells, 15 reps

Lat pulldown: 80 pounds, overhand grip, 15 reps

Leg press: 45-pound plate on each side, 15 reps

Treadmill: 5 percent incline, 3.2 mph, 6 minutes

Chest fly: Cybex machine, 60 pounds, 15 reps

Single-arm row: 25-pound dumbbell, with one arm and leg on a bench for support, 15 reps

Rear delts: Cybex machine, 40 pounds, 15 reps

Leg curl: 40 pounds, 15 reps

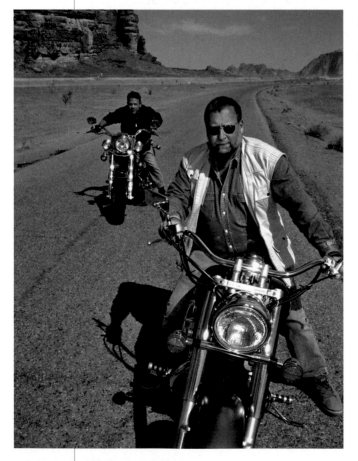

## So How Did I Do?

Between May 2005 and August 2005, I went from 284 pounds to 264 pounds. That November 2005, Lang measured me again: I had lost $2^1/_2$ inches from my chest and 6 inches from my waist! My level of cardio exercise was definitely improving. Not only could I do 30 minutes on the elliptical, I could do it at a constant level 13, which burned around 450 calories per session.

By the middle of February 2006, after my weight plateaued, it started to drop again and kept dropping, down to 252. The key, as always, was consistency in my workouts and diet. However, I quickly learned in one bad stretch that if I didn't allow myself to cheat once a week, I was likely to cheat all the time. Abstinence is hard in the real world. So once a week, especially on the road, when I'm offered a dessert, I indulge in a small portion. That's the deal. Period.

By the time this went to press, I had lost another 2 inches from my chest and 2 inches off my waist. And my weight? Down to 244 pounds! That's 40 pounds lighter than when I started.

And my health has improved, too. My blood pressure is a remarkable 105/70; my total cholesterol level is down to 165; and my LDL (bad) cholesterol has dropped to 65 from nearly 95. My triglycerides plummeted as well, from 148 to 98.

Admittedly, I will never become a gym rat.

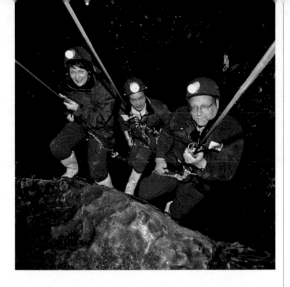

I'm not a planner. To me, a plan is something to depart from. And part of that stems directly from the travel experience. After all, so much of travel is about unexpected change and keeping your options open. Still, I was able to get into a semigroove with exercise. I just needed to get my body moving more, and Lang accomplished that by giving me a flexible program with options.

Were the workouts tough and was the diet challenging? Sure. Was it worth it? Absolutely. I feel better about myself. Not only do I have more confidence but I also look better, dress better, and feel more fit and energetic. When I used to go horseback riding at 284 pounds, the horses would get angry with me. (No kidding; they knew I weighed too much.) And I had to use a ladder to get in the saddle. Embarrassing. Not anymore. I can reach the stirrup and pull myself aboard. And the horses look much, much happier to see me.

BY ADAM CAMPBELL

# Lose Your Gut

No one likes
abdominal fat.
But you'll hate it
even more now
that you know it's
trying to kill you

There may be days when you look in the mirror at your prodigious abdomen—built over many years through a strict regimen of foie gras and Trappist ale—and wonder whether it might not be better suited for a sumo wrestler. You would be wrong: A sumo wrestler's belly is much healthier than the one you're toting around.

Here's why: There are two kinds of potbellies—soft ones and hard ones. And which kind you have may make all the difference in how long and how well you're going to live.

According to a Japanese study, the fat on the bellies of sumo wrestlers is almost entirely subcutaneous. That means it's located just under the skin, in front of the abdominal muscles—which is why the wrestlers' bellies jiggle about like Jennie Finch's sports bra. If you're like most American men, however, you have a very different kind of belly—solid and round, as if you swallowed a hard hat or a miniature Volkswagen Bug. A belly like that is composed of visceral fat, which resides behind the abdominal muscles, surrounding your internal organs (viscera). That fat pushes the abdominal muscles outward, making them protrude into a hard, round gut.

And over the past decade, scientists have concluded that the rounder and harder your belly, the more it puts your health in danger.

For that to make sense, it's important to understand that fat—any fat, subcutaneous or visceral—isn't just lifeless tissue whose only duty is to make you cringe at the idea of taking your shirt off in public. "Fat is an endocrine organ that secretes numerous substances, collectively called 'adipokines,' many of which are harmful," says Robert Ross, PhD, an exercise physiologist at Queen's University in Canada who's been studying the effects of lifestyle on visceral fat for 15 years. Adipokines include resistin, a hormone that leads to high blood sugar; angiotensinogen, a compound that raises blood pressure; adiponectin, a hormone that regulates the metabolism of lipids and glucose (amounts of this hormone decrease with increased visceral fat); and interleukin-6, a chemical associated with arterial inflammation. Of these substances, interleukin-6 is perhaps the most dangerous, because inflammation in your arteries can trigger pieces of plaque to break off and block the flow of blood to your heart. And because visceral fat is significantly

## Waists and Measures

Tracking your waist circumference is the easiest way to gauge your progress—and your risk for heart disease. Here's how to do it: Wrap a measuring tape around your abdomen—or better yet, have your wife help you—so that the bottom of the tape touches the tops of your hip bones. (Your belly button moves as you lose fat, but your hip bones don't, so this method ensures that you always take the measurement at the same location.) The tape should be snug but shouldn't compress the skin. If the tape measures 36 inches or greater, you need to take action—today. Today.

## The Belly-Busting Workout

Here's how to flatten your gut in less than 30 minutes, three times a week.

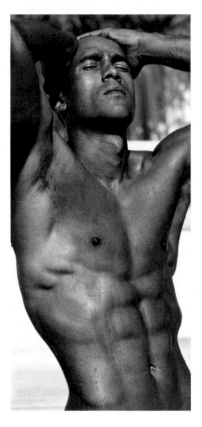

### Weight Workout

Choose four upper-body exercises, two lower-body exercises, and two core (abs and lower back) exercises. Do them as a circuit—performing one after the other with no rest in between—but arrange them so that you alternate upper-body exercises with those for your lower body and core moves. Resting and working your muscles in this way will allow you to work harder in less time, says Jean-Paul Francoeur, owner of JP Fitness, a health club in Little Rock, Arkansas. Try this circuit: bench press, squat, seated row, stepup, chinup, situp, shoulder press, and back extension. Complete two circuits, resting 2 minutes between them, and do 10 to 15 repetitions of each exercise.

Time: 18 minutes

### Cardio Workout

Use this interval method. Start out at an easy pace for 90 seconds (about 40 percent of your best effort). Then increase your speed to the fastest pace you can maintain for 30 seconds (about 95 percent of your maximum). That's one interval. Repeat five times, for a total of six intervals. It's short but intense, so it'll save you time. And unlike traditional steady-state aerobic exercise, it'll keep your body burning fat at a higher rate for hours after you're finished. You can perform it on the road or treadmill, but if you're packing more than an extra 20 pounds, opt for an exercise bike to reduce the stress on your knees.

Time: 12 minutes
Total: 30 minutes

more active than subcutaneous fat, it produces more of these hazardous secretions. Size also matters: The larger a visceral fat cell grows, the more active it becomes.

You might liken the difference between subcutaneous and visceral fat to that of a dormant volcano compared with one that's active. The latter is spewing out nasty stuff all the time; the other is just part of the landscape.

**Now, here's what all this means to you:** If your belly is bulging with visceral fat, it's likely that you have metabolic syndrome. Metabolic syndrome is a condition in which a person is inflicted with a cluster of heart-disease risk factors—specifically, a 36-inch (or greater) waist and any two of these four maladies: high triglycerides (the fat in your blood), high blood sugar, low HDL cholesterol (the good kind), and high blood pressure. This combination increases the likelihood you'll develop diabetes by 500 percent, have a heart attack by 300 percent, and die of a heart attack by 200 percent. (Become diabetic, and there's an 80 percent chance you'll die of heart disease.)

And that brings us back to the sumos.

Despite having waists that far exceed 40 inches, most sumos don't exhibit any of the three blood markers for metabolic syndrome—high triglycerides, high blood sugar, or low HDL cholesterol. Again, it comes down to the jiggle factor—more subcutaneous fat, less visceral fat, less risk of diabetes and heart disease. So that prompts the question: How do you know whether your belly houses dangerous levels of visceral fat or if you have the internal makeup of a sumo wrestler?

The first step is taking that waist measurement (for how-to instructions, see "Waists and Measures" on page 55). If it's more than 36 inches, your immediate plan of action—besides a new diet-and-exercise regimen—should be a visit to the doctor. There, you'll want to request a full "metabolic profile." If you have an increasing waistline and any two of the aforementioned requirements for metabolic syndrome, you most assuredly have high amounts of visceral fat. It's probably more likely than you think: Recent estimates suggest that metabolic syndrome affects nearly 17

percent of men over 20 and more than 40 percent of men over 40.

Unlike subcutaneous fat, visceral fat can't be liposuctioned away. But it's also easier to target by less-invasive means. If you understand how it found its way inside you and why it's humping up against your internal organs, you'll have a pretty good idea of how to send it packing. Some tips:

**Go to bed earlier.** A study in Finland looked at sets of identical twins and discovered that of each set of siblings, the twin who slept less and was under more stress had more visceral fat.

**But have just one drink first.** In a study at the University at Buffalo, the men with the most visceral fat drank only once or twice every 2 weeks but consumed more than four drinks each time. Those with the least visceral fat, on the other hand, drank small amounts of alcohol every day— usually about one drink.

**Have the meat, skip the potato.** A study at the University of Connecticut found that men on low-carb diets lost three times more abdominal fat than those on low-fat diets, while lowering their risk of heart disease.

**Take a walk.** Research shows that the body prefers to use visceral fat for energy, says Ross. In a study that he published in the *Annals of Internal Medicine*, Ross and his team asked obese men to walk briskly or jog lightly daily for 3 months, while eating

# How Stress Makes You Fat

## 1. Stressor (divorce lawyer, mean-spirited boss)

**Hypothalamus:** responds to stress by secreting corticotrophin-releasing hormone (CRH), which travels through the capillaries to the pituitary gland

**Pituitary gland:** reacts to the CRH by releasing adrenocorticotrophic hormone (ACTH)

**Adrenal glands:** respond to the ACTH by flooding the bloodstream with two stress hormones, epinephrine (commonly called adrenaline) and cortisol

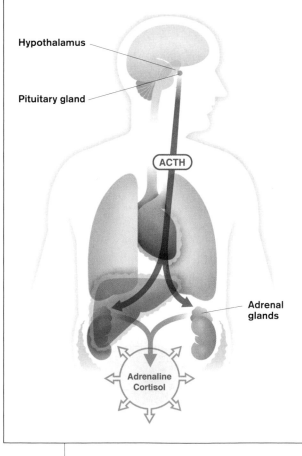

Hypothalamus

Pituitary gland

ACTH

Adrenal glands

Adrenaline
Cortisol

## 2. Adrenaline

Adrenaline switches on the body's primordial fight-or-flight response.

- Heart rate and pulse quicken to send extra blood to the muscles and organs.
- Bronchial tubes dilate to accept extra oxygen to feed the brain and keep us alert.
- Blood vessels constrict to stem bleeding in case of an injury.

## 3. Cortisol (your friend)

Cortisol and adrenaline release fat and sugar (glucose) into the bloodstream for use as energy to deal with the stressor in an emergency. That works perfectly during short-term stress, such as when you need to fend off the angry Rottweiler chasing your bike.

## 4. Cortisol (your enemy)

Cortisol can also signal your cells to store as much fat as possible and inhibit the body from releasing fat to burn as energy. This occurs when cortisol levels remain high due to long-term mental stressors, such as a lunatic boss, a pesky divorce attorney, or a teenager who insists on smoking dope in the living room. Chronically elevated cortisol disrupts the body's metabolic control systems: Muscle breaks down, blood sugar rises, appetite increases, and you get fat! What's worse, the fat tends to accumulate in the abdominal region and on the artery walls because visceral fat, which resides behind the abdominal muscles, has more cortisol receptors than does fat located just under the skin.

—Heather Hurlock

enough to maintain their weight. The result: They reduced their visceral fat by 12 percent.

**Go hard.** Mild exercise whacks away at visceral fat, but strenuous activity has an even greater effect. Canadian researchers found that losing just 11 percent of your body weight can result in a 4 percent reduction in visceral fat; thus, a guy who weighs 205 pounds can cut his visceral fat in half by losing 23 pounds. The best weight-loss plan: cardio and strength training, each performed three times a week. Korean scientists found this formula resulted in 4 more pounds of weight loss and 11 percent more visceral fat loss than cardio alone.

**And keep working out.** Sumos consume up to 7,000 calories a day, but as long as they exercise—and their fat stores remain subcutaneous—their risks of heart disease and diabetes remain small. But if they stop exercising and continue eating heavily once they retire, their risk of diabetes shoots up. The lesson: Don't sweat the jiggles. Just sweat.

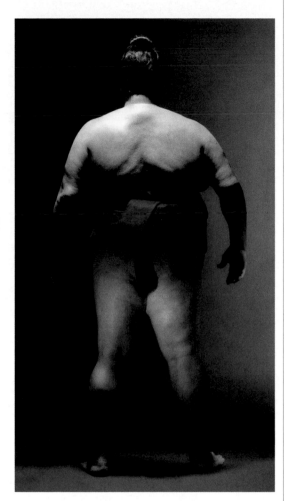

BY MYATT MURPHY

# Win the Fat War

Just 30 minutes a day is all you
need for a leaner, meaner body

**H**ere's a total-body workout that'll leave you leaner than ever and takes less than half an hour a day.

To help you combat weight gain—and prime your body for future muscle growth—we turned to Juan Carlos Santana, MEd, CSCS. As CEO of the Institute of Human Performance in Boca Raton, Florida, Santana works with high-performance athletes and builds South Beach bodies year-round. By not allowing the calendar to determine the shape you're in, he can position you for your best fitness year ever.

Santana's principles are simple but effective: (1) Work large amounts of muscle to rev up your metabolism. (2) Strengthen your core and hone your balance to safeguard injury-prone areas. (3) Apply both of these precepts to one fat-torching routine, performed 3 days a week with at least a day of rest between workouts.

## The Payoffs

**Faster fat loss:** Your body must burn an additional 50 calories a day to maintain every new pound of muscle you build. This routine targets areas where you can add mass fast. For instance, the squat works the largest muscles of your lower body, while the bench press and seated row develop your upper body.

**Harder abs:** This workout may appear devoid of ab exercises; it's not. The Swiss-ball pushup forces your abs to contract to keep you balanced, the medicine-ball chop

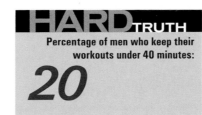

**HARD** TRUTH
Percentage of men who keep their workouts under 40 minutes:

*20*

and torso rotation both engage your core fully, and the squat challenges your abdominals throughout the entire movement.

**Bigger muscle:** By working all your major muscle groups in one session three times a week, you'll give each muscle more frequent attention than conventional bodybuilding workouts do. Studies show that this leads to greater growth—while reducing the overall time you spend in the gym.

## Benchmark of Success

### How do you measure up?

The single-leg squat touchdown is one of the most natural athletic movements: You bend at the knees while balancing on one leg. Even if you've never done the exercise, you'll find yourself in similar positions in sports. As a timed test, the move measures your ability to stay strong while keeping a stable base, an important factor in almost any activity and key to building muscle.

Balance on your right leg with your knees slightly bent. (See Circuit 3 on page 64 for photos.) Start your stopwatch. Slowly bend your knee to lower your body toward the floor while reaching toward the outside of your right foot with your left hand. Push through your heel and squeeze your glutes to return to the starting position, then repeat as many times as you can. Stop the clock when you lose balance and have to stand on both feet. Then restart the clock and repeat on your left leg. Track your progress using the chart on page 65.

# CIRCUIT 1

Do each exercise in this circuit without resting between moves.
Rest for 45 to 60 seconds, and repeat the circuit twice more.
Then move to the next circuit.

## BARBELL SQUAT

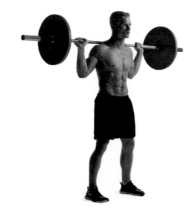

Place a barbell at chest height in a squat rack.
Grab the bar with an overhand grip slightly
more than shoulder width and rest it across
the back of your shoulders. Lift the bar off the
rack and step back.

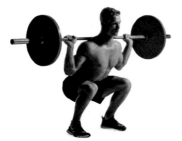

Keeping your back naturally arched, bend at
the hips and knees until your thighs are
parallel to the floor. Press yourself back up into
a standing position.

**The plan:** Perform 8 to 15 repetitions.

## SWISS-BALL PUSHUP

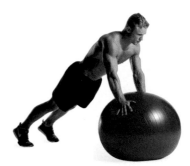

With the balls of your feet on the floor, assume
the standard pushup position, but place your
hands on the sides of a Swiss ball directly
under your shoulders. Spread your fingers,
with your thumbs pointing forward.

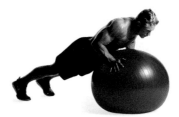

Keeping your body in a straight line from your
head to your heels, bend your arms until your
chest touches the ball. Pause, then push
yourself up to the starting position.

**The plan:** Perform 10 to 15 repetitions.

## TORSO ROTATION

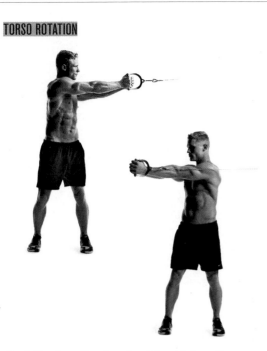

Grab the handle of a shoulder-high pulley cable (or resistance bands) with both hands. With your left side to the weight stack and both arms extended toward the stack, step away until you feel tension.

Keeping your arms straight, rotate your shoulders to the right, then return.

**The plan:** Do 15 to 20 repetitions, then turn around and repeat.

## CIRCUIT 2

Do each exercise in this circuit without resting between moves.

Rest for 45 to 60 seconds, and repeat the circuit twice more.

Then move to the next circuit.

## BARBELL BENCH PRESS

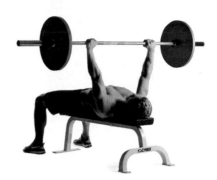

Lie on a bench with your feet flat on the floor. Grab the bar with your hands slightly more than shoulder-width apart and hold the weight with your arms extended over your chest.

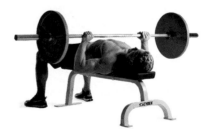

Pull your shoulder blades back and together, then lower the bar to your chest. (Tuck your elbows in—don't let them flare out to the sides.) Pause, then push the weight back up.

**The plan:** Perform 8 to 15 repetitions.

### ALTERNATING ROW

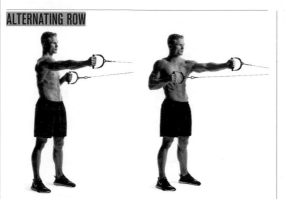

Grab a pulley handle in each hand and step back so there's slight tension in the cables. Quickly pull the left handle in toward the left side of your chest.

Allow your arm to straighten as you draw your right arm in.

**The plan:** Perform 10 to 15 repetitions with each arm.

### MEDICINE-BALL CHOP

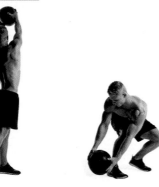

Stand holding a medicine ball with your arms straight and over your left shoulder. Pivot to the left so that your right heel rises off the floor and your torso faces left. This is the starting position.

Quickly bend your knees and rotate your torso to the right as you draw your arms across your body and down. Once the ball is outside your right lower leg, quickly reverse the motion to return to the starting position. Complete your repetitions, then switch positions to work the opposite side.

**The plan:** Perform 10 to 15 repetitions in each direction.

## CIRCUIT 3

Do each exercise in this circuit without resting between moves.

Rest for 45 to 60 seconds, and repeat the circuit twice more.

### SEATED ROW

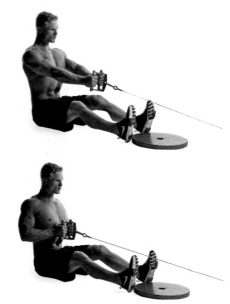

Sit at a seated-row station or on the floor a couple of feet from a low pulley cable, your feet on the footrests or a weight plate. Attach a handle that allows you to use a neutral grip (palms facing each other).

Grab the handle and slowly draw it toward your midsection while keeping your back perpendicular to the floor. The handle should touch just below your chest. Pause, then slowly allow your arms to straighten.

**The plan:** Perform 8 to 15 repetitions.

## SINGLE-LEG SQUAT TOUCHDOWN

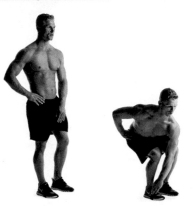

Balance on your right leg with your knees slightly bent and your hands on your hips.

Slowly bend your knee to lower your body toward the floor while reaching toward the outside of your right foot with your left hand. Push through your heel and squeeze your glutes to return to the starting position.

**The plan:** Perform 15 to 20 repetitions on each leg.

## DUMBBELL CROSS PUNCH

Stand holding a pair of light dumbbells in front of you, palms angled in.

Punch your left fist forward and slightly to the right, rotating your wrist as you go.

Draw your arm back as you punch with your right fist.

**The plan:** Perform 15 to 20 repetitions with each arm.

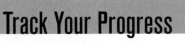

# Track Your Progress

Add up the total time it takes to perform the single-leg squat touchdown with both legs and the total number of reps you did. Divide each number by two, and record the resulting averages in this chart. Follow the workout, and retest yourself every week.

Start (average time/average reps) _____

Week 1 (average time/average reps) _____

Week 2 (average time/average reps) _____

Week 3 (average time/average reps) _____

Week 4 (average time/average reps) _____

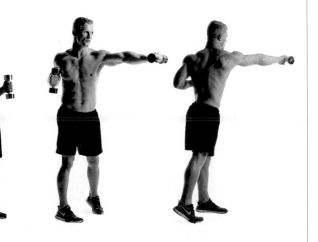

BY MATT GOULDING

# Shop Once, Eat Right All Week

You might not use the terms "pizza box" and "serving dish" interchangeably, but if you're like most guys, you probably could. That's because 64 percent of men spend little or no time preparing their meals. Their excuses? Time and money constraints. Unfortunately—and perhaps not coincidentally—that number parallels the 64 percent who are overweight. It's no wonder: The inexpensive, time-saving foods that guys choose most often are also the ones that are the highest in sugar, fat, and calories, according to a recent study from the University of Washington.

Thankfully, we have a culinary solution that'll perfectly fit your budget, schedule, and diet. The plan: Set aside 20 minutes on the weekend to fulfill our 16-item shopping list, then forget about your wallet—and collection of takeout menus—for the rest of the workweek. By following our 5-day menu, you'll have the precise number of ingredients to create 10 fast, flavorful meals, all of which are designed to help you build muscle and melt fat while saving you money. (The average price of 10 meals eaten out: $85; the total price of our meals: $47.96.) Each night, you'll simply prepare a quick and easy dinner, and

# The Grocery List

A balance of protein-packed meats, fresh produce, and a few versatile extras are all you need to feed yourself well.

Frozen shrimp: 1 pound uncooked, medium size

Rotisserie chicken: 1 cooked

Pork tenderloin: 1 herb-flavored or lemon-garlic marinated (about ¾ pound)

Bell peppers: 1 tray tricolor (or pick out 1 red, 1 yellow, and 1 orange)

Yellow onions: 4 medium

Baby mixed greens: 4-ounce bag, washed

Portobello mushrooms: 2 large caps

Asparagus: 1 bunch

Garlic: 1 head

Sun-dried-tomato pesto: 8-ounce jar

Avocado: 1 ripe

Mozzarella: 8-ounce bag, shredded

Instant brown rice: 1 pound box

Black beans: 12-ounce can

100 percent whole-wheat fettuccine: 16-ounce box

10-inch 100 percent whole-wheat tortillas: 1 package

Cumin: ground, 1 jar

Peanuts: 1 small jar

Orange juice: 1 small box

## The Pantry List

Buy these crucial building blocks every couple of months so they're always on hand to construct meals around the clock.

Canola or other cooking oil

Reduced-fat mayonnaise

Low-sodium soy sauce

Peanut butter

Extra-virgin olive oil

Balsamic vinegar

Parmesan cheese

Salsa

Tabasco or other hot sauce

Salt and ground black pepper

then creatively use the leftovers to assemble the next day's lunch. Call it the mixologist's guide to eating. The best part: While the other guys are stuck on hold in drive-thrus, you'll be rolling through the express line with your next 10 meals in tow.

## Sunday Night's Dinner

### ROTISSERIE CHICKEN WITH ROASTED VEGETABLES

¾ bunch asparagus (about 8 medium spears)

2 portobello mushroom caps, sliced ¼" thick

1 medium onion, cut in ¼"-thick rings

½ tablespoon extra-virgin olive oil

Salt and ground black pepper

1 rotisserie chicken breast or leg

Preheat the oven to 400°F. Remove the woody ends of the asparagus by gently bending each stalk until it breaks—it'll naturally snap off at the right spot. In a baking dish, toss the asparagus, mushrooms, and onion with the oil and season with salt and pepper to taste. Roast for 12 to 15 minutes, or until the vegetables have developed a light brown crust. Serve half the vegetables with the chicken. Reserve the other half of the vegetables for other meals this week.

430 calories, 36 g protein, 18 g carbohydrates, 25 g fat (7 g saturated), 5 g fiber

*Serve with a simple mixed-greens salad tossed with olive oil and vinegar.*

## The Next Day's Lunch

### CHICKEN PORTOBELLO WRAP WITH BALSAMIC AIOLI

1 cup chopped rotisserie chicken (left over from Sunday's dinner)

3 bell peppers

1 clove garlic, minced

1 tablespoon reduced-fat mayonnaise

1 teaspoon balsamic vinegar

1 whole-wheat tortilla

2 tablespoons shredded mozzarella cheese

1 small handful mixed greens

1 cup roasted vegetables (left over from Sunday's dinner)

To chop the chicken, remove the skin and use a fork to pull the meat from the bones. Place the meat on your cutting board and cut it into bite-size pieces—it should yield about 3 cups' worth. Use 1 cup for the wrap and save the other 2 cups for later in the week. Chop the peppers into ½" pieces. They should yield about 4 cups; use ½ cup today and save the rest in a plastic bag for dinner.

In a bowl, mix the garlic, mayonnaise, and vinegar together to make the aioli. Brush the tortilla with the aioli, then put the cheese down the middle, followed by the greens, chicken, and vegetables. To make a tight wrap, fold the bottom of the tortilla up first, then roll it from the side.

400 calories, 43 g protein, 29 g carbohydrates, 15 g fat (4.5 g saturated), 5 g fiber

## Monday Night's Dinner

### SHRIMP FAJITAS

¼ cup instant brown rice (measured dry)

½ can black beans, drained and heated

½ tablespoon canola or other cooking oil

1 medium onion, sliced

1½ cups chopped bell peppers (left over from prepping the Chicken Portobello Wrap you had for lunch)

2 cloves garlic, chopped

8 ounces frozen shrimp, defrosted

Hot-pepper sauce to taste

½ teaspoon ground cumin

Salt and ground black pepper

½ avocado, thinly sliced

1 whole-wheat tortilla, warmed

Cook the rice according to the package directions, then add the beans. Heat the oil in a large skillet over high heat. Add the onion, bell peppers, and garlic, and cook for 5 to 7 minutes, or until the vegetables begin to brown. Mix in the shrimp, hot-pepper sauce, and cumin and season with salt and black pepper to taste. Cook for another 3 minutes, or until the shrimp are pink and firm. Serve half of the shrimp fajita mix with a small scoop of the rice and beans, the avocado, and the tortilla.

Reserve the rest of the rice and beans in a microwaveable bowl or plastic container along with the leftover fajita mix, and use it for tomorrow's lunch.

602 calories, 42 g protein, 71 g carbohydrates, 22.5 g fat (3 g saturated), 15 g fiber

## The Next Day's Lunch

### FIESTA RICE BOWL

Rice, beans, and fajita mix (left over from Monday's dinner)

½ avocado, thinly sliced

Salsa (optional)

Heat the leftovers in a microwaveable bowl for 60 seconds. Top with the avocado and salsa to taste, if desired.

650 calories, 37 g protein, 85 g carbohydrates, 20 g fat (3 g saturated), 16 g fiber

## Classic Kitchen Skill: Mincing Garlic

You can buy the jarred stuff, but precut garlic lacks many of the essential oils that give this classic vegetable its intense (and addictive) flavor. For the full garlicky effect, you need to mince it yourself. Here's how: Lay a clove, still in its papery skin, on a cutting board. Place a heavy knife flat on top and whack it with a tight fist to flatten the clove. Peel off the skin and slice the clove lengthwise into thin planks. Rotate the slices 90 degrees and repeat for a fine mince.

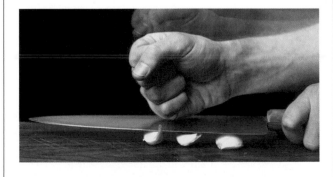

## Tuesday Night's Dinner

### FETTUCCINE WITH CHICKEN, ROASTED VEGETABLES, AND SUN-DRIED-TOMATO PESTO

6 ounces 100 percent whole-wheat fettuccine

Canola oil

1 cup chopped rotisserie chicken (left over from Sunday's dinner)

1 cup roasted vegetables (left over from Sunday's dinner)

1½ tablespoons sun-dried-tomato pesto

Salt and ground black pepper

Parmesan cheese

Cook the fettuccine in a large pot of boiling, salted water until al dente, about 10 minutes. Toss half of the pasta with some canola oil and reserve in a container for Thursday's lunch. Combine the chicken, vegetables, and sun-dried-tomato pesto with the remaining pasta. Season with salt and pepper to taste. Grate some Parmesan and sprinkle on top.

490 calories, 46 g protein, 34 g carbohydrates, 20 g fat (5 g saturated), 6 g fiber

*Serve with 1 cup of mixed greens, dressed with olive oil and balsamic vinegar.*

## The Next Day's Lunch

### ITALIAN QUESADILLA

1 tablespoon sun-dried-tomato pesto

1 whole-wheat tortilla

½ cup shredded mozzarella cheese

½ cup chopped rotisserie chicken (left over from Sunday)

1 cup roasted vegetables (left over from Sunday)

Spread the pesto on the tortilla. Top with the cheese, chicken, and vegetables, and microwave open-faced for 1 minute, or until the cheese has fully melted. Fold over and slice into quarters. If you have time, cook it over low heat in a skillet or sauté pan for a crispier result.

440 calories, 38 g protein, 32 g carbohydrates, 19 g fat (8 g saturated), 4 g fiber

## Wednesday Night's Dinner

### SPICY SHRIMP-AND-ASPARAGUS STIR-FRY

½ cup instant brown rice (measured dry)

1 teaspoon canola or other cooking oil

½ medium onion, chopped

1 cup mixed chopped bell peppers (left over from Sunday's lunch)

2 cloves garlic, chopped (see "Classic Kitchen Skill" on page 69)

1 cup chopped raw asparagus

8 ounces frozen shrimp, thawed

1 tablespoon soy sauce

Hot sauce

Salt and ground black pepper

Prepare the rice according to the package directions. Add the oil to a large skillet and place over high heat. When the oil is smoking, add the onion, bell peppers, garlic, and asparagus and cook, stirring constantly, for 5 minutes, or until the vegetables have browned slightly. Stir in the shrimp, soy sauce, and hot sauce to taste and cook for an additional 3 minutes. Season with salt and black pepper to taste. Serve half of it over the rice, reserving the remaining stir-fry for lunch tomorrow.

592 calories, 36 g protein, 88 g carbohydrates, 11 g fat (2 g saturated), 9 g fiber

## The Next Day's Lunch

### THAI PEANUT NOODLES

1 cup shrimp stir-fry (left over from Wednesday's dinner)

3 ounces cooked whole-wheat fettuccine (left over from Tuesday's dinner)

1 tablespoon peanut butter

½ tablespoon soy sauce

1 tablespoon water

Splash of vinegar or orange juice

¼ teaspoon ground black pepper

Hot sauce

1 tablespoon chopped peanuts (optional)

Toss the stir-fry with the pasta. In a separate bowl, whisk together the peanut butter, soy sauce, water, vinegar or OJ, and pepper. Add hot sauce to taste to the stir-fry and pasta, and mix thoroughly. Top with the peanuts, if desired. Eat cold or at room temperature.

530 calories, 43 g protein, 63 g carbohydrates, 12 g fat (2 g saturated), 7 g fiber

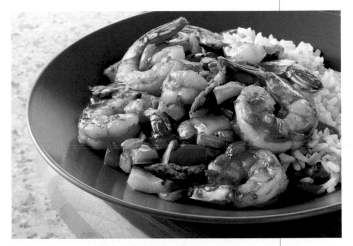

**With 36 grams of protein, this spicy shrimp stir-fry is a biceps builder.**

## Thursday Night's Dinner

### ROASTED PORK LOIN WITH PEPPERS AND BALSAMIC ONIONS

 1 pork tenderloin, about ¾ pound (herb or lemon-garlic marinated, if available; check the meat section of your grocery store)

 1 medium onion, quartered

 1 cup mixed chopped bell peppers (left over from Sunday's lunch)

 2 cloves garlic, crushed

 1 tablespoon extra-virgin olive oil

 1 tablespoon balsamic vinegar

 Salt and ground black pepper

Preheat the oven to 450°F. In a baking dish, toss together the pork, onion, bell peppers, garlic, oil, and vinegar. Season with salt and black pepper to taste. Bake for 20 to 25 minutes, depending on the thickness of the tenderloin (to an internal temperature of 150°F, if using a thermometer). Enjoy half the pork and vegetables tonight, and save the rest—storing both together in a sealed container—for lunch tomorrow.

350 calories, 37 g protein, 12 g carbohydrates, 17 g fat (3.5 g saturated), 2 g fiber

*If you want a bigger meal, prepare ¼ cup of instant brown rice, measured dry. It'll add 170 calories, 4 grams of protein, 36 grams of carbohydrates, 1 gram of fat, and 2 grams of fiber to the nutrition information.*

## The Next Day's Lunch

### ROASTED PORK WRAP

 ½ tablespoon sun-dried-tomato pesto

 ½ tablespoon reduced-fat mayonnaise

 1 whole-wheat tortilla

 2 tablespoons shredded mozzarella cheese

 Pork tenderloin, thinly sliced, and vegetables (left over from Thursday's dinner)

In a small bowl, combine the pesto and mayonnaise, and spread over the tortilla. Layer the cheese, pork slices, and leftover vegetables on top, and wrap it up.

480 calories, 48 g protein, 37 g carbohydrates, 16 g fat (5 g saturated), 3 g fiber

# Rev Your Metabolism

**BY MIKE MEJIA, CSCS**

This grueling four-drill sequence incinerates pepperoni pizzas and other indulgences. Do each exercise for 30 seconds, then break for 1 minute. Repeat the circuit, this time performing each move for 45 seconds. Rest for 90 seconds, then repeat once more, doing each move for 60 seconds.

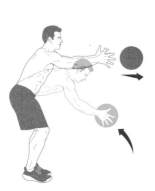

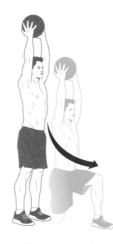

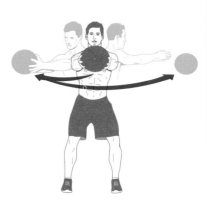

**Side-to-side shuffle:** Stand facing a wall from 5 feet away, holding a medicine ball at chest height. Throw the ball at the wall 3 to 5 feet to your left and at eye level. As the ball bounces off the wall, shuffle sideways and catch it on a hop before firing it back to your right.

**Overhead lunge walk:** Stand holding a medicine ball overhead at arm's length. Keeping your arms straight, take a large step forward until both knees are bent 90 degrees and your back knee is an inch or two off the floor. Stride forward with the opposite leg.

**Medicine-ball 180:** Stand with your side facing a wall about 5 feet away. Hold a medicine ball in front of your chest, arms straight. Rotate your torso away from the wall slightly, then rotate forcefully toward the wall, throwing the ball at the wall and slightly behind you. Turn around and catch the ball, then repeat the move in the opposite direction.

**Pushup shuttle:** Assume the classic pushup position, but instead of placing both hands on the floor, place your left hand on a medicine ball. Bend your arms to lower your body toward the floor. Push yourself up with enough force to propel your hand off the ball. Land with your right hand on the ball and your left hand on the floor, to the left of the ball. Repeat to the other side.

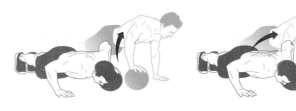

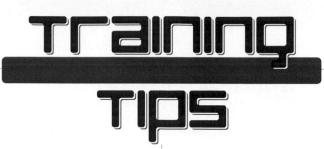

## What kind of exercise spurs the most weight loss?

The kind that works the most muscle—whether it's weight training, cardio, or a combination. For instance, you might do intervals of sprints and agility drills for 20 minutes with minimal rest. Or try a resistance-training circuit of total-body movements, such as the one listed below. Do 8 to 12 repetitions of each move and rest only as long as you need to after the circuit. Repeat for a total of three circuits.

**Dumbbell front squat to press:** Stand holding a pair of dumbbells at shoulder height, with your elbows down and your palms facing each other. Lower yourself into a squat until the fronts of your thighs are parallel (or nearly so) to the floor. Pause, then drive the weights up and over your head while you straighten your legs. Return to the starting position.

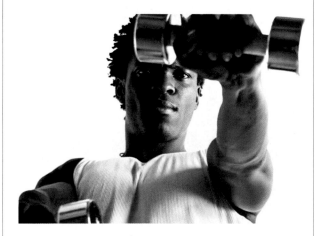

**Romanian deadlift:** Stand with your feet shoulder-width apart, your knees slightly bent, and a pair of dumbbells hanging down at arm's length in front of your thighs. Retract your shoulder blades and pull in your stomach. Bend forward at the hips until the weights are at about shin level and your torso is as close to parallel to the floor as possible. Pause, then press your heels against the floor as you lift your torso back to the starting position.

**Dumbbell row:** Stand holding a pair of dumbbells in front of your thighs. Bend forward at the waist until your torso is almost parallel to the floor. Pull the weights to the bottom of your rib cage, then slowly lower them.

**Dumbbell bench press:** Lie on a flat bench holding a pair of dumbbells up over your middle chest with an overhand grip and straight arms. Pinching your shoulder blades back, bend your elbows and slowly lower the weights until they're right next to your armpits, a few inches higher than chest level. Pause, then press back to the starting position.

**Lunge:** Stand holding a pair of dumbbells, arms at your sides. Step forward with one foot and lower your body until your front thigh is parallel to the floor. Push back up and repeat with your other foot.

**Dumbbell curl to press:** Stand holding a pair of dumbbells with an underhand grip (palms facing forward) at arm's length next to your thighs. Without moving your shoulders forward, move your arms slightly back behind you. Curl the weights up to your shoulders, then rotate your arms as you press the weights overhead so that your palms face forward at the top of the move. Pause for 2 seconds, then return to the starting position.

**The harder my workout, the larger my appetite. Is it okay to pig out, since my body's in fat-burning mode?**

No. Your body does need carbs and protein within 15 minutes of your last rep, but spreading out your eating will make better use of your elevated metabolism. Overloading your fat-burning engine can shunt extra calories to fat reserves.

**How can I stop my postwork food cravings?**

Worker bees eat lunch around noon or 1 p.m., but dinner might not come until 8 o'clock. A snack will blunt the craving and allow for a sensible dinner without the junk-food binge. Our advice is to eat better earlier in the day (but don't gorge), and take advantage of a midafternoon break to down a quick snack, such as yogurt, an apple with a thin layer of peanut butter, or some string cheese.

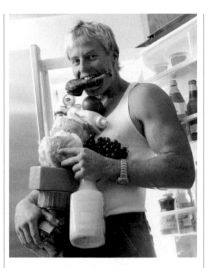

**What can I eat after an evening workout that won't weigh me down?**

Don't worry about eating anything too heavy. Nutritionists advise most people to avoid calorie-laden meals in the evening because that's when the body's metabolism begins to slow down. But your situation is different: Exercising late in the day kicks your metabolism into high gear for at least 4 hours, so after your workout, eat a full meal as soon as possible. Your muscles need that nutrition for repair and growth.

A 400- to 500-calorie meal using a 40-30-30 approach (40 percent of calories from protein, 30 from fat, and 30 from carbohydrate) is ideal. One of our favorite

postworkout dinners: 6 ounces of lean steak, a generous portion of broccoli or green beans, and 2 cups of brown rice (or a yam).

**When I stand up, I'm thin. When I sit down, I'm fat. What's up with that—and what can I do about it?**

The rolls that appear when you sit down are partially a result of how you're sitting. Like many guys, you probably spend the bulk of your day staring at a computer screen—a situation that conditions your body to slouch. When your spine hunches, it compresses your midriff, accentuating any abdominal fat you might have, says Thomas Fahey, PhD, professor of kinesiology at California State University, Chico.

Try to be conscious of your posture every time you take a load off—imagine there's a string at the top of your head attached to the ceiling and that you're being pulled upward. Another tip: If you drive a lot, adjust your rearview mirror so you have to sit straight up to see out the back. Both tactics will help train your body to maintain good posture and help reduce those unsightly rolls.

If you really want to get industrious about things, substitute a Swiss ball for your office chair a few days a week. Sitting on the ball will force your core to balance your body, strengthening every muscle in your torso, says Jim Youssef, MD, an orthopedic surgeon at Durango Orthopedics in Colorado.

Maintaining good posture is critical for any guy over the age of 40. Once into their fifth or sixth decade, men gradually lose bone density. This loss—called osteoporosis—is most pronounced in the spine, where microscopic fractures can cause you to shrink up to 2 inches by the time you're 70. (The drying of gelatinous tissue between your vertebrae can have the same effect.) As your vertebrae and

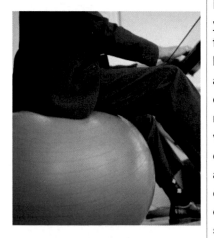

disks age, their alignment changes, making your stomach appear larger, says Andrew Casden, MD, associate director of the Spine Institute at Beth Israel Medical Center in New York City.

You can reverse the process by engaging in bone-stressing activities, such as running and weight lifting, and popping some $B_{12}$. Researchers at Tufts University in Boston recently found that levels of the vitamin below 6 micrograms facilitate bone loss. Get your 6 micrograms by taking a daily multivitamin or eating a fortified breakfast cereal.

**I've lost 20 pounds by walking 5 to 10 miles a day, but the weight has stopped coming off. What happened?**

It's simple math: There's less of you to move, so you're burning fewer calories than you did at the higher weight. If your activity level and diet remain the same, your calorie intake will eventually match your output, and your weight will stabilize. This especially happens with low-impact activities, such as walking. By contrast, it's easier to increase effort with running, cycling, or swimming as you become fit. You

may need to eat less, exercise harder, or both. Add some hills to your walk, or mix in some jogging or short sprints. You'll become fitter and boost your calorie burn.

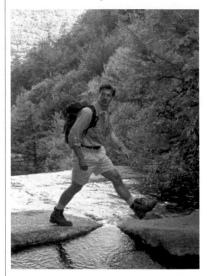

**I eat right and exercise, so why do I hit weight-loss plateaus?**

Weight-loss plateaus have many causes. Let's assume you've ruled out undereating (which triggers fat storage) and excessive stress (which releases cortisol, inhibiting fat loss). Your metabolism could just need a workout of its own.

One intriguing plateau buster comes from a 2004 University of Colorado study, which linked increased "energy flux," or the total amount of calories your body processes in a day, to increased metabolism. Working out harder and eating more—while keeping the overall balance the same—could improve your ability to break down food.

## If I stop lifting, will my muscle turn to fat?

No. Your body composition could eventually shift more toward fat because you'll store calories that aren't being burned off at the gym, but one doesn't "turn into" the other.

## Should I eat less in the winter?

If you bike and swim in the summer, and now you only sit and watch sports, you may need to cut your daily intake by 300 to 500 calories or more. Start by downsizing portions: Trade the 8 ounces of sirloin you eat in July for 6 ounces, and that three-egg

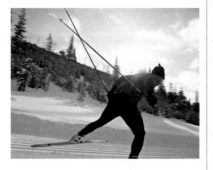

omelet for two scrambled eggs. The best advice: Find a winter exercise—snowshoeing, cross-country skiing—or do some extra time at the gym.

## What fruits aren't loaded with carbs?

Fruits pack healthier carbs than cookies, but not all fruits are created equal. Sure, bananas, pears, and most dried fruits are good for you, but they offer relatively few nutrients for the carbs in each. When possible, opt for blackberries, raspberries, and papaya, which are loaded with fiber and other powerful nutrients and carry far fewer carbs per serving.

## I heard we should eat most of our carbs in the morning. Is this true?

Yes. Skew your morning meal in favor of complex carbohydrates (think steel-cut oats), the glycogen-producing, long-burning muscle fuel. You essentially fasted all night while you were asleep, and your body needs quick energy to attack the day. Avoid breakfasts high in fats (such as your typical fast-food fare), because they interfere with carbohydrate metabolism and

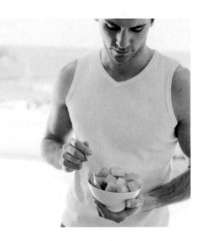

deny your muscles glycogen. A better time to eat fats (in moderation) would be later in the day, so they can fill you up and curb evening cravings.

## When I'm hungry, I want starches. How can I fill up without all the carbs?

There are plenty of satisfying substitutes for the usual pasta and potatoes. I love roasted squash—particularly butternut, acorn, and spaghetti—because it's easy and works well with meat and fish. Cauliflower works as a healthy stand-in for mashed potatoes. Simply boil or steam a whole head, then blend or mash with a bit of milk and a pat of butter. If you must have grains, try quinoa—with more protein and fiber, and fewer carbs, it's a healthier carb choice.

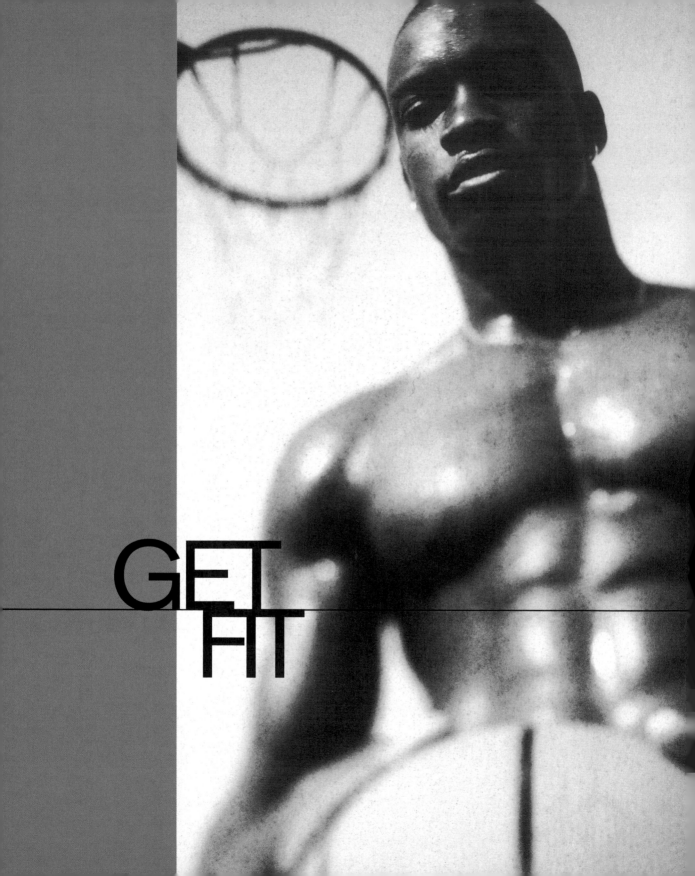

GET
FIT

Almost two-thirds of adults get no vigorous physical activity. And we're not talking marathons here! The experts who keep these stats define "vigorous physical activity" as "lasting 10 minutes or more." The cost of all this sitting to our overall society could be as high as $24.3 billion!

What, besides the force of gravity, is keeping all those folks on the couch and out of the gym? The American Council on Exercise posed this question in an informal survey on its Web site. "I'm too out of shape to work out" said 19 percent of respondents. "I don't know what to do at the gym" said another 21 percent. "Gyms are too crowded," said 46 percent. "People at the gym are too rude," said 11 percent. "I don't know what questions to ask once I get there," said the remaining 3 percent.

If any of those excuses sound familiar to you, we're here to dispel them—and any others you might have come up with. You'll eliminate every excuse and rebuild your entire body with our three-step plan. Then, following the examples of five of the world's best athletes, you'll unleash your faster, stronger self. Next, you'll get a glimpse inside the NFL's secret training camp to steal their best muscle, speed, and agility workouts.

So, lest you fall into that two-thirds of Americans whose posteriors are taking on the shape of their La-Z-Boys, let's get moving.

BY SCOTT QUILL

# Eliminate Every Excuse

With this three-step plan, you'll rebuild your entire body

**T**here are plenty of good reasons not to work out: job pressures, family commitments, and painfully long workout sessions that are equal parts boring and complicated.

Our solution: a three-step fitness plan backed by science but built around your life—to conquer your time constraints, speed your progress, and simplify your workouts. It's designed to increase muscle size and strength; improve flexibility and endurance; and, of course, burn fat—all in less than 90 minutes a week. Start now, and you're the odds-on favorite to be fit in 5 weeks.

## Measure Your Success

Before you start, use the following fitness tests to gauge your current levels of strength, flexibility, and endurance. After 5 weeks, repeat the assessments. "You can expect improvements of 15 to 20 percent across the board," says Michael Mejia, CSCS, coauthor of *Scrawny to Brawny*. As for muscle gain and fat loss, our plan works for both. Snap a digital photo now and another after 35 days, and your new body image will be all the proof you'll need.

**Test your strength.** Do as many classic pushups as you can without stopping, but use this precise execution: Take 2 seconds to lower your body until your upper arms dip below your elbows; pause for 1 second; then take 1 second to push your body up. This ensures that you'll perform the test identically each time you take it.

**Test your flexibility.** Place a yardstick on the floor and put a foot-long piece of mask-ing tape across the 15-inch mark. Sit with your legs out in front of you and your heels at the edge of the tape, one on each side of the yardstick. Put one hand on top of the other and reach forward over the yardstick as far as you can by bending at your hips. The number your finger-tips touch is your benchmark.

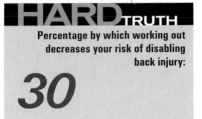

**Test your endurance.** On a treadmill or on a flat outdoor course, run or walk 1.5 miles as fast as you can, and record your time. (Warm up first by walking or jogging at an easy pace for 5 minutes.)

## Step 1: Adopt a 3-Day Standard

In a recent survey, the National Center for Health Statistics found that only 19 percent of Americans do three or more intense workouts a week. Given these hard numbers, it's unrealistic to expect that you'll suddenly start exercising for 6 or 7 days straight. Fortunately, that level of commit-ment isn't necessary. "You'll see most of the benefits of exercise by working out hard just three times a week," says Mejia. "And that's especially true if you're out of shape." Use these strategies to make sure you stick to the plan.

**Save one workout for the weekend.** "Even if Saturday and Sunday are packed with family commitments and various home-improvement projects, it's likely that you'll still have more free time then than on any given weekday," says John Raglin, PhD, an exercise psychologist at Indiana University. And that means you'll have to fit in only two sessions between Monday and Friday.

**Track the ancillary benefits.** Keep a job-performance journal on the days you exercise and the days you don't. Each day, rate these three categories on a scale of 1 (poor) to 7 (excellent):

1. Your ability to work without stopping to take unscheduled breaks

2. Your ability to stick to your routine or plan (your "to do" list) for the day

3. Your overall job performance

## Start Today

**Write down your primary goal.** Be specific: Whether you want to lose 20 pounds of fat, gain 10 pounds of muscle, or complete your first triathlon, give yourself one major objective and put it on paper.

**Schedule your first three workouts.** Plan the date, time, and place of each session on your computer's calendar or in your day planner. You'll be less likely to allow meetings or social events to interfere with your workouts. Be sure to block off a big enough chunk to account for any time needed to change your clothes, shower, or travel to the gym—the forgotten factors that doom workouts.

**Create a workout log.** Provide space to record the number of sets and repetitions and the amounts of weight you use, as well as the duration and distance of your cardio session and your total exercise time. This will give you tangible numbers to improve on with each workout.

"It's likely you'll find that you score higher and do more on the days you exercise, despite taking time out for your workout," says Jim McKenna, PhD, a professor of physical activity and health at Leeds Metropolitan University in the United Kingdom. (Make sure you compare days that are similar in workload.) And this'll reinforce your motivation to keep at it.

**Keep your streak intact.** Research shows that when men skip a workout, there's a 62 percent chance they'll miss an exercise session the following week. Worse, "a single lapse can result in feelings of failure that are so overwhelming that a person will just quit, even though he successfully followed through with exercise 99 percent of the time," says Raglin. Institute this policy: If you don't have time for your entire workout, take 10 minutes and do a portion of your routine—even if it's only a couple of sets of pushups and lunges.

## Step 2: Go Hard, Not Long

Cap your exercise sessions at 30 minutes. YMCA researchers found that men were twice as likely to stick with an exercise program when they did shorter workouts—30 minutes or less—than when they did longer sessions. "They also gained more muscle and lost more fat because they worked at a higher intensity, instead of just going through the motions of a long workout," says Wayne Westcott, PhD, CSCS, coauthor of the study. Here's how to streamline your routine.

**Work every muscle every workout.**
University of Alabama researchers found
that men who trained their entire bodies
each session, 3 days a week, gained 10
pounds of muscle in 3 months. In fact, they
packed on four times more muscle and lost
twice as much fat as men who worked each
muscle group only once a week. It doesn't
take a lot; the big gainers did just nine total
sets in each session, about the same as two
sets each of five exercises.

**Use a modified circuit routine.** Do one
set of each exercise in a consecutive fashion,
but—unlike with a classic circuit—rest after
each. "You'll improve recovery between sets,
which will allow you to give your best effort
each time, the key to optimal gains," says
Bill Hartman, PT, CSCS, a strength coach
in Indianapolis. Why the circuit approach?
Your rest periods will be shorter than if you
performed back-to-back sets of the same
exercise—so you'll save time.

Use this simple trick to gauge the ideal
downtime: "Rest between exercises only as
long as it takes for your breathing rate to
return to normal," says Hartman. As you
become better conditioned, you'll automati-
cally take less time between sets. This
ensures that your workout is as challenging
in week 5 as it was in week 1.

**Finish with cardio.** After your weight
session, dedicate the remainder of your time
to running, cycling, or rowing. Don't worry
about the clock: "You'll improve your
conditioning more by running at a high
intensity for 15 minutes than with the slow
30-minute jog that most guys do," says Mejia.

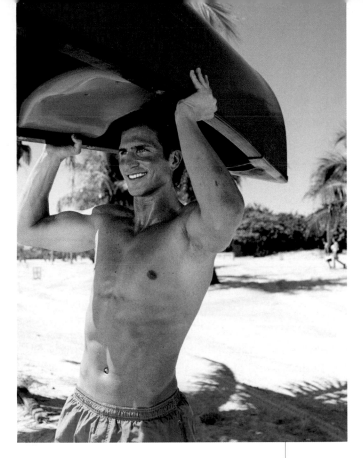

## Step 3: Keep It Simple

Forget about target heart rates and three-
digit lifting tempos. "Working out isn't
rocket science," says Mejia. "You just need to
challenge your body a little bit more each
session." The keys to doing just that, without
thinking twice:

**Trust your lungs.** In a recent study at the
University of Wisconsin–La Crosse, researchers discovered that running at a pace that
allows you to talk—but only in short spurts
of three or four words at a time—is approximately the same as exercising at your
"ventilatory threshold," or the highest
intensity you can sustain for the duration of
your cardio session. By gauging your effort

# The Transformation Workout

This plan was created by Michael Mejia, CSCS, using the concepts on the accompanying pages. Complete the routine 3 days a week, resting a day after each session. Do the exercises as a modified circuit, performing one after another in the order shown and resting only as long as it takes for your breathing rate to return to normal. Repeat once, for a total of two circuits, then spend the rest of your time running or cycling.

## 1. Reverse Overhead Lunge

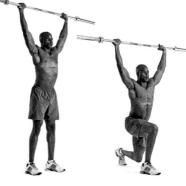

Grab a broomstick using a grip that's twice shoulder width and hold it directly above your head, elbows locked. Take a step back with your left foot and lower your body until your left knee almost touches the floor. Push yourself up and repeat, this time stepping back with your right leg. Do 10 to 12 repetitions with each leg.

## 2. Pushup

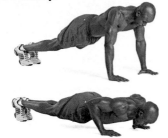

Get into standard pushup position. Keeping your body in a straight line from your head to your ankles, lower yourself until your upper arms dip below your elbows, then push your body back up. Do 10 to 12 repetitions. If it's too hard, do the incline version, with your hands placed on a bench or step. If it's too easy, place one foot on top of the other's heel as you perform the movement.

## 3. Contralateral Stepup

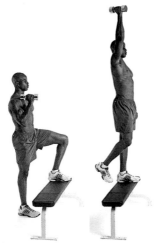

Place your left foot on a step or bench that's about knee height and hold a dumbbell in your right hand at shoulder height. Simultaneously lift your body onto the step and press the weight over your shoulder. Lower both back to the starting position, then repeat. Do 10 to 12 repetitions on each side.

## 4. Twisting Single-Arm Row

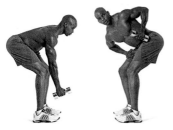

Hold a dumbbell in one hand, your palm facing in. Keeping your back naturally arched, bend forward until your torso is almost parallel to the floor and let the dumbbell hang straight down. Pull the weight to your rib cage as you rotate your upper body toward the ceiling. Reverse the move back to the starting position. Do 10 to 12 reps with each arm.

## 5. Superman

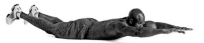

Lie facedown with your legs straight and your arms lying on the floor straight forward. Simultaneously lift your shoulders, legs, and arms off the floor. Try to hold this position for 60 seconds.

this way, you exercise as hard as possible without running out of gas too early.

**Trust your judgment.** "Without counting, lower the weight slowly and lift it fast," says Mejia. George Washington University researchers showed that lifters who used this technique gained twice as much strength as those who performed each repetition at a slow speed from start to finish. Don't worry about taking an exact amount of time: Just think "slow" or "fast" as you move the weight; your body will react accordingly.

**Trust your muscles.** In general, use the heaviest weight that allows you to perform all your repetitions without reaching failure. One caveat: Instead of defining "failure" as the point at which you can't complete one more repetition ("absolute failure"), employ the concept of "technical

failure," says Hartman. That's the point at which your body posture changes—you have to cheat by leaning forward or back to complete the movement—or you can't control the speed of the weight you're lifting. For instance, if the rate at which you perform a pushup starts to slow as you press yourself to the starting position, you've achieved technical failure. Consider that the end of your set. The reason: Once you've hit technical failure, fewer target muscle fibers are firing during each repetition thereafter—so you've achieved maximal benefit from that exercise.

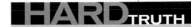

**HARD TRUTH**

Percentage increase in distance covered when men walked for 6 minutes in a group, compared with walking alone:

## 12.5

BY TED SPIKER

# Unleash Your Stronger Self

Everybody has the potential
to do extraordinary things.
Here's how you can maximize yours

Have you ever truly tested your athletic limits? If you're like most men, the answer is no. Sure, you go to the court and dribble till you're winded or head to the track and run till you're dripping wet. But you won't find your limits there. Team sports and workout routines are all about, as the adage goes, "playing within yourself." Testing your limits is about playing beyond yourself. It's about actively seeking your physical boundaries, pushing down those walls, and raising your game to a level you never thought possible.

On the following pages, you'll meet five of the world's best athletes, each representing a pillar of peak performance. For these men, success would never have come had they stopped pushing when they met resistance. Learn their strategies, and you'll soon be busting through your personal barriers. You may not earn a ticket to training camp, but you will end up in the best shape of your life.

## Speed: The Great Equalizer

You might say it's better to be fast than good. If you're too slow to beat your man, you'll never have a chance to showcase your skills. And for those short on talent, speed can level the playing field. But sports speed isn't just about maximum velocity. It's also about how fast you can accelerate and decelerate—that is, go from standing still to your top speed and vice versa. And because every 10th of a second matters, even small improvements can make a major impact on your performance.

## TEST YOUR LIMITS

The 40-yard dash is one of the best measurements of speed and acceleration, which is why it's a highly regarded test at the NFL combine.

**How to do it:** You'll need a partner and a stopwatch. Mark off 40 yards on a track or grass field. Get into a comfortable stance—a four-point sprinter's stance is typical—and instruct your timer to start the clock as soon as you move. The clock stops when any part of your chest crosses the finish line.

In "Score Yourself" on page 97, tally your scores from this and the other tests in each category.

3 points: 4.49 seconds or less
2 points: 4.5 to 4.99 seconds
1 point: 5.0 seconds or longer

## PUSH YOUR LIMITS

**Get a running start.** Mark a starting line and a finish line 20 yards apart. Begin running about 20 yards behind the starting line, and progressively build up speed so you're at top speed as you pass it. Maintain that intensity until you cross the finish line. Rest for 3 minutes, then repeat for a total of two to four sets. "This drill reinforces the running mechanics and acceleration you need to switch gears and pick up speed when you're already in motion," says Bill Hartman, PT, CSCS, a sports-performance specialist in Indianapolis. Do this workout twice a week, resting at least a day after each session.

**Step on the gas.** To develop fast starts, try this ball-drop drill from Tom Shaw,

CSCS, speed coach of the New England Patriots. Have a workout partner stand on a hard surface, holding a tennis ball at eye level. Stand about 5 yards away in a three-point stance. When he drops the ball, sprint and catch it before it bounces a second time. Have him move back a yard or two and repeat the drill until you can't get to the ball in time. The biggest gap Shaw's ever seen closed? Fifteen yards, by Deion Sanders.

**Sock it to your core.** Abs are critical to speed. Strengthen yours with this situp routine: Lie on your back and rest your heels on a wall so that your legs are straight

## Dwyane Wade

### Shooting Guard: Miami Heat

Ask Dwyane Wade who's the best player in the NBA, and he'll tell you LeBron James. That's not humility. It's strategy. "I like it better that way," says Wade. "I need a rabbit to chase. Because if I keep fighting, I'll only achieve greater success."

Before Wade entered the NBA, his rabbit was the league. College recruiters labeled him a kid from the ghetto who couldn't pass the ACT test, and his failing grade (by a point) scared off all the big schools. Still, Tom Crean, head basketball coach at the small and academically driven Marquette University, paid Wade a visit.

He was one of only three coaches who recruited the future fifth pick in the NBA draft. "He saw I had character and the will to be someone, to do something others didn't expect," Wade says of his mentor. So Wade became the first partial qualifier in Marquette's history—meaning he was accepted to attend class but couldn't play ball until his sophomore year, grades permitting.

It was that year of ineligibility—of being relegated to the practice squad—that prompted

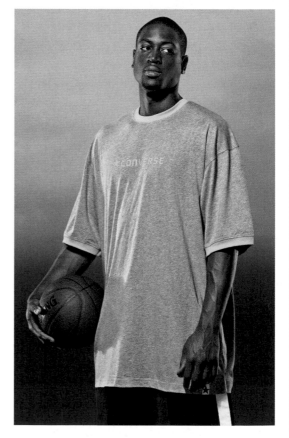

Wade to explore his boundaries. "I played the role of our upcoming opponent's star in every practice," he says. "One day I had to be a point guard, the next a post player, the next a three-point shooter." Wade learned every position on the court, which is why he excels at every location today.

—David Schipper

# Wade's Breakthrough Strategies

**Embrace deception.** You can make yourself seem quicker if you master the holdback. "I can't always go 100 miles per hour because defenders will get used to my speed," Dwyane Wade says. "But if I go slow at first, they'll get caught when I decide to blow by them."

**Beware of hesitation.** There's a difference between patience and hesitation, and it depends on confidence. "You can't be underconfident when your teammates are putting the ball in your hands," Wade says. "Remind yourself that others are depending on you."

**Be a quick study.** "No matter how bad or good you are, if you're a great listener, you're going to respond to coaching and surpass your limits," says Wade. "During practice, I always want the coach to say I picked up the play quicker than anyone else."

and at a 45-degree angle to the floor; extend your arms straight above your head. Lift your torso and touch your toes, then rotate to the right and touch both hands to the floor. Now rotate to the left and touch the floor on that side. That's one repetition. Do as many as you can in 30 seconds, rest 30 to 60 seconds, and repeat. Stop when you can't match the reps of your previous set. Perform this workout two or three times a week.

## Strength: The Unstoppable Force

Whether it's turning on a fastball or posting up in the paint, pure strength is hard to defend. But size is only part of the equation; strength is more dependent on your ability to activate the muscle you have. Learn to tap the full capacity of your muscles, and you'll become a dominant force in any sport.

### TEST YOUR LIMITS

The squat was recently ranked the single most important exercise for sports, according to a survey of NFL, NBA, NHL, and MLB strength coaches. "Squat performance is the best predictor of total-body strength," explains Hartman. The classic measure: the one-repetition-maximum squat.

**How to do it:** The safest way is to estimate it. Set the safety bars on your squat rack and grab a couple of spotters. Then load the barbell with the heaviest weight you can squat at least six times but no more than eight. Lower your body as if you were sitting back into a chair until your

thighs are parallel to the floor. To figure out your one-rep max, multiply the weight you used by the appropriate conversion factor below, then add that number to your test weight.

| NUMBER OF REPETITIONS | CONVERSION FACTOR | ONE-REP MAX |
|:---:|:---:|:---:|
| 6 | 0.17 | 3 points: More than 200 pounds |
| 7 | 0.19 | 2 points: 150 to 199 pounds |
| 8 | 0.22 | 1 point: Less than 150 pounds |

### PUSH YOUR LIMITS

**Prep your muscles.** If you're new to weight training, you'll need to strengthen your connective tissue and improve your muscular endurance before you take on the heavy weights—both to prevent injury and to improve performance. Shaw suggests this game: Pick a card from a deck. If you draw an 8, do eight pushups, eight crunches, and then eight split jumps (from a lunge position, jump straight up, switch legs in midair, and land back in a lunge). Rest for 30 to 60 seconds, then pick another card. Repeat until you've gone through 15 to 20 cards. "Do this for a week before lifting heavy," says Shaw.

**Get more rest.** To grow stronger, you have to train more muscle fibers to fire. Yes, that means heavier weights, but it also means giving your muscles longer breaks. "Your muscles need to recover fully between sets to perform at their max," says Michael Mejia, CSCS, coauthor of *Scrawny to Brawny*. Try the 5 × 5 method. For any exercise, use the heaviest weight that allows you to do five sets of five repetitions. Rest for a full 2 to 2½ minutes between sets.

**Train like you play.** In sports, your leg muscles have to support your body weight in a variety of positions, whether you're lunging to your left or planting on your right. Use the single-leg squat to develop sport-specific lower-body strength, suggests Hartman. Stand on a bench with your left foot planted firmly and your right foot hanging off, your toes pointing up. Hold your arms straight in front of you and bend

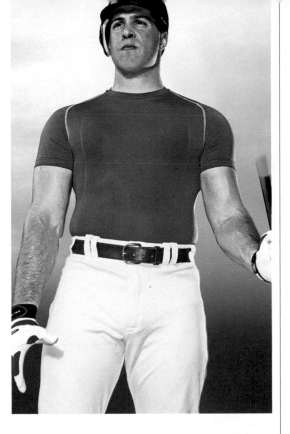

## Mark Teixeira

### First Base: Texas Rangers

In the sixth game of the season during his junior year at Georgia Tech, Mark Teixeira's cleat got stuck in the turf as he chased a fly ball. The resulting broken ankle required surgery and 3 months of rest. "Having to watch your team play and your body go in the toilet is not fun," says the 26-year-old Texas Rangers slugger, who knocked in 144 runs last season. "My whole right leg basically lost its muscle. I couldn't walk, I felt lethargic, I gained 10 pounds. You go from being on top of the world one minute to not knowing if you'll ever be the same the next."

What followed was a feat of strength—and character—as Teixeira rebuilt his legs, arms, and core. Every day, he did an hour of ankle-only rehab moves, 90 minutes of total-body conditioning, and batting and fielding sessions to get back into baseball shape. It took almost 2 years to return to his preinjury form.

"I tried to keep the big picture in mind, and that was to be a big-league baseball player. So you have to mentally break through the pain, the fatigue, the frustration," Teixeira says. "From the time I knew I had a chance to be a big leaguer as a teenager, my motto has been, 'If someone is better than me, fine. But no one is going to outwork me.'"

## Teixeira's Breakthrough Strategies

**Trump talent with hustle.** When you're younger, you can cruise on talent alone, says Mark Teixeira. But talent can take you only so far. "As you move up, the talent gap narrows, so everybody is really good," he says. "You have to work that much harder to push yourself to the top."

**Train your mind, too.** When you're rehabbing or just training to break barriers, remind yourself why you're doing it—especially on that last rep or lap, when your muscles feel as if they're full of battery acid. "Your mind will shut down before your body," Teixeira says. "Don't let it."

**Check a map.** Recovering from an injury is a long road. After his broken ankle, Teixeira was off his feet for 3 months, but it took a lot longer for him to get his body back. "Heck, I wasn't the same for 2 years," he says. What could your body look like in 2 years?

your left knee, keeping your torso as upright as possible. Lower your body until your right heel almost touches the floor. Push yourself back to the starting position and repeat as many times as you can. Do four or five sets with each leg, resting 3 minutes after each.

## Endurance: The Secret Advantage

The fittest not only survive, they also excel. The ability to resist fatigue longer than your opponent ensures you'll outperform him when you need that little extra, whether you're hustling after a loose ball, sprinting for the finish line, or driving hard for the last shot. The better your physical condition, the bigger your edge in every sport.

### TEST YOUR LIMITS

The 300-yard shuttle run is a great measure of sports endurance. Compared with traditional tests of stamina—a 2-mile run, for example—it's a better gauge for the type of endurance that's required for most sports. How to do it: Set up two cones 25 yards apart. Sprint from one to the other, then back again. That's one repetition. Do six continuous repetitions, for a total of 300 yards, as fast as you can. Then rest for 1 minute and repeat. The slower of your two times is your score.

3 points: Less than 60 seconds

2 points: 60 to 65 seconds

1 point: More than 65 seconds

**Build endurance for competition.** Run 10 "plays" of random length for 2 minutes, says Shaw: a 10-yard run to the right, hustle back

for a 10-second huddle (read: short rest), then a 30-yard post pattern, and so on. Integrate this drill into your workout once or twice a week, and work up to three 2-minute sets of 20 to 30 plays, resting for 30 seconds after each set.

## Landon Donovan

### Forward: Los Angeles Galaxy

Landon Donovan got his first real chance at soccer stardom before most guys get a driver's license. At age 16, he was invited to a camp for the under-17 national team—a place where he'd finally be able to gauge whether he was an elite national player or just a darn good regional one. The day before, playing with his club team, he made a slide tackle and broke his fibula and tibia.

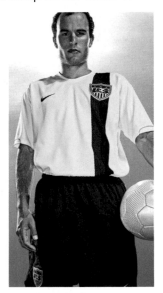

At first, the injury crushed him. Soon, however, he came to realize this was an endurance test: Could he outlast his own misery? His impatience? Four months after his injury, he found out when he got another shot at the national team—and nailed it.

Donovan, 24, now realizes that that obstacle was an opportunity, because he's not so sure he would've made the team had he gone to that first camp. "I was still developing," he says. "At the second tryout, I think my body was more on par with the other guys" at that camp.

## Donovan's Breakthrough Strategies

**Forget the other guy.** There are always people your age who are faster, stronger, and better than you, but "you need to progress at your own pace," says Landon Donovan. "Plenty of athletes don't develop until they're in their twenties. And then they're in the World Cup when they're 30."

**Understand true endurance.** It means simply to outlast. Can you perform at a higher level for a longer time than your opponent? But it also applies to the opponent in the mirror. Can you outlast your own self-destructiveness, such as pride and anger? That's some heavy mettle.

**Cage your ego.** When you're peaking as an athlete, you risk becoming cocky. "I used to see people get hurt and miss games, and I thought they were stupid guys getting into stupid tackles," he says. "But when I got hurt, it drastically changed my perspective."

**Build endurance for distance.** Set a goal—2 miles in 12 minutes, for example, which is a 6-minute-mile pace. Then find the longest distance over which you can maintain that pace—it could be 1 mile in 6 minutes, $1/2$ mile in 3 minutes, or $1/4$ mile in 90 seconds. Run the appropriate distance, and then rest for the same amount of time you spent running. Repeat the process until you can no longer maintain the target pace. Each workout, reduce your rest periods by 15 seconds.

**Build endurance in your basement.** Strapped for time? Try this body-weight exercise from Dan John, a National Masters champion in track and field. Stand with your feet shoulder-width apart, your arms hanging in front of you. Keeping your lower back naturally arched, squat quickly until your fingers touch the floor, then push yourself up to the starting position. Perform as many reps as you can in 20 seconds, then rest for 10 seconds. Aim for four sets in 2 minutes, and work your way up to eight sets.

## Power: The Ultimate Weapon

From Mickey Mantle to Jim Brown to Michael Jordan, explosive power is the stuff of legends. Simply defined, it's the combination of strength and speed, and it results in 500-foot home runs, broken tackles, and 40-inch verticals. Though the best athletes are born with natural explosiveness, any man can boost his power by training his muscles to activate faster. Do so, and you'll instantly become a better athlete.

### TEST YOUR LIMITS

The standing long jump is one of the best measures of total-body power, says Shaw, because it requires dozens of muscles to fire at the same time.

**How to do it:** Stand with your toes on a line and your feet shoulder-width apart. Dip your knees, swing your arms forward, and jump as far as you can. To obtain your score, measure from the starting line to where the backs of your heels landed.

3 points: More than 10 feet
2 points: 8 to 10 feet
1 point: Less than 8 feet

## PUSH YOUR LIMITS

**Tackle the box.** Boost your leaping ability with box jumps, says Hartman. Place a sturdy knee-high box 6 to 12 inches in front of you. Set your feet shoulder-width apart and jump onto the box. Step back down to the starting position, and repeat for a total of six repetitions. Rest for 3 minutes, then do another set. Perform two or three sets every 4 days.

**Run the throwback drill.** To improve total-body power, try the reverse scoop toss, says Shaw. Stand holding a medicine ball with your arms hanging straight in front of you. (Use a ball that's roughly 10 percent of your body weight, or substitute a piece of firewood.) Squat, and then quickly explode up

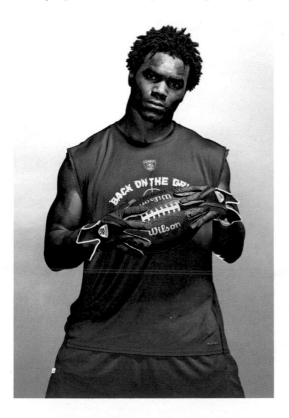

# Edgerrin James

## Running Back: Arizona Cardinals

Standing alongside crack addicts on a downtown sidewalk, a teenage Edgerrin James was after a different score—male guidance. "I found some of life's most valuable lessons in the strangest places," says James, who was raised by his mother in the small Florida Everglades town of Immokalee. "When you don't have a father around, it's easy to get lost in the shuffle. So I had to learn from an uncle or cousin or just a dude on the corner." After a junkie asked him for money, James sat and talked with the man. "He said some powerful things," remembers James. "I couldn't figure out how he got so messed up, because he was so smart."

The lessons he picked up from the transient male role models in his life added up to a bigger formula for power: long-term vision. He banked on something better happening. It did. After being named a *Parade* High-School All-American (suiting up at running back, linebacker, and kicker for Immokalee High School), James became the first player in University of Miami history to post consecutive 1,000-plus-yard rushing seasons. After he'd put in 2 years at UM, the Indianapolis Colts selected the explosive back as the fourth overall pick in the 1999 NFL draft. Replacing superstar Marshall Faulk, the rookie ran for 1,552 yards to win the NFL rushing title. Payday had arrived. "I was taught that you won't know until you try, so see it all the way through to the end, to give yourself the best chance," says James. "That's all I did."

—David Schipper

## James's Breakthrough Strategies

**Maintain a hustler's mentality.** Says Edgerrin James, "A hustler is always looking to see if the police are after him. I have to be aware of my surroundings as well, looking for those trying to bring me down or take my spot. It pushes me to improve." After all, staying one step ahead means you'll be harder to tackle.

**Forget about glory.** Greed brings isolation. Let the team be your power base. "When you have happy teammates, they'll be in your corner, ready to tell you the truth," says James. "On the field, it made me better, because if Marvin [Harrison, the Colts wide receiver] was getting double-teamed, I knew I had to step up."

**Don't feel cornered.** In high school, James played three positions, wherever he was needed, no complaints. Even if you feel that your role in the company or team is unfair, "be up for any situation, because that's the vehicle that's eventually going to get you where you want to go," he says.

with your legs, swinging your arms up as you heave the ball over your head as far as you can behind you. Do three reps, 2 days a week.

**Sprint short hills.** Contrary to popular belief, hill sprints don't just improve leg strength. "They're a great way to build explosiveness because you have to drive upward with your whole body," says Neil Chasan, PT, director of the Sports Reaction Center in Bellevue, Washington. Your sprints should last no more than 10 seconds—it's difficult for your muscles to maintain their maximum power output any longer than that—on hills inclined no more than 10 degrees. (Steep hills slow step time, decreasing power production.) Build up to 10 sprints, resting 20 seconds after each, three times a week.

## Agility: The Game Breaker

Think of agility as the ability to defy inertia. Because it allows you to change direction at any moment, to stay on your feet when you should have fallen, agility creates highlight films (see "Sanders, Barry"). But it's not just the domain of the genetically gifted. It requires balance, quick reactions, and body control—all skills that can be systematically improved.

### TEST YOUR LIMITS

The T drill measures your ability to change directions while you're moving at your top speed, explains Juan Carlos Santana, CSCS, director of the Institute of Human Performance in Boca Raton, Florida.

## Score Yourself

How fit are you?

**14 or more points:** Congratulations—you're a world-class athlete.

**11 to 13:** Nice job. You're the best athlete on your block. Integrate a few of our drills into your workout, and you'll be the best at your community center, too.

**9 or 10:** You're an above-average athlete. That's okay. Larry Bird was above average all the way to the hall of fame.

**8 or below:** You'll never be like Mike, but you knew that. Do one drill from each of our categories regularly, and you'll be in the best shape of your life within weeks.

**How to do it:** Set up cones or towels in the form of a T: 10 yards for the stem and 5 yards out to each side. Start at the base of the T, sprint to the top, side-shuffle 5 yards to the left, side-shuffle 10 yards to the right, side-shuffle 5 yards back to the middle, and then backpedal down the stem.

3 points: Less than 10 seconds
2 points: 10 to 12 seconds
1 point: More than 12 seconds

### PUSH YOUR LIMITS

**Practice the unexpected.** Try this drill from Jim Liston, CSCS, owner of C.A.T.Z. Sports in Pasadena, California. Find a partner and stand facing each other, 15 feet apart. Ask him to run forward, backward, and side to side randomly for 15 seconds. Your task: Mirror him. Do six sets, resting for 45 seconds after each, every other day. After 2 weeks, add two sets.

# Vincent Lecavalier

## Center: Tampa Bay Lightning

True agility combines speed, dexterity, and balance. More important, it helps you win when you're physically over-

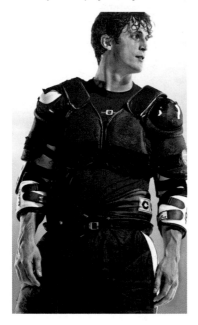

matched. Vincent Lecavalier learned this plastered up against the Plexiglas, slapping at the puck. The first overall pick (by the Tampa Bay Lightning) in the 1998 draft, Lecavalier entered the NHL at age 18, 6'4" and skinny as a stick blade. Playing against more experienced guys who were also more physically mature was his toughest professional challenge. Speed and stick-handling tricks got him through, but sleight of hand would take him only so far. He had to get bigger—without losing his agility.

"I knew that next summer was a big one," Lecavalier says. "I wanted to get heavier and stronger, but I didn't want

to feel like I'd gained 10 pounds." He ate six or seven meals a day and spent the first 2½ months focused on packing on muscle mass. By the end of that phase, he'd put on 12 pounds. He then spent the next month working on explosiveness (with plyometrics) and footwork to maintain his speed and quickness. The results are in the books: 28 points that rookie season, 73 points in '02–'03, and another 66 in '03–'04, when the Lightning won the Stanley Cup. Not only has his body grown, but so has his stature as one of the league's elite. "You can always push harder," he says. "Your body can really take a beating."

**Reverse course.** Go to a basketball court and stand at one side of the free-throw lane. With knees bent at 45 degrees, shuffle to the side, touch the line, and return. Go as hard as you can for 10 seconds, and count your touches. Rest for 30 to 60 seconds and repeat. Continue until your number of touches decreases by two. "You're training to absorb force when you decelerate and stop and to generate force when you reaccelerate," says Hartman.

**Improve your footwork.** Mark off 10 consecutive 2-foot squares with tape. Now hop as fast as you can through the squares for 10 seconds. Mix it up—one- and two-legged hops, forward, backward, and sideways—each time through. Do 10 sets, resting for 45 seconds after each, several times a week.

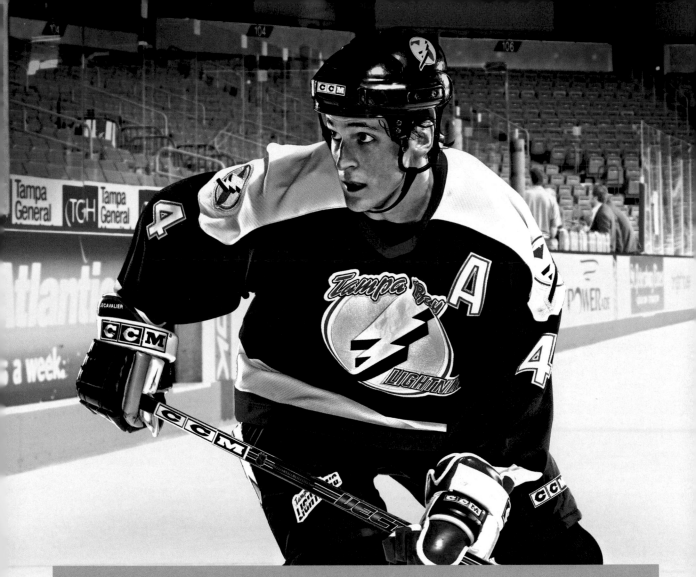

# Lecavalier's Breakthrough Strategies

**Play to your strength, not to his.** If you're overmatched, there's no point going muscle-to-muscle with a guy. Instead, neutralize him. That's what Vincent Lecavalier had to do in the corners before he added size. "Fake him out, get a step on him," he says. "Change speeds to beat him."

**Remember the good old ways.** Sure, Lecavalier put on some beef and grew into his lanky frame. But he never forgot the stick-handling tricks he'd learned as a smaller man. Strength and size simply became additional weapons in his athletic arsenal.

**Break the big goal into small challenges.** When he's in the corners, Lecavalier isn't thinking about the Stanley Cup; he's thinking about controlling the puck. To reach your big goals, focus only on the next step, workout, or repetition. "Just beat the guy in front of you," he says.

# Balance It Out

Like many things, your workout should be about balance. If yours is out of whack, here's how to get back on the right path

BY BILL HARTMAN, PT, CSCS

**A**s a physical therapist, I'm the go-to guy when my buddies' bodies start to fail them. Just last week, my friend Tony called, complaining of upper-back pain after his last few workouts. When he described his weight-lifting program, the problem was obvious to me.

Tony was packing on muscle in a completely unbalanced fashion. Not only did 80 percent of his routine consist of pushing motions (bench, incline press), but most of his gym time was directed at his chest and shoulders. And he'd been doing it for years. The back pain was his body's way of begging for a new workout.

As I explained to him, your body and its joints are held in place by opposing muscle groups (for example, chest and back, quads and hamstrings). These groups work together to control movement. If one becomes stronger or tighter than normal, that dominant muscle group will overwork its counterpart—that is, you'll have a muscle imbalance. You don't want a tug-of-war between muscles every time you move. Nagging discomfort can mean you're at a much greater risk of injury.

Tony came to me too late. He needed a ton of time and work to undo the damage he'd done. For you, the key is to check yourself before you wreck yourself. You must identify and repair imbalances before they cause pain. That's what the following self-tests and corrective strategies are for.

For each muscle imbalance the self-tests reveal, perform the stretches twice a day—for instance, first thing in the morning and after your workout. Complete the entire corrective program for each imbalance three times a week until you can pass the test. You can also do these as a warmup before your regular workout.

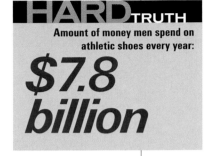
## Supine Pec Test

Lie on your back on the floor with your hands behind your head. Let your arms relax. They should lower to the floor and rest comfortably. If they don't...

**Your problem is:** protracted shoulders. You look more like Notre Dame's hunchback than like one of its defensive linemen.

**The cause:** You've spent too much time training your "mirror muscles" (pectoralis major and minor) on the front side of your body, while neglecting your upper-back muscles (middle trapezius and rhomboids).

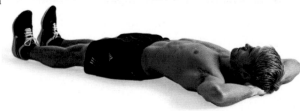

## FIX YOURSELF

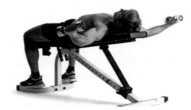

**Step 1:** Stretch your pecs. Holding a pair of 5- or 10-pound dumbbells, lie faceup on a 10-degree incline bench and lower the weights out to the sides with your arms extended. Hold for 30 seconds.

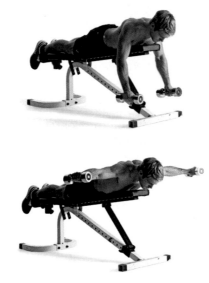

**Step 2:** Strengthen your middle trapezius and rhomboids. Follow the above stretch with a prone dumbbell lateral raise. Lie chest down on the same bench you just used to stretch your pecs.

Raise the dumbbells out to the sides and squeeze your shoulder blades together. Hold for a count of six, and lower the weights to the starting position. Do a total of six repetitions.

## Thomas Test

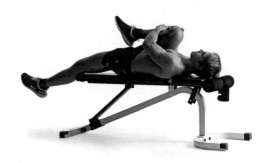

Lie faceup on a bench and bring both knees to your chest. Grab your right knee and hold it at your chest. Let your left leg straighten, then lower it by relaxing your hip. Test both legs, and if either leg can't lower to the bench...

**Your problem is:** tight hip flexors, which can result in hamstring strains and back pain.

**The cause:** Prolonged sitting and avoidance of single-leg exercises, such as lunges, have caused your hip flexors and butt muscles to weaken. Hip-flexor tightening has made your pelvis tilt forward, which places more stress on your lower spine. If the front of your belt sits lower than the back, consider yourself a sufferer of this most common muscle imbalance.

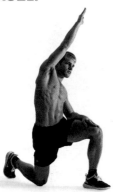

**Step 1:** Stretch your hip flexors. Kneel on your right knee with your right arm extended overhead. Contract your right glutes until you feel a comfortable stretch in the front of your right hip and thigh. You can intensify the stretch by bending your torso directly to the left. Hold the stretch for 30 seconds, then repeat on the other side.

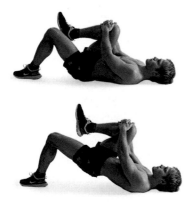

**Step 2:** Activate your gluteus maximus (butt) muscles. Lie on your back with your knees bent and your feet flat on the floor. Grab your right knee with both hands and pull it to your chest.

Then lift your hips by driving your left heel into the floor. Hold the up position for

a count of 6 seconds, then lower your hips to the starting position. Repeat six times. Perform the same sequence on the other side if it tests tight.

## Single-Leg Squat Test

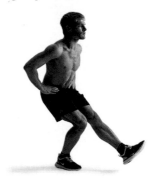

Balance on your right foot and suspend your left foot out in front of you. Keeping your right foot flat, lower yourself as far as possible into a squat while reaching forward with your left foot. If your right knee shifts inside of your big toe as you lower into the squat position…

**Your problem is:** a knock-kneed posture. This causes your knees to drift inward when you squat, putting you at great risk of suffering a noncontact knee injury because your ACL is under maximum tension.

**The cause:** You have tight adductors (groin muscles) and weak gluteus medius muscles (smaller muscles in the buttocks).

## FIX YOURSELF

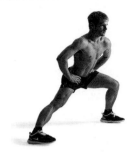

**Step 1:** Stretch your adductors. Spread your legs wide and, keeping your right leg straight, lower yourself into a side lunge by bending your left knee and pushing your hips back until you feel a comfortable stretch in your right groin area. You can intensify the stretch by turning your shoulders to the left. Hold this position for 30 seconds. Repeat the stretch on the other side as needed.

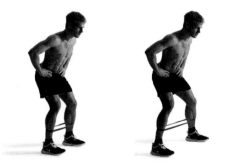

**Step 2:** Strengthen your gluteus medius muscles. Place a stretch band (available at www.performbetter.com or www.elitefts.com) around your lower legs, and perform side steps for 10 steps to the right and 10 to the left.

Repeat for six sets in each direction. You also need to perform single-leg exercises, such as lunges, split squats, and stepups, while keeping your kneecap in line with your big toe.

## Apley's Scratch Test

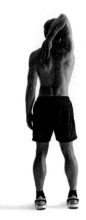

Reach behind your head with your right hand and try to touch your left shoulder blade. Then put your the arm down and bend it behind your back, again trying to reach your left shoulder blade. Complete the same movements with your left hand touching your right shoulder blade. If you fail to reach a shoulder...

**Your problem is:** tight internal or external rotators, a common ailment for men who lift weights. The tightness reduces shoulder rotation and can cause pain.

**The cause:** Stiff latissimus dorsi and pectorals will reduce your shoulders' external rotation (reaching behind your head). If your rotator-cuff muscles are stiff, it will hamper your internal shoulder rotation (reaching behind your back with your arm down).

## FIX YOURSELF

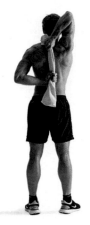

**Step 1:** Hold a towel with two hands behind your back—one hand near your head, the other midback. Walk your hands as close together on the towel as you can. Then try to rip the towel, pulling with both hands for a count of 10. Relax, then try to move your hands even closer together and pull for another 10 count. Reverse hand positions and repeat. This move fixes both external- and internal-rotation problems.

## Wall Test

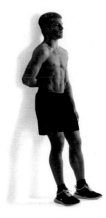

Stand with your feet about 12 inches from a wall and rest your back against it. Place your right hand on the small of your back, palm facing the wall. Then tighten your abs until your palm is pressed against the wall. In this position, your body should have four points of contact with the wall: your tailbone, palm, upper back, and head. If you have to tilt your head back to reach the wall…

**Your problem is:** kyphotic posture—also known as slouching.

**The cause:** Your abdominal and chest muscles have shortened, while your back extensor muscles and spine have weakened. Sitting for extended periods of time leads to this imbalance.

## FIX YOURSELF

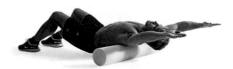

**Step 1:** Mobilize your spine. Lie across a foam roll (available at www.performbetter.com) or a thick PVC pipe so that it's perpendicular to your spine at the lower part of your rib cage. Reach overhead so your spine extends over the roll and hold for a count of 10. Move the roll up your spine about 2 inches, then repeat. Continue this process until the foam roll reaches the base of your neck.

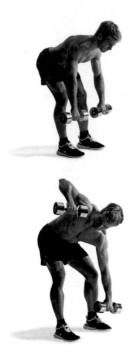

**Step 3:** Perform a single-arm dumbbell row with external rotation. Stand with your back almost parallel with the floor, holding lighter-than-normal dumbbells.

However, instead of pulling the dumbbell to your rib cage, pull it to a position by your ear, allowing your torso to rotate upward. Repeat for a total of 15 repetitions with a lighter-than-normal dumbbell. Then switch arms and repeat.

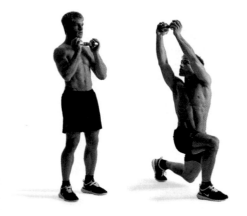

**Step 2:** Use this dynamic backward lunge to stretch your abdominal, groin, and chest muscles. Hold a single 10-pound dumbbell with both hands.

Step back with your left foot until your left knee nearly touches the floor. As you lunge, turn your torso to the right and reach up over your right shoulder with both hands. Then return to a standing position. Repeat for a total of 15 reps on both sides.

## The Go-Anywhere Workout

Jumping rope isn't just for wannabe boxers. It's a go-anywhere exercise that can help you prevent injury and increase your power, coordination, balance, agility, speed, quickness, cardiovascular fitness, and explosiveness. Need we say more? This simple program by Mark Roozen, CSCS, owner and director of the Performance Zone Fitness and Training Center in Granbury, Texas, ups the ante by adding the four-quadrant grid below (draw or imagine it on the floor), which forces you to stay agile by moving your feet between quadrants while jumping.

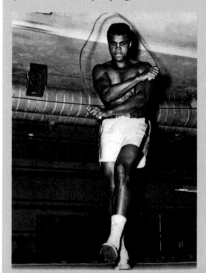

| DRILL | LOCATION OF FEET | REPETITIONS |
|---|---|---|
| Regular jumps | Any | 50 |
| Side to side—land on both feet | 4 to 3 and back | 25 |
| Forward and back—land on both feet | 4 to 1 and back | 25 |
| Boxer shuffle—land twice on your right foot, twice on your left | Any | 30 |
| Forward and back—land on one foot | 4 to 1 and back | 20 on the right foot, then 20 on the left foot |
| Side to side—land on one foot | 4 to 3 and back | 20 on the right foot, then 20 on the left foot |
| Triangle—land on both feet | 1 to 2 to 4 (or 4 to 3 to 2) | 25 |
| Double jumps—land on both feet, passing the rope underneath twice | Any | 25 |
| Running in place—alternate landing on your right and left foot | Any | 30 seconds |
| Bonus jump—as many regular jumps as you can do without breaking form | Any | 30 seconds |

1 2
4 3

BY GRANT STODDARD

# Can Hypnotherapy Help You Build a Better Body?

Experts were skeptical. So were we.
Then we sent a 150-pound weakling to head-shrinker Pete Siegel

**Close your eyes.
You are feeling sleepy.
Very sleepy. When I snap my
fingers, you will awaken. You will
have a sharper mind. Rock-solid
confidence. And killer biceps.**

I met hypnotherapist Pete Siegel at a luxury hotel in Santa Monica. I can't tell you which one; Pete issued a gag order. Because he outweighs me by 150 pounds, and because he can manipulate my brain at will (even over the phone), I'll keep his secret. Or, rather, the secrets of his client list. When a pro athlete arrives for a session—Siegel's job is to tweak their minds so their bodies perform better—hotel security guards form a perimeter around the star and escort him to a penthouse suite. That's where the mind/muscle meld happens.

But I met Pete in the lobby, sans security guards; the paparazzi couldn't care less who was messing with my brain. Pete shook hands with a hit man's crunch and asked, intensely, "Are you ready for what's about to happen to you?" Everything Pete does is intense.

"I hope so," I said, unconvincingly.

Pete gave my physique a disparaging look. "I hope so, too."

You would never peg this guy for a mental-health counselor. Not many hypnotherapists possess a 23-inch neck or can leg-press 1,100 pounds. Pete is 5'8", 275, and his demeanor is just like his body: unapologetically blunt. "I'm not here to make people like me," he sneered. "I'm here to help you do your job better. If people don't like me, too bad."

Hypnotism has been used to elevate athletic performance for quite a while. The Soviet Olympic team took 11 hypnotists along to the 1956 games in Melbourne. The Soviet athletes won 98 medals; the unhypnotized U.S. team scored only 74. Yet, 5 decades later, there is still a stigma attached to hypnotism. You picture head cases like ARod on the couch, not champions like M.J.

But maybe that's why nonbelievers—like me—aren't performing so well in the clutch. Maybe we should all have a little more mental gymnastics in our lives.

"The trend to get the mental edge is happening and will continue," says Joan S. Ingalls, EdD, a sports counselor and the author of *The Reframing of Performance Anxiety*. "Athletes will call their local psychologist. Universities will put mental-training specialists on staff, available for athletes. But I don't think sports hypnosis will catch on any time soon. It's controversial."

There's good reason for her skepticism: According to Shawn Arent, PhD, CSCS, a professor of exercise science at Rutgers University, no large-scale studies have been conducted on hypnotherapy in athletic performance. "That's not to say that it may not be extremely effective for some people; we just don't know enough about the processes involved. So, from a purely scientific standpoint, the jury is still out."

Not that everybody is going to wait for

the official verdict. "Hypnosis can bypass the critical mind," explains Ingalls. "The conscious mind is constantly evaluating what is and isn't b.s. We put that critical mind to sleep."

That's one way to blast past your self-imposed limits: Sleepwalk on by.

By the time I flew to L.A. to meet with Pete, we had already logged 5 hours on the phone. He claimed he had identified my core issues after only 6 minutes of our first conversation. "It usually takes me 3," he added. So either he was off his game with me, or I'm twice as messed up as his average client. Essentially, Pete's diagnosis was that I

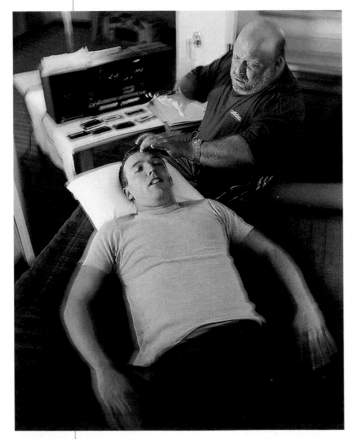

have retained my androgynous physique since adolescence because of a lack of resolve, poor self-control, and, most worryingly, zero self-respect. So I couldn't help feeling sheepish as Pete shut the door to his hotel suite and told me to make myself comfortable.

His first question, alarmingly, was, "Who is Grant Stafford?" I didn't have time to correct Pete on my last name—it's Stoddard—before he cleared his throat and treated me to The Who's "Who Are You?" a cappella and at considerable volume: "Who the f— are you? . . . I really want to know. . . . Who are you?" He finished singing, took a breath, and jabbed his meaty index finger into my sternum, accusingly. "So, seriously, Grant, who the f— are you?"

I was speechless; Pete mimicked my gaping mouth. "You don't know who you are because you don't have a sense of self yet. I am going to help you remedy that." After talking, singing, and yelling for another 90 minutes, Pete asked me to lie down for hypnosis.

With a tape of the ocean playing in the background, he began talking in a slightly different tone: slower, more deliberate. He repeated the word "easy," elongating the first syllable. He told me to visualize my eyelids as closed window blinds and then asked me to try to open them. I couldn't. In minutes, I'd gone from hypnosis skeptic to compliant zombie.

Now Pete could help me with the first task: exorcising negative thoughts about myself. He had me talk about three different and, to my mind, benign events that happened to me between the ages of 3 and 5. Then I talked about my girlfriend. The next thing I remember, my fists were clenched, and I was telling my parents off and screaming that my girlfriend should "kiss my balls!"

Now Pete changed tapes, and the sound of a heartbeat filled the room; my heart rate matched it. With my eyes still closed, Pete slapped me loudly on the forehead. Then he commanded, "Now tell me: WHO IS GRANT STAFFORD?"

The last person you want to get your name wrong is the man rewiring your psyche.

"I . . . I don't know," I said.

"YOU DO KNOW! THE ANSWER IS INSIDE OF YOU!"

Before I could address Pete's question, a siren started blaring, and a prerecorded voice yelled, "ATTENTION! ATTENTION!"

Was the siren on Pete's hypnosis tape? In my mind? Was this part of the therapy?

"Focus!" Pete shouted, thumping my forehead again. The heartbeat got louder and faster. "ATTENTION! ATTENTION!" the prerecorded voice demanded. I felt vulnerable, lying there, eyes locked shut. Pete had taken me from total relaxation to volcanic rage to the verge of an anxiety attack.

Then the siren stopped, and all was calm.

TOUGH TALK

Create a fan base. Build a muscle by using your mind. Hit the gym at 6 p.m.; Arizona State University researchers found that men bench-press an average of 41 pounds more under the gaze of spectators.

Pete began rousing me to full consciousness. As I got up from the bed, he was on the phone. "Some moron kid set off an alarm," he said; that explained the "ATTENTION!" scream. Then he told me that he had already dealt with my major psychological blocks: "I put some deep stuff in there," he explained. "The eggs are still cooking. You won't realize the extent of the changes until you're back home."

After leaving Pete, I called my girlfriend to apologize. She took it all right, considering.

How do you become "the best peak-performance hypnotherapist in the world," as Pete calls himself? Believe you are, and tell people. It's a form of self-hypnosis: Pete's belief in himself is off the charts.

He told me about his 1,900 inspirational quotes that he unapologetically boasts are "up there with Confucius, Plato, Socrates, Aristotle . . . all those f—in' guys." He is so assured of this that he has labeled it absolute truth, so I guess he can hand down encyclicals, like the pope.

Pete long ago pulled the plug on his critical, limit-setting mind, and he's seemingly undeterred by conventional thought and the limitations that go with it. For example, Pete has just penned 17 songs for perma-buff hip-hop legend LL Cool J to record for his next album. "They are mostly about working out, fitness, inner power. I visualize them being played in every gym in the country," he said. Now, a rational voice might point out, gently: Pete, you do not know Cool J, so he will not record these songs. But Pete believes that if he can get in a room with the rapper, the album is a done deal. "That's the way Siegel operates," he said. "Pete Siegel makes sh— happen." (Pete often speaks about Pete in the third person, a veritable flock of Siegels flying past his lips.)

He was even a hard-charging, self-motivating go-getter while, um, homeless. In the early '90s, he said, he spent a year sleeping on the streets, thanks to a business downturn. "You know when people say that their life was in the gutter?" he asked. "Well, Pete Siegel was underneath the gutter. I was the lowest of the low. I don't just dispense advice like these psychologists. I've had intense and traumatic experiences. I've lived in a way Dr. Abraham Q. F—stick can't imagine. I'm living proof. There's no issue I haven't overcome myself."

The night after Pete hypnotized me, I met him at World Gym in Marina del Rey. It seemed as if the Gold's Gym graduating class of '79 was all there, including Pumping Iron character Eddie Giuliani. Oh, and the sullen-looking bald dude in the corner? "Stone Cold" Steve Austin.

After I logged a few seconds on the stationary bike, Pete had me do "warmup"

**TOUGH TALK**

Think bigger. Build muscle by using your mind. Before a set of arm curls, knock out a set in your mind. Dutch scientists found strength gains in men who just thought about lifting heavy weight.

cable crossovers that were about as heavy as my final sets back at my gym in New York.

"I'm going to work you hard," he warned. "But you should tell me if you're about to puke or pass out."

Now I was really worried.

Pete loaded up weights on a barbell for bench presses. He had to spot me. I was instantly emasculated—I couldn't get it up. Pete stripped 25-pound plates off the bar, and I could at last perform the first reps by myself.

Every set Pete had me do followed this protocol: 10 reps on my own, three to five with his assistance, three with the negative part of the exercise (the "down" of an up/down movement) performed at a rate almost imperceptible to the human eye, then a full 5-second exertion during which I would strain to move the bar an inch or two.

After the first five reps of each set, I was sure I was going to fold, but Pete got in my face, barking, "Focus!" "Concentrate!" or simply, "SQUEEEEZE!" To put me over the top, he ordered me to visualize the muscle working. Okay, Pete's a bit of a madman, but the white coats agree: Even thinking about exercise fires up the neural pathways that activate muscles. So you can build muscle without lifting a finger.

I willed myself through the workout. Amazingly, I completed all three four-part sets. "See?" said Pete, slapping me on the back. "You far exceeded what you thought you could do. What we're doing is teaching the muscle that it can be worked much more intensely than before."

He was right: My muscles were getting a bigger pump than ever. Midway through the session, my pecs felt heavy and tight and looked noticeably larger in the mirror. "I've been sore before, but never during the actual workout," I said to Pete. He chuckled maniacally. "Take a very long, hot bath tonight and get some rest. You are going to be feeling this for the rest of the week."

After the workout, Pete and I sat outside the gym in the cool night air and talked. Well, he mostly talked, and I mostly listened. It was a homespun mix of philosophy, misogyny, and off-color remarks, all delivered with a vim befitting the dictator of a very small country. Which he is, of course.

"People will be in the gym for hours and hours, doing whatever it takes to get a little bit bigger," he sighs. "But at what expense? You should want bigger muscles, greater power, but it should translate into wanting a bigger life. Turn that power into money, parlay that strength into building strong and valuable relationships with people. Twenty-three-inch biceps don't look so good tucked into a rusted-out Chevy Nova or a shoebox apartment. I work out because that's where I get my power to do other things."

Pete's philosophy about the muscle-success connection may have history on its side. I had been watching HBO's *Rome* religiously. In one scene, Julius Caesar's niece Atia has her waif son, Octavian,

tutored in masculinity by veteran soldier Titus Pullo. Atia wants her son to learn to "fight, copulate, and skin animals."

When Pete and I were not at the gym or in a hypnotherapy session, he would take on the role of a mentor, posing rhetorical questions, illustrating points with anecdotes from his own life. I felt like the young Octavian during these chats. Not a bad precedent, considering that the scrawny boy later became Augustus Caesar, the first emperor of Rome. I could feel Pete's eggs cooking inside me.

I was still incredibly sore by my next training session with Pete, a couple of days later. But this time, it was different. We were training biceps and back, and then doing some ab work. Pete made me look at my biceps with every curl, focusing on the idea of growth, recalling that feeling of power from the previous session, and the pain began to fade. My arms pumped almost

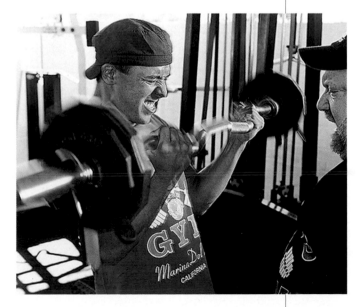

independently of the rest of my body.

With Pete's coaching, my final and heaviest set of each exercise was often my best. He was almost fatherly in his support, using phrases like "that-a-boy" or calling me "sport" after a good set. Grant Stafford was nowhere in sight. But why, exactly? I wasn't really sure how much my gains in the gym were related to hypnosis and how much they were rooted in my wanting to impress this force of nature.

"With hypnosis, there's a kind of placebo effect for a lot of people," says Arent. "If people are achieving more from this placebo effect, well, that's great, though it doesn't necessarily give more credence to hypnotherapy. As you told me, you had a desire to impress your hypnotherapist. That's a huge factor in the work you were prepared to do."

My final hypnotherapy session was much more intense than the previous two. My defenses were down, and Pete stormed in.

"You are in a room that contains body parts," Pete intoned in his hypnotherapy voice. "Start by finding a pair of legs that your perfect, confident being would have." I imagined a cross between Dr. Frankenstein's lab and a Costco and picked out a pair of legs and set them on the floor.

"Good," Pete said, as though he were approving my purchases at the checkout stand. "Now find the torso that your perfect, confident being would have."

I picked out a shredded frame that Bruce Lee would have envied.

"That's right," said Pete. "Now set the torso on the legs and notice how they fit perfectly." We continued building Mr. Potato Head from top to bottom. Next, Pete urged me to think about how my perfect creation would think and feel and act.

Then Pete asked me to name my creation. "Maximus," I replied instantly, after the protagonist in *Gladiator*, my favorite movie.

Pete had me clench my right fist and imagine melding Maximus with myself. "You and Maximus are standing feet away from each other, but you are inching closer and closer." After another 5 minutes, he had us standing nose to nose, and I became extremely worried that Pete was going to ask me to make out with him. Luckily, he just asked me to step into Maximus until we were the same person.

"You look like Maximus, you think like Maximus, all the positive attributes Maximus imbues, you feel like Maximus, you are Maximus!" The music on his tape player was cranked up very loud, sounding like a Keith Emerson synth solo.

Then, silence.

When I became fully conscious, Pete was staring off into space in the silence. "Wow! That was f—ing intense, right?" he asked. Pete was so into his performance that he'd been taken along for the ride.

We sat down for our postsession briefing, and Pete had me make a fist and repeat my alter ego's name to myself: Maximus, Maximus, Maximus. As I did so, I was filled with a sense of relaxed confidence and complete well-being.

"Now look in the mirror," said Pete.

I did so, and for the first time in ages felt really pleased and proud of the handsome brute looking back at me.

During my last gym session with Pete, whenever he would see me flagging, he'd press my mantra button: "Clench your right fist and repeat, 'I am Maximus,'" he instructed. I cleared my head, took a deep breath, and said the words, feeling that wonderful rush of power and well-being fill my torso, as it had before. I started my set, realizing that the weight was increased but that my attitude toward the weight had somehow changed. My form felt right; my body worked like a piston.

"That was your best set by far," said Pete, dropping a muscled hand on my

## Self-Help through Hypnosis

Hypnosis is a state of profound relaxation that induces you to switch off your critical mind and yield to the behavioral suggestions of a therapist. He might use it to help you quit smoking, lose weight, or ditch a phobia. Here's a primer on the process, adapted from *Illustrated Method for Self-Hypnosis*, by Barbara DeBetz, MD. The American Society of Clinical Hypnosis provides referrals at asch.net.

(ONE) Sit in a comfortable armchair in front of a blank wall in a quiet room. Rest your arms, palms down, on the arms of the chair. Now relax your body and gaze at the wall. Comfortable? Good—that's the prime requirement for hypnosis.

(TWO) Now, without moving your head, slowly roll your eyeballs upward. You'll feel a pleasant, almost ticklish sensation in the middle of your forehead. Now slowly close your eyelids.

(THREE) Inhale deeply through your nose. Hold that breath for 10 seconds or so. Now slowly exhale through your mouth, letting your eyeballs roll back to their normal spot behind your still-closed eyelids. Your breathing should be slow, comfortable, and rhythmic. Relaxing, isn't it?

(FOUR) Relax successive body parts so that you feel first your arms, then your back, then your butt and legs sinking into the chair cushions. You'll begin to feel as if you're floating.

(FIVE) This is where the magic happens: You're in a hypnotic state, which may mean that your critical, decision-making mind has pretty much shut down. You're very open to behavior modification, and in the hands of a skilled hypnotherapist, that can be a powerful thing.

(SIX) Ready to return to the world? Keeping your eyes and mouth closed, take a slow, deep breath through your nose and roll your eyeballs back toward your forehead. Hold your breath for a few seconds; exhale…and slowly open your eyes. Welcome back.

By Charles Hirshberg

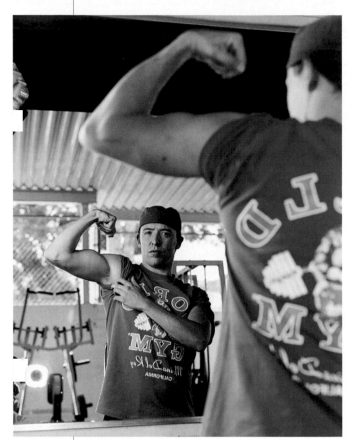

explains sports psychologist and trainer Jack N. Singer, PhD. "Alpha, beta, theta, and delta. Alpha is the optimal state in which to achieve peak physical performance. It's the relaxed state of mental being, and hypnosis impacts alpha brain activity. However, a level of anxiety is also required to achieve peak efficiency." And if that doesn't explain the polar opposites in Pete's working method, nothing does.

"Think of it as your mind being made up of networks of tracks," says Singer. "Some of these tracks have been poorly laid with repeated notions of negative thoughts, self-doubt. Utilizing positive thought is like laying new, stronger tracks that, through repetition, will start to replace the older tracks entirely and become permanent."

Did Pete's hypnotherapy work for me? It's hard to tell—as Pete might say, my eggs are still cooking. Or, what the hell, maybe they've hatched by now. All I know is that I went into this thinking that Pete wouldn't even be able to hypnotize me, but there I was, rebuilding myself into an imaginary man of superior strength, lifting more weight and working harder in my workouts than I ever thought was possible for me.

Now, when I head over to the gym, I leave Stafford behind. Maximus is my workout partner. With his help, I will fight; I will copulate; I will skin animals.

shoulder. "It was also your heaviest by 30 pounds."

As stupid as it sounds, it was true: I had become Maximus.

The incredible gains left me with some burning questions. What exactly had Pete Siegel done to my brain? Was it permanent? Pete stressed that my Maximus persona was relaxed. But how was a feeling of relaxation helping me throw steel around?

"There are four types of brain waves,"

BY THE EDITORS
OF *MEN'S HEALTH*

# The Ones to Beat

Find fitness inspiration in the routines of these big-name bodies

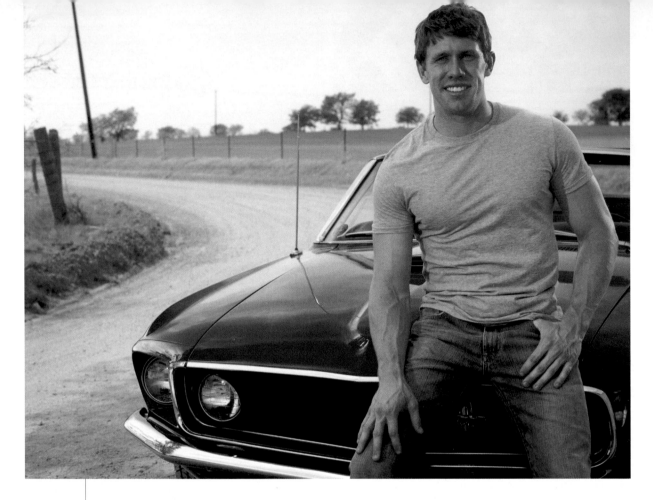

## Carl Edwards

Once fueled as much by beer as by gasoline, NASCAR has always lagged Indy when it comes to fitness. But as the prototype for a new breed of driver, Carl Edwards is changing that perception. He does backflips after victories, he lifts weights four times a week, he snacks on fresh fruit and vegetables, and he explores cycling and running trails at every NASCAR tour stop. Even his private plane has been retrofitted for the driving athlete. "I actually took two seats out of it so I could put my mountain bike in there," he says.

Edwards insists that six-pack abs aren't a prerequisite for racing, but his high level of fitness clearly offers an advantage in a sport where drivers make split-second decisions under extreme stress and fatigue. "It gives me a little extra something," says the 26-year-old Missouri native, who won four races in 2005, his first full year on the Nextel Cup circuit.

No doubt a "little extra something" can work wonders for you, too. Indeed, we all operate in the same high-pressure, fast-paced world as Edwards, even if we spend our days behind a desk, rather than behind the wheel of the No. 99 Office Depot Ford Fusion. The benefits of this lifestyle, Edwards believes, extend beyond the physiological adaptations: "You feel like you're doing something to help yourself." And, after all, perception is reality.

**Play a sport that multitasks.** Although Edwards spends plenty of time exercising outdoors and in the weight room, his most effective training takes place in a tightly enclosed space: "Racquetball mimics racing by requiring you to focus on sustaining your hand-eye coordination under intense physical demands," he says. For you, that could translate into an improved ability to think and react better under pressure. Call it the science of the unexpected: Texas A&M researchers found that regularly participating in unpredictable sports trains you to handle mental stress, while providing all the physical benefits of intense exercise. Just ask Edwards—if you can catch him.

## Chris Evans

The *Fantastic Four* star laughs at workout programs. "The key is dedication."

On camera, Chris Evans is known for the cocky swagger he's brought to roles in *Fantastic Four* and the 2007 sci-fi film *Sunshine*. But he's known offscreen for his self-deprecation, from his "crap" diet to his loathing of treadmills ("like pulling teeth"). Even though Evans professes to be unscientific about exercise, he has been pushing iron with regularity since high school. The 6', 170-pound actor's disdain for the treadmill is offset by basketball, tennis, and even football whenever possible. The lesson: You don't need a meticulous workout plan. "The key is just dedication," Evans says.

**Take your workout anywhere.** Researchers in France found that exercise frequency and duration are the best predictors of body-fat levels. On the road or on set, Evans does pushups, pullups, and situps. Do a set of each—as many reps as you can in 30 seconds—without resting. Take a 1-minute breather, and repeat until you can't match the same number of reps.

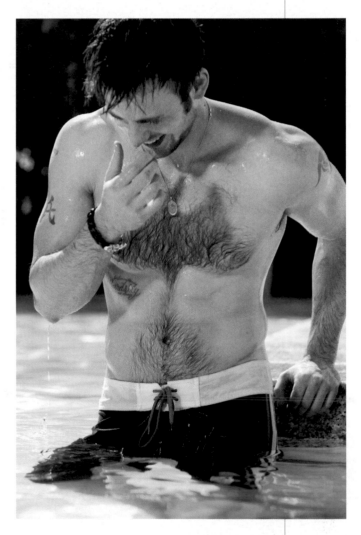

## Daniel Dae Kim

Unlike so many men in their thirties, Kim has never lost his way when it comes to keeping his body in game shape. If you were confined to a diet of fish and mangoes, like Daniel Dae Kim's marooned character on ABC's *Lost*, you'd be stripped-down lean, too. Alas, he looks this good all the time, thanks to faithful workouts designed to accommodate a crushing schedule. He runs 3 to 4 miles 3 or 4 days a week and trains with weights on the same days. Most important, he keeps his workouts moving at peak efficiency. "I don't take long breaks between sets," says Kim.

**Make the most of your gym time.** Scientists at the University of Southern Maine found that just one set of 10 to 12 reps burns as many as 28 calories. So the key is to pack as many total sets as you can into each weight-training session—even if you have only 15 minutes. Try an eight-exercise circuit in which you alternate upper-body with lower-body and core exercises without resting. Because you're targeting different areas of your body with each set, you'll be able to perform each exercise intensely, despite the lack of downtime. Do just two circuits, and you'll have incinerated 450 calories.

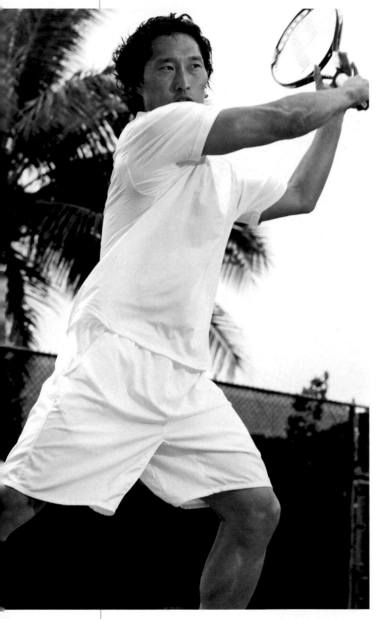

## Jared Padalecki

He went from string bean to star. Supernatural? No, just big weights and big shakes.

Jared Padalecki was a skinny kid when he landed a role on *Gilmore Girls*. Now, in his twenties, he's the star of his own CW series, *Supernatural*, and has the body of a leading man. His transformation began after a 4-inch growth spurt, to his current 6'4". "Suddenly I really needed to add muscle mass," he says. He packed on 35 pounds of muscle while staying lean. He credits Scot Mendelson, a two-time world bench-press

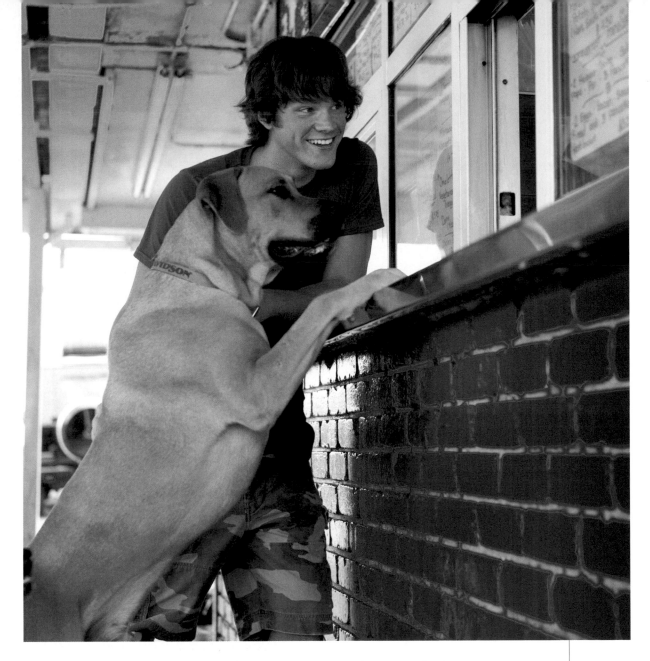

champion who guides Padalecki through short but intense workouts and encouraged him to snack on 600-calorie protein shakes.

**Pack on plates to pack on size.**
Mendelson goes old school on guys like Padalecki: Get strong to get big. "The heavier weights you use, the more muscle fibers you'll activate, leading to greater growth," he says. Research shows that for experienced lifters, muscle fibers grow the most when you use weights that are 80 to 95 percent of the amount you can lift once. Beginners, go lighter: You'll gain the most strength at 60 percent of your best effort.

## James Denton

This guy fought his slowing metabolism and won. It took James Denton nearly 2 decades of hard work to become an overnight sensation, as Mike Delfino on *Desperate Housewives*. An accomplished stage actor, he shed about 20 pounds to land the role, which he likens to "winning the lottery." Denton credits dietary vigilance for his ability to carry less fat now, in his forties, than he did in high school. "Everybody reacts differently to diets, but the universal downfall seems to be sugar," says Denton.

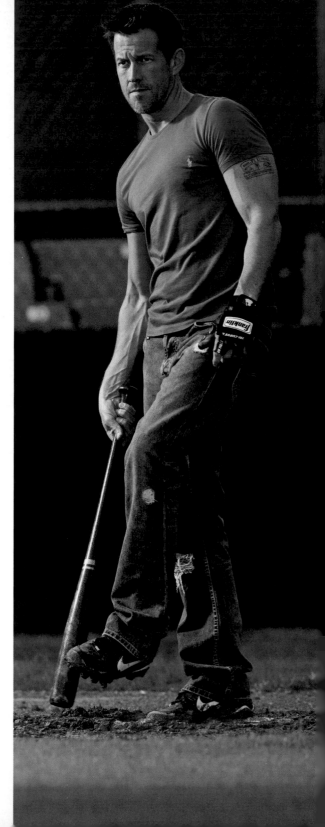

**HARD** TRUTH

Percentage faster exercisers' wounds heal than sedentary people:

## 25

Like Denton, you can reclaim the waistline of your youth, simply by decreasing your intake of sugar and other fast-digesting carbs. Keeping your gut in check does pay off, and not just because you can wear 32-inch-waist pants: Men with flat stomachs are half as likely to develop heart disease as those with sloppy midsections.

**Weed out weak foods.** Bread, pasta, white rice, potatoes, cereal, and baked goods spike blood-glucose levels and signal your body to store fat. Simply limit these high-carb foods to one or two meals a day—say, breakfast and lunch—and your body will spend more time burning fat, rather than storing it.

## Nick Cannon

The kid actor is now a hip, ripped rap mogul. His way: Keep trying something new.

Nick Cannon knows something about transformation. As a teenager, he was the face of Nickelodeon—writing, producing, and starring in hundreds of kids' programs before he was old enough to drink. Now, he's successfully transitioned from aging teen idol to budding hip-hop mogul, complete with his own record label. Just as his career has matured, so has his physique, which he's defined by spending an hour in the gym 5 days a week. "People say, 'Okay, he's starting to look like a man,' " Cannon says, laughing. The work is in private. The results are there for all to see.

**Try a new exercise.** Cannon experiments in the gym. His top abs choice: the bicycle crunch. Lie on your back, fingertips behind your ears, feet 6 inches off the floor. Crunch your torso and touch an elbow to the opposite knee, bringing that knee toward your chest. Do the same with the other elbow. That's one repetition. Do two sets of 25 reps, resting 1 minute between sets.

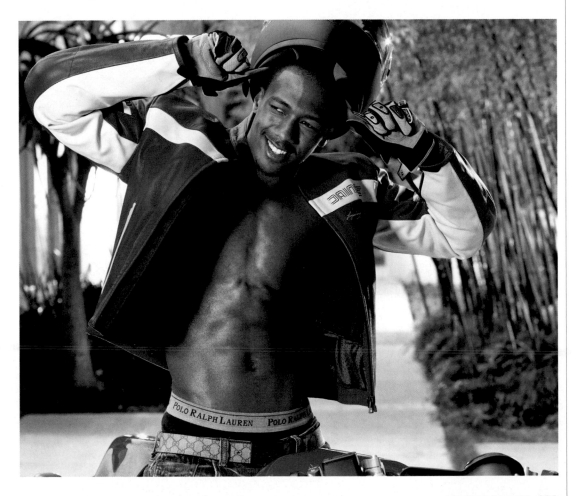

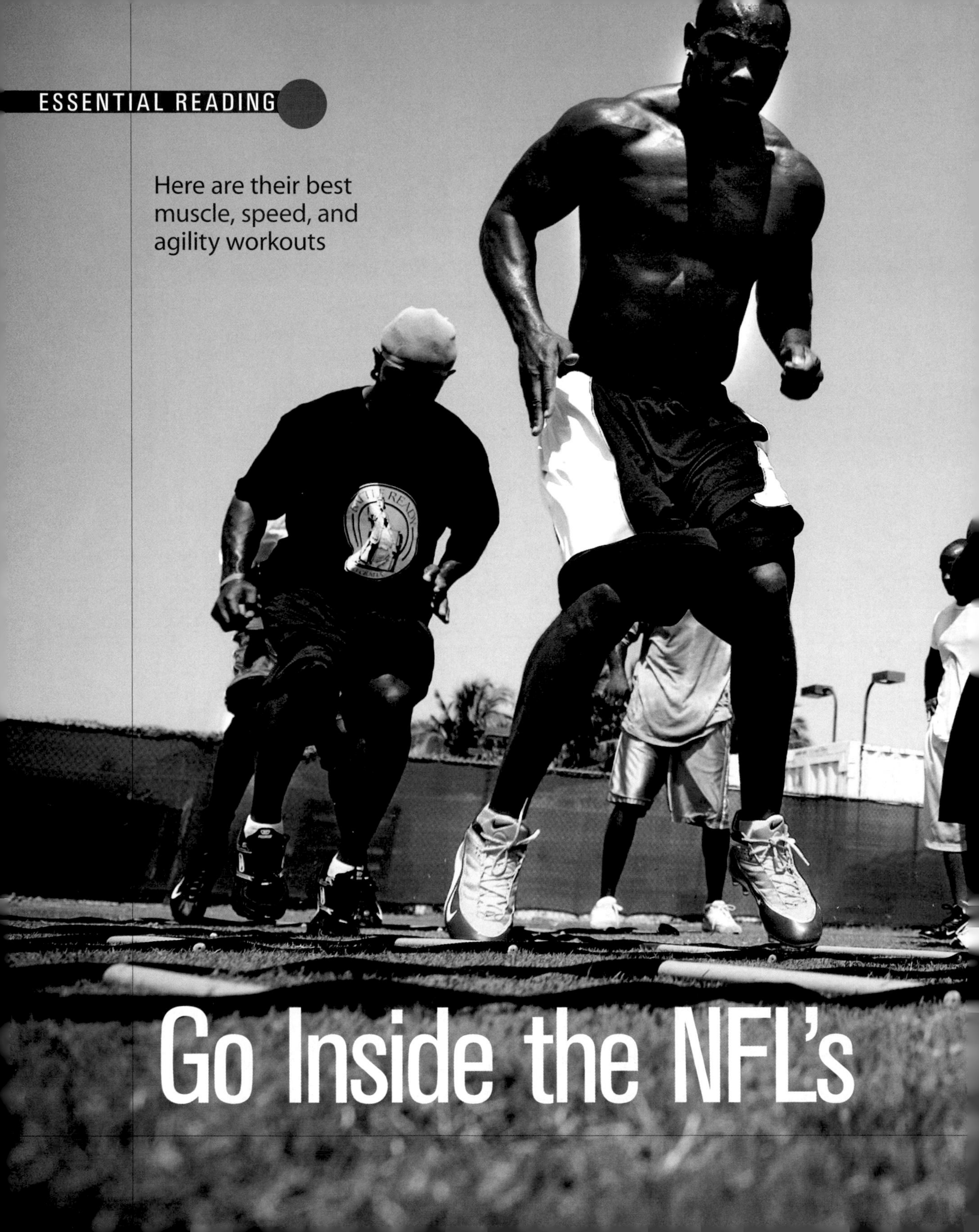

Here are their best
muscle, speed, and
agility workouts

# Go Inside the NFL's

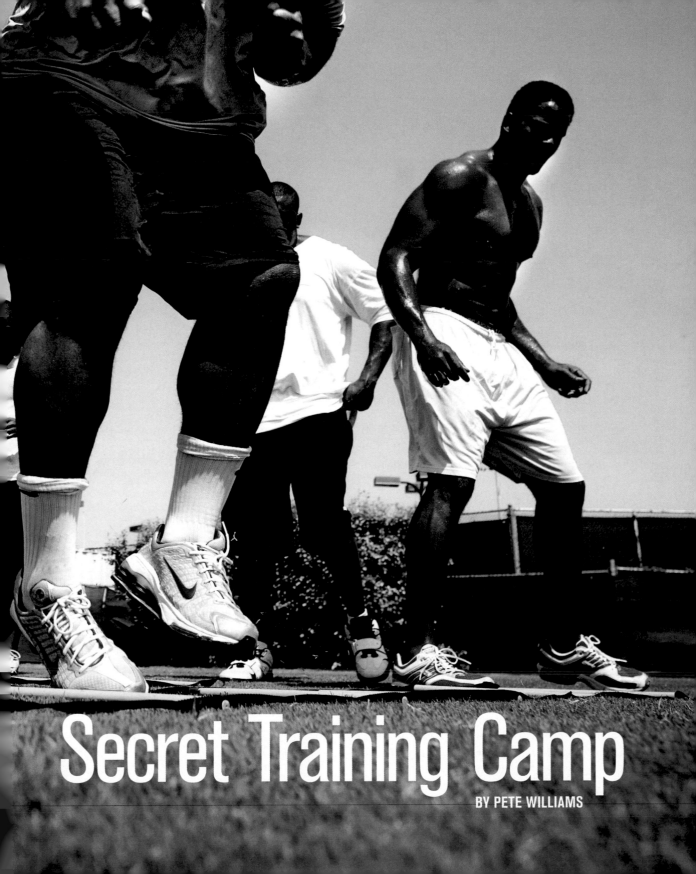

# Secret Training Camp

BY PETE WILLIAMS

All-pro middle linebacker Jonathan Vilma cringes as he crunches his body into a V to complete the last of 100 toe touches. Vilma, of the New York Jets, squints, exhales, barks an expletive, and looks over his shoulder.

"Keep fighting it, Frank," he says.

San Francisco 49ers running back Frank Gore grunts an acknowledgment and continues crunching, his toes near the windows of the University of Miami weight room. Were this not 6:25 on a late April morning, these windows would provide a panoramic view of the Hurricanes football team on their practice field. Now, all is darkness.

Ten feet away, Andreu Swasey watches these NFL players as he finishes a set of biceps curls. It's the only time the UM strength coach can lift, what with five groups of current Hurricanes to train, a five-person staff to oversee, and a dozen NFL veterans returning for preseason conditioning to the place they affectionately call "the U."

Vilma is usually the first to arrive. The New York Jets, like most teams, prefer their players to spend the off-season training at team headquarters. It builds camaraderie, the theory goes, reinforces the team concept, and, if nothing else, motivates those less than committed to the weight room. It's a philosophy ignored by Vilma and many other Hurricane alumni in the NFL.

"I understand where the Jets are coming from, but I've always gotten a good workout down here," Vilma says, nodding at the unoccupied 12,000-square-foot collegiate training facility. "This is what took me to the NFL."

Swasey nods. "Anyone who thinks guys are just down here hanging out at South Beach should come and watch."

At 7 a.m., the first wave of 20 current UM players trudges out to one side of the practice field, cleats leaving footprints on the dew-soaked grass. Vilma and Gore line up with them and, at Swasey's command, sprint 100 yards. They rest briefly and sprint back.

After the sixth sprint, the players are

## Get Back in Shape

You don't need ladders, tires, and tackling dummies to get in football shape. "Doing a jump-rope circuit helps with conditioning, coordination, and quickness," says Swasey. Try completing, in continuous fashion, 20 repetitions of each of the following seven jump-rope drills. If you can complete all 140 repetitions without resting, you're ready to suit up.

**1.** Keep your feet together and hop straight up and down.

**2.** Keep your feet together and alternate hopping forward and backward.

**3.** Keep your feet together and hop side to side.

**4.** Hop in place on your right leg.

**5.** Hop in place on your left leg.

**6.** Alternate hopping on your right and left legs each repetition.

**7.** Start in a split stance—one foot forward, the other back—and switch leg positions as you perform each rep.

# Recover Faster

When you bend over from fatigue, you restrict airflow to your lungs and bloodflow to your muscles and heart. But by standing upright with good posture, your body can better deliver oxygen to all areas of your body, speeding recovery. Physiologically, raising your hands above your head might be slightly better than placing them on your hips, since it helps blood travel from your muscles back to your heart and lungs—where it's replenished with oxygen—even faster.

So why does University of Miami strength coach Andreu Swasey prohibit it? "It looks lazy," he says.

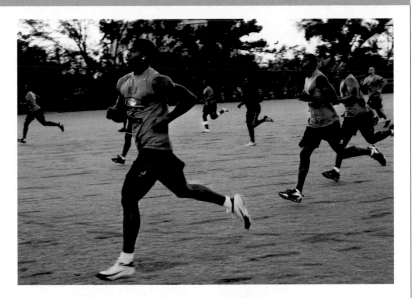

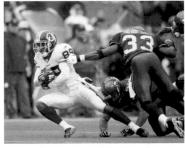

Santana Moss cuts downfield after a catch. His advice for sure hands: Make a diamond with your thumbs and index fingers. "When your hands meet the ball, that's how they should catch it," he says.

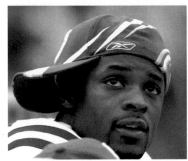

Reggie Wayne

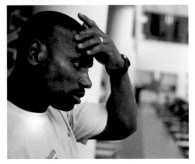

Andreu Swasey

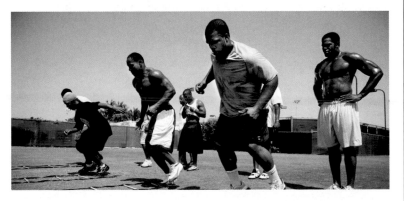

# Be a Big-Game Receiver

## Three no-fail pass routes for breaking away from your opponent

Santana Moss is a small man in a big man's league. At 5'10", 190 pounds, the Washington Redskins wide receiver regularly battles taller cornerbacks and bulkier safeties—and wins. His secret? Simple routes. Check out his three favorites below, then rotate through them in your next flag-football game. "No matter what high-tech defense is being used against you, these classic plays work," says the Pro Bowl wideout.

### "7"

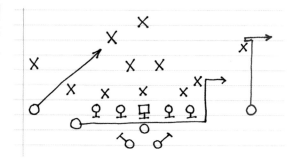

**How to run it:** Go 10 yards, then make a sharp step to the center of the field. Once your closest defender breaks inside with you, cut back toward the sideline. "You'll get the defender to move his feet inside with you," says Moss. "When you break back, he'll be leaning the wrong way."

### "Attack"

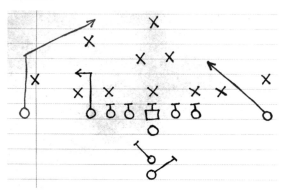

**How to run it:** Head downfield at full throttle, letting your opponent know that you're challenging him. At the 12-yard mark, break off on a left or right slant. "The defender is going to relax and wait on your next move if you sit on the line playing patty-cake with him," says Moss.

### "Comeback"

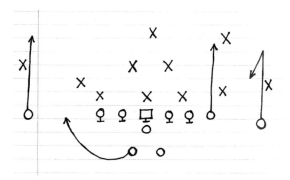

**How to run it:** Sprint 12 yards, make a sharp 180-degree turn, then sprint back toward the quarterback. "It puts the defender on his heels," says Moss. "He's left not knowing anything about what you're running, whether you're going inside or outside."

gassed, but nobody takes a knee, bends at the waist, or places hands on his head. The only acceptable posture is hands on hips. Players must even ask permission to tie their shoes.

Gore leads a military cadence. "Don't stop . . . won't stop . . . feels so good . . . real good."

Swasey, 34, smiles. He wants his college players to invest themselves in the program. And it helps when they have NFL million-aires setting the example. Miami has produced at least one first-round draft pick each season since 1995 and boasts more active NFL players than any other school.

There are glitzier off-season conditioning centers, full of athletes from all sports who pay big money for training. But nowhere else attracts as much NFL talent.

Many still live in South Florida during the off-season, either for tax purposes or because they have homes or family here. They believe in Swasey's program and remember as students seeing men like Warren Sapp and Michael Irvin returning to train in the off-season. Then there's the everlasting bond with the U.

Reggie Wayne, a wide receiver for the Indianapolis Colts, explains the allure while sitting in Swasey's office before his workout. "Look at this," he says, pointing to a school-logo tattoo on his shoulder. "It's like our own fraternity, our brand. When you get that tat, you've made it. You're a brother. You've been through the blood, sweat, and tears."

At 10:30 a.m., the parking lot begins to fill with exotic vehicles. Washington Redskins

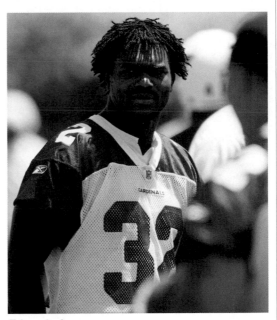
**Edgerrin James**

wide receiver Santana Moss arrives in a burgundy Mercedes S550. D.J. Williams, a linebacker for the Denver Broncos, parks a BMW 760Li with oversize tires and rims. The players and their vehicles cause no particular stir; it's just another day in sunny South Florida.

A few minutes later, Swasey lines up the NFL veterans in the end zone, along with another wave of current Hurricanes. It's an impressive group of NFL talent. Besides Moss and Williams, there are wide receivers Wayne of the Colts and Roscoe Parrish (Buffalo Bills) and defensive linemen Kenard Lang (Broncos) and William Joseph (New York Giants).

It's actually a slow day for Swasey. Ed Reed, safety for the Baltimore Ravens, is usually on hand. Alex Rodriguez, a Miami native who would have played baseball for the Hurricanes had he not turned pro out of high school, trains alongside the football players before spring training. In recent years, Swasey has welcomed back Clinton Portis, Bubba Franks, Willis McGahee, and Jeremy Shockey.

"What's this?" Swasey asks as the players line up. "The Pro Bowl team working out?"

The players start with 100-yard sprints, followed by a series of exercises designed to improve explosiveness. For 20 minutes, they high-step and sprint through rope ladders and, with shirts and shoes removed, move on to Swasey's notorious sandpit. Here they square off in rigorous lateral shuffle drills, struggling against the sinking sand, which quickly saps them of energy.

Not exactly a day at the beach. "We don't have hills, so we use the sandpit for resistance," Swasey says. "The speed of the game is multidirectional. You need quick feet and change-of-direction ability, and the sand helps with that."

Soaked with sweat, their calves dusted with sand, the players retreat to the weight room. It's nearly noon now, and they have the place to themselves.

For a younger guy, Swasey is old-school when it comes to lifting weights, developing strength, and training elite athletes. You won't find Bosu balls, balance boards, foam rollers, or other new training tools in his gym. There are only a couple of Physioballs. Don't expect to see his football players—past or present—spending much time on weight machines, either.

Instead, Swasey—who played defensive back at Baylor University—focuses on traditional weight exercises, such as the bench press, Romanian deadlifts, squats, and Olympic lifts, which many NFL teams and trainers have abandoned for trendier movements and methods.

"I'm not going to be sitting around with a

## Hit the Sand

Because sand absorbs virtually all the force you apply with your feet, your muscles have to work harder than when you exercise on a more solid surface, such as concrete, hardwood, or grass. And performing sand drills barefoot provides the additional benefit of reducing your risk of injury while playing sports. That's because, without shoes, the muscles of your feet and ankles learn to better work in unison with your knees. This helps distribute the stress of repeated impact throughout your body, instead of just on your knees. Try running barefoot on the sand to protect your lower body from injuries, and practice broad jumps, squat jumps, and skipping to build explosive power.

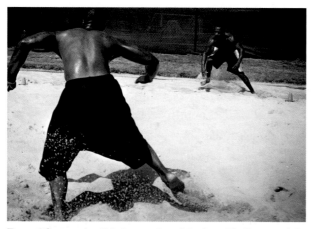

Two of Swasey's athletes go head-to-head in the sandpit.

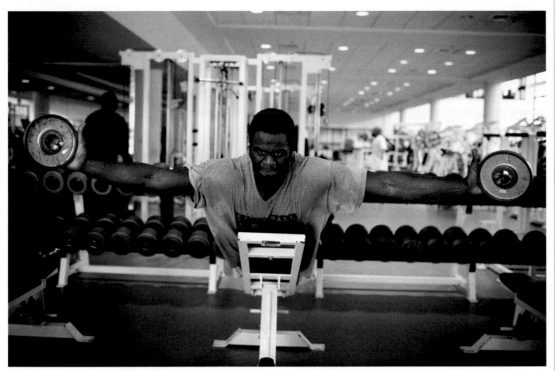

Here, Kenard Lang of the Denver Broncos performs a lying rear lateral raise. This exercise emphasizes your rear deltoids, your rotator cuffs, and the muscles that stabilize your shoulder blades. If these muscles are weak, almost every upper-body lift—bench press, arm curl, pullup—will suffer. Here's how to make sure they don't: Set an adjustable bench to a low incline. Grab a pair of dumbbells or weight plates and lie chest down against the pad. Let your arms hang straight down from your shoulders, your palms facing out. Keeping your arms straight, raise the dumbbells out to your sides until they're in line with your shoulders. Pause, then slowly lower the dumbbells back to the starting position.

bunch of guys on Physioballs," Swasey says. "We're going to stand up, like in a game, doing a lot of stuff on our feet." His overriding philosophy is simple: "The old stuff always works and always will."

The players pair up or work alone at weight stations, all within shouting distance of one another, as rap music blares from the sound system. Running back Edgerrin James, now with the Arizona Cardinals, sets up shop in the middle of the room. On one side of James, his former Colts teammate,

Wayne, is working with Moss. Williams loads a bar on James's other side.

As James finishes a set of squats, he searches for his favorite verbal sparring partner. Lang is entering his 10th NFL season, his first with Denver, and James is already eyeing the late-season matchup between the Broncos and Cardinals. "I can't wait to see you coming on the blitz, Kenard," says James.

Lang takes a look at James's weight rack. There are four 45-pound plates on either side, for a total of 405 pounds. "That's a warmup set, right?" Lang deadpans. "Please tell me that's a warmup set. You'd better do more than that if you want to get by me coming around the corner."

"I'll just stiff-arm your ass," James says.

Williams, who has been training virtually nonstop since last season ended, stays clear of the smack-talk crossfire, concentrating on an intense workout. The others leave him alone, other than offering a few words of admiration.

The chance to work out with his all-pro buddies is why James comes back to Coral

## Train Like a 'Cane

### You, too, can make explosive gains in any sport

Try this modified version of the old-school plan that Swasey uses with elite athletes. It's been tweaked slightly to better fit a nonpro's schedule and fitness level, but without compromising your results. Do each exercise on the day and in the order shown, using the prescribed scheme of sets, repetitions, and rest periods.

| DAY | EXERCISE | SETS | REPS | REST (MINUTES) |
|---|---|---|---|---|
| Monday | Snatch-grip jump shrug | 3 | 3–5 | 3–5 |
| | Barbell squat | 5 | 4–6 | 3–5 |
| | Push press | 3 | 6–8 | 2–3 |
| | Back extension | 2 | 10 | 1–2 |
| Tuesday | Bench press | 4 | 4–6 | 3–5 |
| | Pullup (or lat pulldown) | 4 | 8 | 2–3 |
| | Dumbbell shoulder press | 2 | 12 | 1–2 |
| | Barbell curl | 3 | 10 | 1–2 |
| Thursday | High pull | 3 | 3–5 | 3–5 |
| | Front squat | 3 | 6–8 | 2–3 |
| | Romanian deadlift | 4 | 6–8 | 2–3 |
| | Lunge | 3 | 10 | 1–2 |
| Friday | Dumbbell row | 4 | 6–8 | 2–3 |
| | Dumbbell incline bench press | 3 | 10 | 1–2 |
| | Lateral raise | 3 | 12 | 1–2 |
| | Lying triceps extension | 3 | 10 | 1–2 |

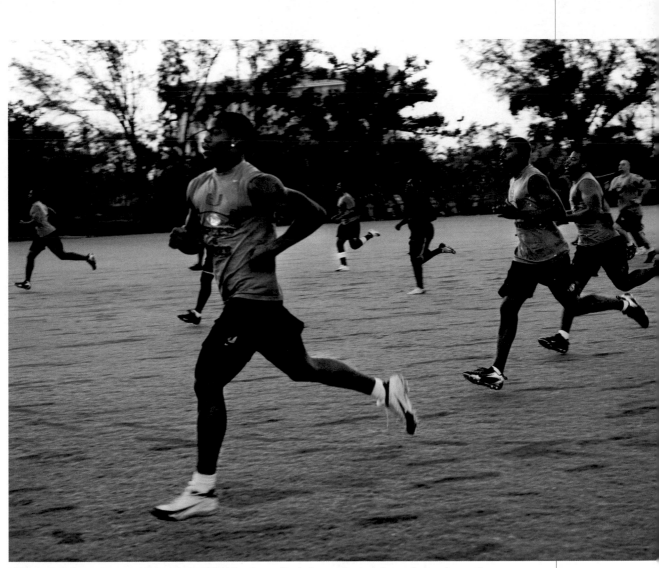

The players head out to the practice field, where their "morning run" consists of grueling 100-yard sprints.

Gables, to the U. They inspire him to work harder. "They are my fuel source," he says. "It goes back to being around successful people, having those healthy habits, and doing the things it takes to maintain success."

By 1 o'clock, the workout is over, and the ex-'Canes relax in Swasey's office. Soon the NFL's endless series of minicamps will begin, breaking them up for another year.

"We'll be ready," Wayne says. "Teams are always waiting to see what kind of condition you're in. If you're in bad shape, you'll be expected to stay in town next summer. But as long as I'm with Coach Swasey, I know I'm going to be in phenomenal shape."

BY PETE WILLIAMS

# Train Like a Pro

From Curt Schilling to Cadillac Williams, the world's top athletes look to one man for better performance. Now you can, too t's an early February morning, and the Athletes' Performance training center looks like backstage at the ESPY Awards—except that the jocks are clad in workout gear and not formal attire.

At one end of the training floor, "performance coaches" direct a group of baseball players that includes Pat Burrell of the Philadelphia Phillies; Carl Crawford of the Tampa Bay Devil Rays; and Brian Roberts, the pint-size but powerful infielder for the Baltimore Orioles.

Curt Schilling is lying on a padded table as a physical therapist examines his famous ankle. Outside, NFL prospects pull weighted sleds across an Astroturf field. Last year, NFL teams drafted eight Athletes' Performance clients in the first round, including top-10 picks Ronnie Brown, Carnell "Cadillac" Williams, and Carlos Rogers.

Roberts, who at 5'9" hit 18 home runs last season, surveys the scene and shakes his head. "Look at the people you see here. You work out all your life, then come here and quickly find out there are more effective ways to train."

It's an impressive show of talent gathered here in Tempe, Arizona, to improve strength, power, and overall performance, under the whip of Mark Verstegen, better known to these pros as the fast-talking, flat-topped hulk of energy who has pioneered the concept of "performance training." At 36, the *Men's Health* "Muscle Guy" columnist still looks as if he could suit up as a linebacker for Washington State, which he did until a career-ending arm injury launched his coaching career.

In his new book, *Core Performance Essentials*, Verstegen shows how anyone can follow the same routines used by the likes of

## Recharge Your Muscles
### Make faster gains—outside the gym

Pros at Athletes' Performance quickly learn trainer Mark Verstegen's mantra: work + rest = success. Work + Rest = Success. They train hard 3 or 4 days a week and use the days in between as "regeneration" days.

That doesn't mean you should shut it down. Verstegen's regeneration plan includes working with a foam roll, the next best thing to a professional massage. By rolling on the foam, working key areas such as your hamstrings, quads, calves, groin, and back, you'll loosen muscle, get the blood flowing, and hasten your body's recovery from all the work you did the previous day. The payoff: Your muscles will grow faster, and you'll perform better in your next workout.

You can buy your own foam roll at select fitness-equipment stores. (We like the 36-inch Foam Roller Plus at www.performbetter.com; $35.) But in a pinch, you can use a basketball. Here's a sample foam-roll routine for your hamstrings, but the same method works for any area of your body. (You'll find instructions for a complete recovery workout at www.menshealth.com/foam.) Place the foam roll under one or both of your hamstrings and roll your body back and forth over the foam.

For added benefit, put all your body weight on the roll. It may be uncomfortable at first, but over time, it'll become considerably easier. It's a great barometer of the quality of your muscle and connective tissue; the less it hurts, the higher the quality of both.

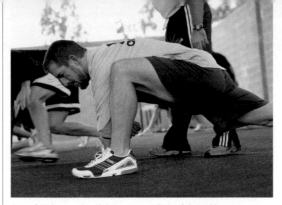

**Jay Gibbons builds strength in his off-season.**

top athletes in almost every sport. You, too, can add your name to his list of all-star success stories.

## Do Your Prep Work

If you could spend 3 minutes at the beginning of your workout to boost production for the rest of your regimen by 20 percent, would you do it? How about if you knew that such chiseled athletes as Crawford and NFL wideout Nate Burleson perform the same exercises?

Verstegen's "movement prep" routine usually consists of six to eight exercises that boot up the body's computer and prepare it for action. But you only have to do two of them.

First, perform 10 hand walks. Start in pushup position: legs straight, hands on the floor. Keeping your knees straight, walk your feet toward your hands. (Your hips will rise toward the ceiling.) When you feel a stretch, walk your hands out until you're in pushup position again. That's one repetition.

Next, do 10 repetitions of what Verstegen calls the world's greatest stretch. Take a large step forward with your left leg to get into a lunge position. Now bend down and

place your left elbow against the instep of your left foot while keeping your right knee off the floor. Pause momentarily, then lift your left hand and place it outside your left foot. From this position, push your hips to the ceiling (your back knee will straighten) and lift the toes of your left foot toward your shin. Finally, stand up and step forward into the next lunge and repeat. That completes one repetition. "You're giving your muscles mobility and stability, which will support the rest of your workout. This is the most important and easiest thing you can do to improve performance," says Verstegen.

## Master Time Management

You'll never see a pro at Athletes' Performance resting between sets. That's because Verstegen believes in workout density—packing as much as possible into a workout for maximum physiological response. "Time is the limiting factor for most of us. Put the work back into working out," says Verstegen. The key: Strategic arrangement of exercises. By alternating between upper- and lower-body exercises, as well as movements in which you either push or pull (see page 138), you'll be able to do set after set at your highest intensity—without resting. You'll double your workout efficiency, and that means you'll save time—or get more done during the same period.

In fact, you'll be better off than if you spent the previous 2 minutes ogling bare midriffs. By activating more muscles, you're increasing the amount of muscle-building and fat-burning hormones released, so you'll grow stronger and leaner.

Here's how to set it up: Organize your workout so that an upper-body pushing movement is always followed by a lower-body pull, and an upper-body pull is always followed by a lower-body push. See the lists below for basic examples.

**Upper-Body Push**
Bench press
Shoulder press
Pushup

**Lower-Body Pull**
Deadlift
Romanian deadlift
Back extension

**Upper-Body Pull**
Pullup
Pullover
Row

**Lower-Body Push**
Stepup
Lunge
Squat

## Train Movements, Not Parts

Good luck trying to find a jock in Verstegen's shop performing a preacher curl or run-of-the-mill row. That's because Verstegen believes in training body movements—not body parts—for maximum gains in strength, as well as mobility, stability, and flexibility.

So, instead of doing a routine bent-over row, try a dumbbell single-leg, single-arm row. This will develop not only upper-back strength and power but also hip stability and flexibility. It's still an upper-body pull, but you're getting lower-body benefits as well. "A lot of guys don't take the time to work on flexibility and stability because they think they don't have time," Verstegen says. "But if you take a common exercise and tweak it, you can accomplish a lot more."

This is part of Verstegen's overriding emphasis on pillar strength, the notion of strengthening and stabilizing the musculature around the hips, shoulders, and midsection. Think of it as training the hub of the wheel, not the spokes.

## Shore Up Weak Spots

When it comes to lifting, muscle imbalances are a prescription for injury. Of course, you've probably spent a lot of time trying to create symmetry, at least the kind that reflects in the mirror—that is, equally impressive-looking pecs, arms, and shoulders. But unless you've established muscle

*(continued on page 140)*

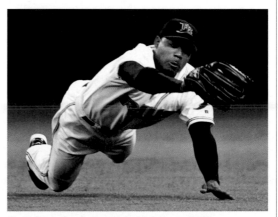

**Carl Crawford showcases his mobility.**

## Elevate Your Game

### Use this 20-minute workout to build a world-class body

Train like a pro with this Mark Verstegen workout, courtesy of his new book, *Core Performance Essentials*. Perform the workout as a circuit—doing one movement after another without resting—3 days a week. Do 8 to 10 repetitions of each exercise, using the heaviest weight that allows you to complete all of the prescribed repetitions. Repeat one time (don't rest between circuits) for a total of two circuits.

**Dumbbell Alternating Bench Press**

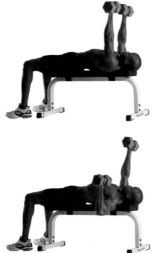

Lie faceup on a bench, holding a pair of dumbbells over your chest with your arms straight, palms facing forward.

Keeping your right arm straight, lower the dumbbell in your left hand to the outside of your chest, then push it back up. Next, keep your left arm straight as you lower the dumbbell in your right hand and push it back up. Continue alternating arms for the prescribed number of repetitions.

**Dumbbell Single-Leg Romanian Deadlift**

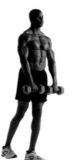

Stand on one foot, holding a dumbbell in each hand with an overhand grip (palms facing your thighs).

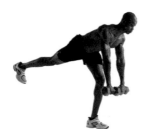

Keeping your knees slightly bent and your lower back naturally arched, push your hips back and lower the weights until they're just below your knees. Push yourself back up to the starting position and finish a set, then switch legs and repeat.

**Single-Leg, Single-Arm Row**

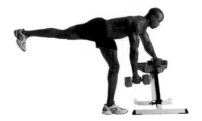

Grab a dumbbell with your right hand and stand on your right leg next to a bench. Holding the bench with your left hand, bend forward at the waist so your right arm hangs beneath your shoulder and your right leg is nearly straight. From the side, your body should resemble the letter T.

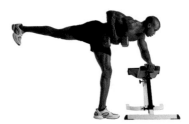

Pull the weight up until your elbow passes your torso, then lower it. Finish a set, then turn around and repeat the move, this time standing on your left leg and rowing with your left arm.

### Bulgarian Split Squat

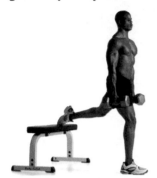

Grab a pair of dumbbells and stand with a bench a few feet behind you, with your left foot on the bench and your arms at your sides.

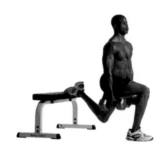

Keeping your torso upright, lower your hips toward the floor. Pause when your front thigh is parallel to the floor, then push yourself back up to a standing position. Complete a set, then switch legs and repeat.

### Standing Single-Leg Lift

Stand on your left leg holding a weight plate at arm's length. Bend your left knee and lean forward and to the left until your upper body is almost parallel to the floor and the plate is just outside your knee.

Raise your torso and pull the plate to your chest as you lift your right knee in front of your body.

Without pausing, twist your torso to the right as you raise the plate over your right shoulder. Now reverse the motion. Finish a set, and repeat on the other side.

### Dumbbell Split Curl to Press

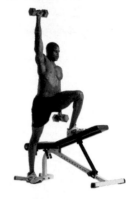

Stand holding dumbbells at your sides (palms facing each other), with one foot on a bench that's about midthigh height.

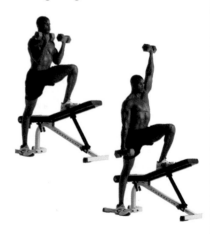

Perform a biceps curl with your right arm, rotating your palm as you go so it faces you at the top.

Press the weight overhead, rotating your palm so it faces away. As you lower your right hand, repeat the motion with your left arm so the dumbbells pass at your torso. Finish your reps, then place the opposite foot on the bench and repeat.

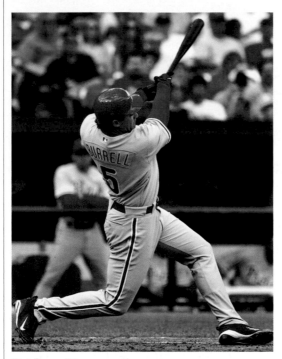

**Pat Burrell turns on the power.**

symmetry throughout your entire body from a strength-and-stability standpoint, you're setting yourself up for injury. (To find out if you have strength imbalances, see "Balance It Out" on page 100.)

The idea is to create balance in your right and left sides, and the easiest way to do that is through unilateral movements, or exercises in which you work one arm or leg at a time. For instance, instead of doing a barbell or dumbbell bench press, try a dumbbell alternating bench press. (See "Elevate Your Game" on page 138.) "This forces you to stabilize your shoulders and pillar the entire time," says Verstegen. "Working unilaterally also keeps the muscles under tension longer, which will improve your size and strength gains."

Verstegen recommends that you spend part of each workout—or even one full workout a week—working unilaterally.

## Jump-Start Your Routine

Step onto the workout floor at Athletes' Performance, and chances are you'll see somebody jumping. That's because Verstegen wants to create elastic power in his athletes. The goal is for your muscles to store and release energy powerfully, like a pogo stick or Super Ball. Whether you're swinging a golf club or reacting to slipping on a patch of ice, all movement has an elastic component. "Elasticity is your body's shocks and springs," Verstegen says. "Even if you have big muscles, they don't necessarily generate much power unless you've trained them elastically."

It's simple: The next time you do a set of squats, follow up with a set of squat jumps. This will heighten your nervous-system activity—improving your mind's ability to communicate with your muscles—and put those movement patterns immediately to work the way you'll use them in real life. "It's like taking the doughnut off the baseball bat and going up to the plate," Verstegen says.

To do it, perform 8 to 10 repetitions of a squat using the heaviest weight you can lift that many times. Then perform the same movement explosively without the weight—quickly lowering your body until your thighs are parallel to the floor, then jumping as high as you can 10 times. Repeat the sequence for a total of two sets of each exercise.

# Ditch the Gym

**BY MIKE MEJIA, CSCS**

**N**obody likes logging hours in the gym when it's beautiful outside. The solution: Replace fat with muscle using this outdoor alternative to traditional cardio. The varying intensities will shake up your metabolism and boost endurance, and the agility and throwing involved also improve athleticism.

Perform one exercise after another for the specified length of time or number of repetitions. Rest for 15 seconds after each exercise and 60 seconds after the circuit. Repeat the circuit twice.

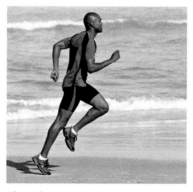

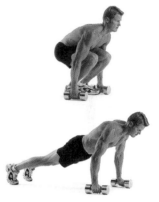

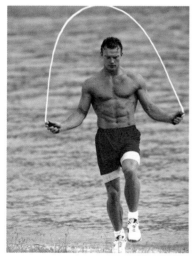

**Jumping rope:** Jump rope for 90 seconds. Try hopping on one leg to increase balance, alternating between legs. So you'll jump once on your right foot, once on your left, twice on your right, twice on your left, and so on, until you're alternating every 10 jumps between right-leg hops and left-leg hops.

**Shuttle run:** Position five small objects—agility cones, tennis-ball cans—in a row approximately 10 to 15 yards away from you. Sprint toward the objects, and retrieve them one by one. The drill is complete once you've brought all five objects back to the starting line as quickly as possible.

**Squat thrust:** From a standing position, bend at the hips and knees to lower yourself into a deep squat. Place your hands on the floor in front of you, then kick your legs back so you're in pushup position. Immediately bring your legs forward again so you're back in squat position and stand up. Perform 10 squats.

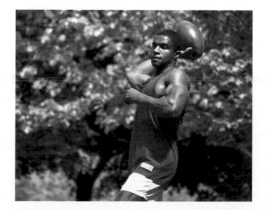

**Football rundown:** On a large field, throw or kick a football as far as you can. Run to retrieve it, then repeat. Do six to eight reps. No ball? Do stairwell sprints: Sprint up 5 to 10 flights, jog back down to the starting point, then repeat once.

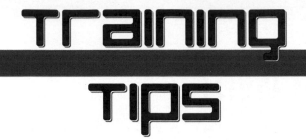

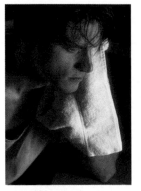

**I know exercise is supposed to give you energy, but I'm always too tired to get moving. How can I boost my energy before a workout?**

You have two choices to break this cycle: Hop up on false energy with caffeine or sugar and trudge through a 30-minute workout, or learn how the body uses and produces energy. Here's what you need to know to have a better workout: During exercise, your body taps into energy stores to contract muscles and adapts to become better at storing and releasing fuel. Exercise teaches your body how to work more efficiently, but it's up to you to work on nutrition, mind-set, and recovery.

**Nutrition.** Stock your office. By now, you know that eating five or six small meals or snacks a day, approximately every 2 to 3 hours, keeps your energy level constant. Load a desk drawer with dried fruit, almonds, jerky, tuna in a pouch, instant oatmeal, condiments, and plastic forks, spoons, and bowls. You'll stay productive and keep from crashing.

**Mind-set.** Think about tomorrow's workout today. A champion's mind-set starts with vision and ends with determination. I didn't read that in a fortune cookie; it's just how this works. If you write down when you're going to exercise (beginning and ending times) and jot down a few objectives, you'll start achieving your goals. All you need is a small spiral notebook. (Keep it in your gym bag or desk.) Try planning your complete workouts a night, week, or month ahead to eliminate uncertainty. Any plan is better than no plan.

**Recovery.** Shake and stretch. A full recovery from one workout gives you energy for the next. Start recovering the minute your workout ends by drinking a shake that's four parts carbohydrate and one part protein while you complete a cooldown consisting of foam-roll moves and static stretches.

## How can I find a good trainer?

Relying on the staff at your local gym can be a crapshoot since not all health clubs employ rigorous hiring standards. Instead, go to www.ustrainersearch.com and plug in your address, and you'll receive a list of trainers in your area. Cull all of those that don't have one of the following certifications: NASM, ACE, NSCA, ACSM, NFPT, or NCSF.

"There are about 75 certifying organizations out there, but only these six are accredited by the National Commission for Certifying Agencies," says Alan Russell, director of the Health Science Institute at the National Academy of Sports Medicine. In other words, these programs abide by a set of national standards that the other 69 do not.

Next, weed out trainers whose specializations (detailed in their profiles) don't match your fitness goals. Once you've narrowed the list to two or three candidates, feel them out over the phone.

"The key is to find someone you're comfortable with," says Russell. Translation: Let your gut decide. You'll know you've picked a winner if he (a) listens to your goals instead of pushing his own, (b) gives you his undivided attention during every workout, and (c) tracks your progress and adjusts your routine accordingly.

### I want to set up a home gym without breaking the bank. Tips?

Start off with a pair of "selectorized" dumbbells. These work like the machines in your gym in that you insert a pin to select the amount of weight. For $369, you can get a pair that ranges from 20 to 60 pounds from www.powerblock.com. Next,

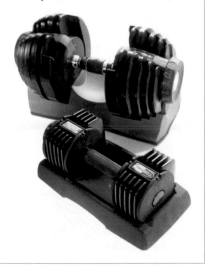

scan the local classifieds for a squat cage with a chinning bar and storage pegs, weight plates, a barbell, and a weight bench. I'd be surprised if you couldn't find the equipment used for under $250. With these few pieces of equipment, you'll be able to perform dozens of exercises—from lunges to pullups.

### What's the difference between fast-twitch and slow-twitch muscles?

The proper terminology is "fast-twitch and slow-twitch fibers," and every muscle contains a mix of the two. Fast-twitch fibers contract rapidly and are used during anaerobic activities, like sprinting and weight lifting, that require short bursts of power. Slow-twitch fibers contract less rapidly and are called into play during aerobic endurance sports, such as distance running and cycling.

We're all born with more of one kind of fiber than the other. To figure out which dominates in your body, look in the mirror. Mesomorphs—guys who are stocky—typically have more fast-twitch fibers. Ectomorphs—those who are tall and thin—generally have more slow-

twitch fibers. You'll get the best results by focusing on exercises that cater to your particular physiological strengths, but don't let that stop you from bulking up your fast-twitch fibers if you're an ectomorph: They're much easier to add than their slow-twitch counterparts.

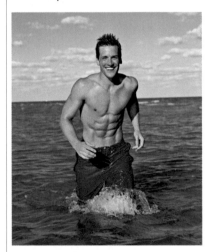

### Give me an exercise that'll help me look great at the beach.

The pullup is the ultimate two-in-one muscle builder for beach-ready biceps and a V-shaped back. This variation, called the mixed-grip pullup, also helps define your midsection. By using an overhand grip with one hand and an underhand grip with the other, you add a rotational component to the exercise, says

Alwyn Cosgrove, CSCS, owner of Results Fitness, in Santa Clarita, California. That is, your core musculature is forced to contract hard to stabilize your torso so your body stays straight throughout the move. The result: abs so solid, she can leave her surfboard at home.

## MIXED-GRIP PULLUP

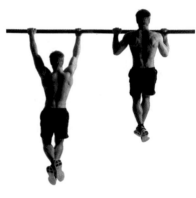

Grab a chinup bar with an alternating grip—one palm facing you (underhand grip), the other facing forward (overhand grip).

Keeping your abs tight, pull yourself up until your chest is even with the bar. Pause, then lower yourself. Do all your repetitions with your hands in this position, then, on your next set, do the reverse.

## What's a workout to make me look lean and tall?

Posture is everything here. Strengthening your core will help you stand tall throughout the day. Do one or two sets of 10 to 15 repetitions of the front bridge, side bridge, and glute bridge every morning. Warm up first with forward and lateral lunges, hand walks, hip-flexor stretches, and chest stretches.

## Is it okay that I vomit after a hard workout?

No. This phenomenon (long enjoyed by sadistic coaches) is a sign of a distressed cardiovascular system. If you're blowing chunks, your workout is too tough. "What happens is, you're training so hard that you're building up very high levels of blood lactate," says Bill Hartman, PT, CSCS, a strength coach in Indianapolis. This overstimulates your brain's vagus nerve, which connects to nerve fibers in the heart, esophagus, and intestinal tract. The result: "It causes a drop in heart rate and blood pressure, promoting nausea and heart stress," says Hartman.

Push yourself during your workouts, but if you start to feel nauseated, back off. Of course, eating an unusual food beforehand could cause gastrointestinal problems. So don't eliminate your preworkout meal—just keep it simple and familiar. An empty stomach will only hurt your workout by limiting your endurance and ultimate gains.

## Will boozing wreck my workout gains?

Yes. Alcohol inhibits protein synthesis and impedes muscle growth. "After a workout is the very worst time to drink," says Cynthia Kuhn, PhD, coauthor of *Pumped: Straight Facts for Athletes about Drugs, Supplements, and Training.* "Heavy alcohol intake decreases muscle mass, even if the alcohol isn't consumed after a workout." Wait until your muscle repair has peaked—about 24 hours after you leave the gym—before having a drink. And don't overdo it.

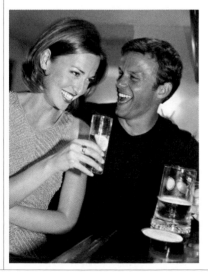

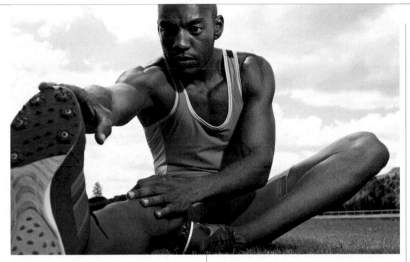

## Do I need to stretch before I lift?

No, you don't, but the right kind of stretching might make you stronger. Most of us, when we think of stretching, think of static stretching (i.e., elongating a muscle to the point of discomfort and holding it). But this type of stretch has limited benefit in weight training; it might even make you weaker by relaxing your muscles and reducing blood flow to them.

Dynamic stretching—moving a muscle in and out of a stretched position—is another matter entirely. It increases your "active" flexibility, which helps your muscles stretch quickly in various positions, and boosts blood flow—beneficial for any sport, including weight lifting.

Here's one of our favorite dynamic-stretch routines: body-weight lunge, squat, trunk rotation, leg swing, and arm circle. Do one set of 10 reps of each exercise before you work out.

## How many exercises per muscle per workout is enough?

One, as long as you're doing full-body workouts. Most guys take the opposite "isolation" approach, focusing on, say, chest and triceps one day and back and biceps the next. Their goal is commendable (i.e., to work each muscle group from multiple angles), but there's no reason to have to pack all of your chest exercises into a single workout. Sprinkle one or two into

each gym session, along with exercises for your arms, legs, and back. Doing so will ensure that you hit more muscles more often, resulting in better overall tone.

## Is it better to perform certain lifts on machines than with free weights?

Yes, but remember, barbells, dumbbells, and cable units are all "free weights." Everything else is a "machine." Unless you're a beginner—in which case, you'll benefit from using just about any type of gym equipment—focus on free weights. The training effect is enhanced when muscles control and stabilize the weights in addition to pulling or pushing them. That said, some exercises, including leg curls and adductor and abductor extensions, work better on machines.

Also, although free weights aren't necessarily more dangerous than machines, certain maneuvers, such as deadlifts and squats, do require a baseline level of skill, so get instruction from a qualified trainer before you attempt them on your own. Those caveats aside, free weights will always be the best way to maximize muscle gain.

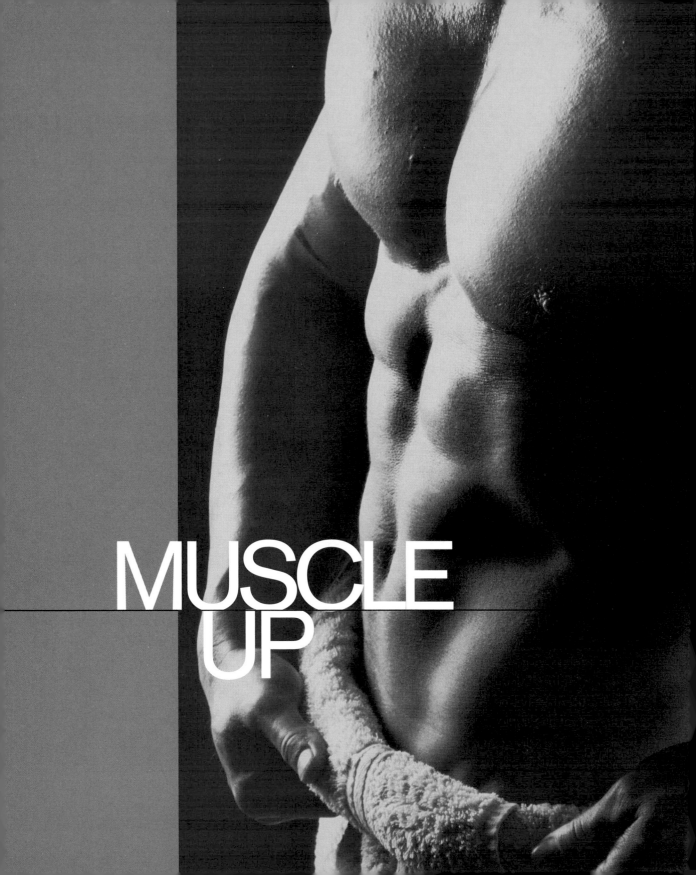

# MUSCLE
# UP

## PART THREE

No doubt you want to build muscle for many reasons—to look equally great in both a business suit and a swimsuit, to sweep your girl off her feet and into your arms without breaking your back, and because a heck of a lot more women swoon at the Rock than at David Spade. But here's perhaps the best reason: Building muscle may turn back the clock.

Here's the theory: If you could offset the natural decline in testosterone levels, you might be able to build more muscle, burn fat faster, and lift your libido. And though scientists have long known that resistance exercise boosts testosterone in young men after a workout, a new study shows that this is true for men of all ages—even into your seventies.

Toward that aim, in this section, you'll find dozens of tips for muscling up. Using the power of Olympic weight lifting, you'll experience the greatest workout known to man. With our four-step lifting plan, you'll transform your workout—and your body. Is poor posture ruining your workout? Could be, and you might not even know it. In this section, you'll learn how to get it straight and build a better body. And then you'll learn from a master bench presser how to press twice as much as you do now, in less than 60 days.

There's no time to waste; let's get growing.

BY ADAM CAMPBELL

# A Glimpse Inside the Muscle Laboratories

Learn why that workout you've been doing is pretty dumb

"Have you had lunch yet?" the rocket scientist asks as he straps me into the Space Cycle. I nod yes, but it wasn't an invitation; he wants to be well informed. You see, I'm about to be spun at 3 g's in a hypergravity exercise gym, a prototype designed for a Mars space station. For a visual, picture doing squats in a weight-room power rack, with one potentially catastrophic difference: The rack—and you—are swung horizontally around a steel pole at more than 40 revolutions per minute, sort of like a human tetherball. "You'll be fine," he says. "But whatever you do, don't look sideways." I don't need to ask why.

Vincent Caiozzo isn't a mad scientist. He's a professor of orthopedic surgery at the University of California at Irvine who's been studying muscle for nearly 30 years. The NASA–funded Space Cycle represents the pinnacle of his lifelong research—and, I think, a great investment opportunity. "Exercising in the Space Cycle is like hanging a barbell on every atom of your body," he tells me. Clearly, it's infomercial gold.

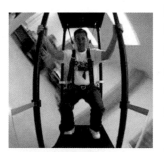

Only, Caiozzo isn't concerned with helping men build bigger biceps; his research interest is far less marketable. Like that of almost all muscle scientists, its purpose is to find better ways to prevent the muscle loss that occurs with

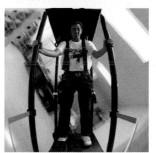

aging, cancer, spinal injuries, and, in the case of the Space Cycle, interplanetary travel.

But the lessons these researchers learn can still benefit those of us who want to look more buff at the beach. In fact, by using their findings to better understand the biology of muscle, you can build your body faster and more simply than ever. The trick, however, is knowing how to apply the hard science to your primary goal: building hard muscle.

Alwyn Cosgrove doesn't claim to be a muscle scientist. But, in a sense, he's become one by default. Since Cosgrove opened his gym, Results Fitness, in 2000, he's kept a detailed account of every single workout session that's been conducted there. "Clients pay for the fastest results," he says. "So to compete with the gym down the street, I had to find out what works best." And that meant collecting workout data on a large number of ordinary men who were using a variety of training methods.

Unlike commercial health clubs, Cosgrove's facility— located in Santa Clarita, California—offers only semiprivate training, meaning each workout is designed, monitored, and recorded by a member of the staff. Consider that in a typical week, it hosts 400 workouts, providing feedback on 20,800 sessions a year. To equal those numbers, a regular guy would have to work out every day for 57 years. In effect, that makes Cosgrove's gym a bona fide research laboratory and his gym-rat clients, it seems, human lab rats.

To explain his real-world findings, he's tried to bridge the academic research of men like Caiozzo with the practical application of exercises, sets, and repetitions. "A 19th-century English biologist named Thomas Huxley once said that 'science is nothing but organized common sense,'" says Cosgrove, "which is what training should be."

The end result of Cosgrove's human experiment is a muscle-building plan that's not just gym proven, it's supported by science. And because it shatters nearly 40 years of bodybuilding dogma, it will probably surprise you.

The biology of muscle isn't, in fact, rocket science. At its most basic level is the SAID principle, an acronym for "specific adaptation to imposed demand." "When a muscle contracts against a large amount of resistance, it adapts by getting bigger and stronger," says Caiozzo. Likewise, if it's regularly forced to contract for long periods of time, it becomes more resistant to fatigue. These adaptations occur to reduce stress on the body, which is why you can perform everyday functions—like walking up stairs or picking up a light object—with little effort.

Now let's apply the SAID principle to your workout. When you lift weights, you cause tiny tears in your muscle fibers. This accelerates a process called muscle-protein synthesis, which uses amino acids to repair

and reinforce the fibers, making them resistant to future damage. And although this happens at a microscopic level, the effect becomes visible over time—in the form of bigger arms, broader shoulders, and a thicker chest.

Understanding this process provides you with a logical rationale for how often you should train your muscles. In multiple studies, researchers at the University of Texas Medical Branch in Galveston have reported that muscle-protein synthesis is elevated for up to 48 hours after a resistance-training session. So if you work out on Monday at 7:00 p.m., your body is in muscle-growth mode until Wednesday at 7:00 p.m. After 48 hours, though, the biological stimulus for your body to build new muscle returns to normal.

On paper, this supports Cosgrove's first assertion: "Performing total-body workouts three times a week is the most effective way to gain muscle." Unfortunately, that advice directly contradicts what most guys actually do. That's because almost everyone subscribes to a leftover from the Stay Hungry days of weight lifting: what Cosgrove calls "body-part training."

The idea is to divide the body into specific muscle groups, or body parts, and dedicate an entire session to working each individually. For example, you might perform exercises for your chest on Monday, your back on Tuesday, your shoulders on Wednesday, and so on. Even though you're training daily, each muscle group is targeted only once a week. So, in essence, those

## The Anatomy of Muscle

Here's a microscopic view of your muscles.

**Muscle fiber:** A single muscle cell, which contains several hundred to several thousand myofibrils

**Sarcoplasm:** A semifluid membrane that surrounds the myofibril and contains structures—such as mitochondria—that provide energy for muscular contraction

**Fascicle:** A bundle of several muscle fibers

**Capillaries:** Tiny blood vessels that deliver nutrients and enzymes to the muscle fibers

**Muscle:** A bundle of fascicles that are enclosed in a sheath of connective tissue called fascia

**Myofibril:** A collection of thousands of tiny proteins that together generate force to help a cell contract

**Tendon:** Tough connective tissue that attaches muscle to bone

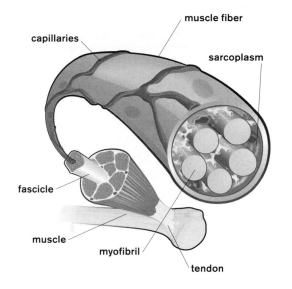

muscles grow for just 2 days out of every 7. With total-body workouts, though, you work each muscle more often. "When you train a muscle three times a week, it spends more total time growing," says Cosgrove.

Anatomically speaking, you can't isolate muscle groups in the first place—which is Cosgrove's other beef with body-part training. Imagine, for a moment, that you could strip the skin away from your muscles. You'd see clearly that they're interconnected, surrounding the body like a unified web. This is because all of your muscles are enclosed in a tough connective tissue called fascia. And since fascia attaches to bone and other muscles, it creates "functional" relationships between seemingly separate muscle groups.

"Even a small movement of your upper arm triggers a complicated network of muscles from your shoulder down to your hip," says Bill Hartman, PT, CSCS, a physical therapist in Indianapolis. Here's why: The latissimus dorsi (or lat), the largest muscle of the back, attaches to the upper-arm bone, shoulder blade, spine, and thoracolumbar fascia—a strong layer of connective tissue that attaches muscles to the spine and pelvis. The glutes, or rear hip muscles, attach to the pelvis. See the connections?

Don't misunderstand: There's no doubt you can emphasize a muscle group by choosing the appropriate exercise; just don't

# From Meat to Muscle

Here's how steak makes you grow.

**1. Breaking down the meat:** The process starts in your mouth with the mechanical digestion of food: Your teeth cut, tear, and mash the steak into smaller particles, mixing it with saliva to form a semisolid lump.

**2. Digesting the protein:** Once swallowed, the pulverized beef moves down your esophagus and lands in your stomach. Here, enzymes such as pepsin chemically break the steak into strands of amino acids. The whole mess is now more of a liquid called chyme.

**3. Creating usable parts:** From your stomach, the chyme passes into your small intestines. Here, additional enzymes—trypsin and chymotrypsin—act on the amino acid strands to break them into even smaller parts, until only single and double amino acids remain.

**4. Preparing for delivery:** The amino acids are then transported through the cells that line the walls of your intestines and into your bloodstream, a process called absorption. They're now ready to be sent to your muscles via your blood vessels.

**5. Building the muscle:** Once they reach your muscles, amino acids are delivered to the cells by way of capillaries. There, the amino acids help repair damaged fibers. In fact, muscle-protein synthesis can't occur unless amino acids are readily available—all the more reason to eat some protein at every meal.

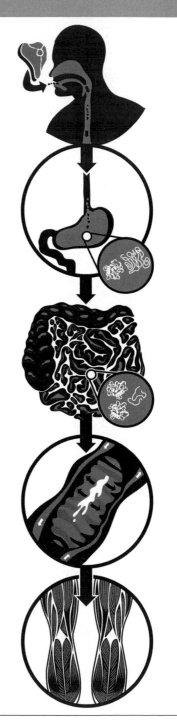

confuse targeting with isolating. To illustrate this point, Cosgrove uses the example of a popular exercise known as the bent-over row. If you subscribe to body-part training, it's a back exercise, since that's the area of your body it emphasizes. But, because of the interconnection between the muscles and connective tissues of the hips and back, your hamstrings and glutes are contracted for the entire exercise. So you're not only working your back, you're challenging your legs as well. And don't forget the involvement of your forearms and biceps in pulling the bar to your chest. "Separating your workouts by body parts is illogical," says Cosgrove. "You're not actually separating anything."

Also, since body-part training is generally performed intensely on consecutive days, it impedes the recovery process. "The nutrients your body needs to repair muscle damage from the previous day are allocated toward providing energy for your workout instead," says Jeff Volek, PhD, RD, an exercise-and-nutrition researcher at the University of Connecticut. "Your muscles grow best when your body is resting, not working." This isn't an issue with Cosgrove's total-body recommendation, since there's a built-in recovery day after each session.

Bodybuilders argue that total-body training doesn't allow you to work muscle groups hard enough. For instance, they claim that if a typical chest workout takes 30 minutes or more to complete, you'd have to spend hours in the gym to adequately train your entire body. "That's based on the assumption that a chest workout needs to take 30 minutes," says Cosgrove. He goes on to explain that a typical chest day might consist of three sets of four exercises, for a total of 12 sets every 7 days. But Cosgrove says you could do the same amount of work—12 total sets—in the same time period by performing four sets 3 days a week. "I've found that training works like a prescription," says Cosgrove. "You wouldn't take an entire bottle of Advil on Monday to relieve pain all week; you'd take smaller doses at regular intervals."

A study at the University of Alabama supports this notion. The researchers had one group of men train each muscle group once a week for 3 months; another group performed the same number of total sets weekly but split them equally among three total-body workouts. The result? The men who worked each muscle more frequently gained 9 pounds of muscle—5 more than those who trained each muscle only once a week.

But, to save even more time, Cosgrove employs another strategy: alternating sets. When possible, he pairs exercises that work opposite muscle groups and cuts the rest period between sets in half.

It's a concept based on the scientific work of Sir Charles Scott Sherrington, who won the Nobel Prize in 1932 for his contributions in physiology and neuroscience. Sir Sherrington's law of reciprocal innervation states that "for every neural activation of a muscle, there is a corresponding inhibition of the opposing muscle." This means when you work your chest muscles, the opposite back muscles are forced to relax, thereby resting.

So, instead of waiting 2 minutes between sets of bench presses, you can perform one set of the bench press, rest for just 1 minute, and then do a bent-over row. After you finish, you'll rest again, and then repeat the entire process until you complete all sets of both exercises. "In an average workout, this technique saves at least 8 to 10 minutes," says Cosgrove, "without sacrificing performance."

There's another piece to this puzzle, though. In analyzing thousands of workout logs, Cosgrove developed a volume-threshold theory. "It seems that growth occurs once a muscle has been exposed to 90 to 120 seconds of total tension," he says.

For example, let's say it takes 5 seconds to complete one repetition. This means one set of eight repetitions would place your muscles under tension for 40 seconds. So, using Cosgrove's theory, you'd need to do only three sets—for a total of 120 seconds—to perform enough exercise to stimulate muscle growth. Likewise with four sets of five repetitions or two sets of 12 repetitions.

However, even Cosgrove admits that this is more theory than fact, primarily for one reason: Human studies simply haven't compared a wide variety of set and repetition ranges or even controlled for the duration of muscle tension. So there's simply no data to draw from. At least not until you look elsewhere in the animal kingdom.

"Some men simply gain muscle faster, easier, and to a greater degree than others, which is why we study rats," says Caiozzo. Compared with humans, rats are a much more homogeneous species, meaning there's little variation from one to another. This allows scientists to more accurately study the enzymes, metabolic pathways, and genes that regulate muscle growth.

Of course, actual lab rats aren't gym rats by nature. So, in 1992, Caiozzo developed a rat-size resistance-training apparatus—a device that looks like a high-tech leg-curl machine. However, since they couldn't simply ask a group of rats to lift weights, there was another step involved.

The researchers permanently implanted a stainless-steel wire in the gastrocnemius muscle of each rat's hind limb and ran the wire under the skin to the skull, where two small screws had been inserted using a handheld drill. By connecting a wire to the outside of the screws, the scientists were then able to stimulate the muscle manually with an electric current, causing it to contract with maximal force. This allowed them to mimic a human weight-lifting workout.

To test the device, the rats were "encouraged" to perform four sets of 10 repetitions, with each repetition lasting 2 seconds—a total tension time of 80 seconds. The result: The group didn't increase muscle size in an 8-week period. This meant that either the machine didn't work or the volume of exercise was too low. So the researchers

tweaked the workout. When the contractions were increased to 4 seconds in duration, doubling the total tension time, the rats gained a significant amount of muscle mass—and in just 4 weeks, not 8.

Of course, this doesn't authoritatively validate Cosgrove's volume-threshold theory in humans, but it does provide a biological precedent that supports it. And it just may be that some of his data is simply ahead of its time.

"Go heavy or go home" is a common saying among bodybuilders. But, while it's crucial that you use a weight that provides a challenging load, the mantra is flawed. That's because muscle fibers can grow in two ways. The first is when the myofibrils— the parts of the fiber that contain the contracting proteins—increase in number and density. This type of growth leads to strength gains and can be accomplished by using heavy weights that allow only one to seven repetitions.

The second type of growth, however, occurs when your muscles are forced to contract for longer periods of time. Typically, this means using lighter loads that allow you to complete 12 to 15 repetitions. This increases the number of energy-producing structures within the fiber. So you don't get significantly stronger, but you do get bigger.

Using a repetition range that falls between the two causes a combination of both types of growth, but each to a lesser degree. And that's why Cosgrove uses all three repetition ranges. For instance, he

# The Minimalist Workout

## Get big results in almost no time

Use this 3-day total-body workout, designed by Alwyn Cosgrove, CSCS, to muscle up in less than 90 minutes a week. By incorporating the laws of functional anatomy, it works every muscle in your body with just five exercises. Building brawn has never been faster—or simpler.

**How to do it:** Perform this workout 3 days a week, resting a day after each session.

Do the same exercises each workout, but vary the sets, repetitions, and rest periods according to the chart below. (One exception: For the Swiss-ball pike, do 12 to 15 repetitions every session.)

For the first exercise (1), use straight sets, so that you complete all sets of the movement before moving on to the next.

Then perform each subsequent pair of exercises (2A and 2B, 3A and 3B) as alternating sets, resting for the prescribed amount of time after each. So you'll complete one set of exercise 2A, rest, do one set of exercise 2B, rest, and repeat. After you've finished all sets of both exercises, move on to the other pair.

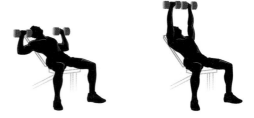

**1. Wide-grip deadlift:** Set a barbell on the floor and stand facing it. Squat down and grab it with an overhand grip that's twice shoulder width. With your back flat and head up, stand up with the barbell, pulling your shoulder blades back. Slowly lower the bar to the starting position.

**2A. Dumbbell incline press:** Lie on your back on a bench that's set to a low incline and hold a pair of dumbbells at the sides of your chest. Press the dumbbells up and together. Pause, then lower the weights back to the starting position.

might prescribe five repetitions of each exercise on Monday, 15 on Wednesday, and 10 on Friday. "It not only leads to better growth but also helps keep you from hitting plateaus," he says.

And indeed, in a 2002 study, Arizona State University researchers discovered that men who alternated their repetition ranges in each of three weekly training sessions gained twice as much strength as men who didn't vary their repetitions. To Cosgrove, it's just another case of a logical approach generating a logical result.

Being in the space cycle is a strange experience. Although my body is nearly parallel to the floor as I exercise, it feels as

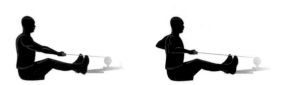

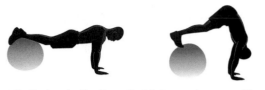

**2B. Cable row:** Attach a straight bar to the cable and position yourself in a cable-row machine. Grab the bar with an overhand, shoulder-width grip. Without moving your torso, pull the bar to your abdomen. Pause, then slowly return to the starting position.

**3B. Swiss-ball pike:** Get into pushup position, but instead of placing your feet on the floor, rest your shins on a Swiss ball. Raise your hips as high as you can as you roll the ball toward your body. Pause, then return to the start by lowering your hips and rolling the ball backward.

For each exercise, take 3 seconds to lower the weight, pause for 1 second, then take 1 second to lift it.

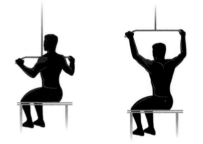

**3A. Wide-grip lat pulldown:** Grab the bar with an overhand grip that's about twice shoulder width and sit up straight. Without moving your torso, pull the bar down to your chest. Pause, then slowly return to the starting position.

| WORKOUT | SETS | REPS | REST |
|---------|------|------|------|
| Monday | 4 | 5 | 90 seconds |
| Wednesday | 2 | 15 | 30 seconds |
| Friday | 3 | 10 | 1 minute |

if I'm upright, and there's no sensation of spinning—provided, of course, that I don't violate the sideways rule. (Doing so, by the way, really sucks.) Caiozzo explains that the laws of physics prevent me from falling off, much as if I were on a roller coaster.

He invented the Space Cycle to help remedy one of NASA's biggest headaches.

"Because of the lack of gravity, an astronaut's muscles waste away quickly," he says.

As a veteran of four space flights, Commander Bill McArthur knows this reality firsthand. When I spoke to him by phone in early 2006, he was living on the International Space Station, a 6-month tour of duty 120 miles above Earth's surface. To stress the physical impact of space travel, he shared this memory from his first mission: "When we landed, I bent over to give my wife a hug, and she had to catch me because the bending wasn't going to stop," he says. "That was after just 14 days." So, in his space station detail, McArthur exercised nearly 2 hours a day—using a specially designed resistance-training machine called the IRED—just to try to maintain his muscle. Hardly a time-efficient solution.

Enter the Space Cycle. Because of its ingenious design, the rotating exercise gym creates artificial gravity, up to seven times the normal amount on Earth. Caiozzo believes this not only will prevent muscle loss in space but also will stimulate growth—without the need for weights. And in just a few minutes a day, not hours. "There's no magic," he says. "It just capitalizes on what we already know about muscle growth."

Granted, most of us aren't worried about bulking up on Mars just yet. But the Space Cycle illustrates an important point: The most effective workout isn't necessarily the longest or the hardest; it's simply the smartest. And the nearly 18 hours a day every guy spends sitting on his keister while commuting, driving the desk, settling into the couch, and hitting the sack isn't a bad approximation of weightlessness. So you may have more in common with Commander McArthur than you think.

"Building muscle takes sweat, guts, and determination," says Cosgrove, who's always eager to help the couch-bound. "So why make it harder than it needs to be?"

ESSENTIAL READING

BY JOHN K. WILLIAMS, PhD

# Ultimate Muscle Meals

## 8 great protein foods (that won't crawl off your plate)

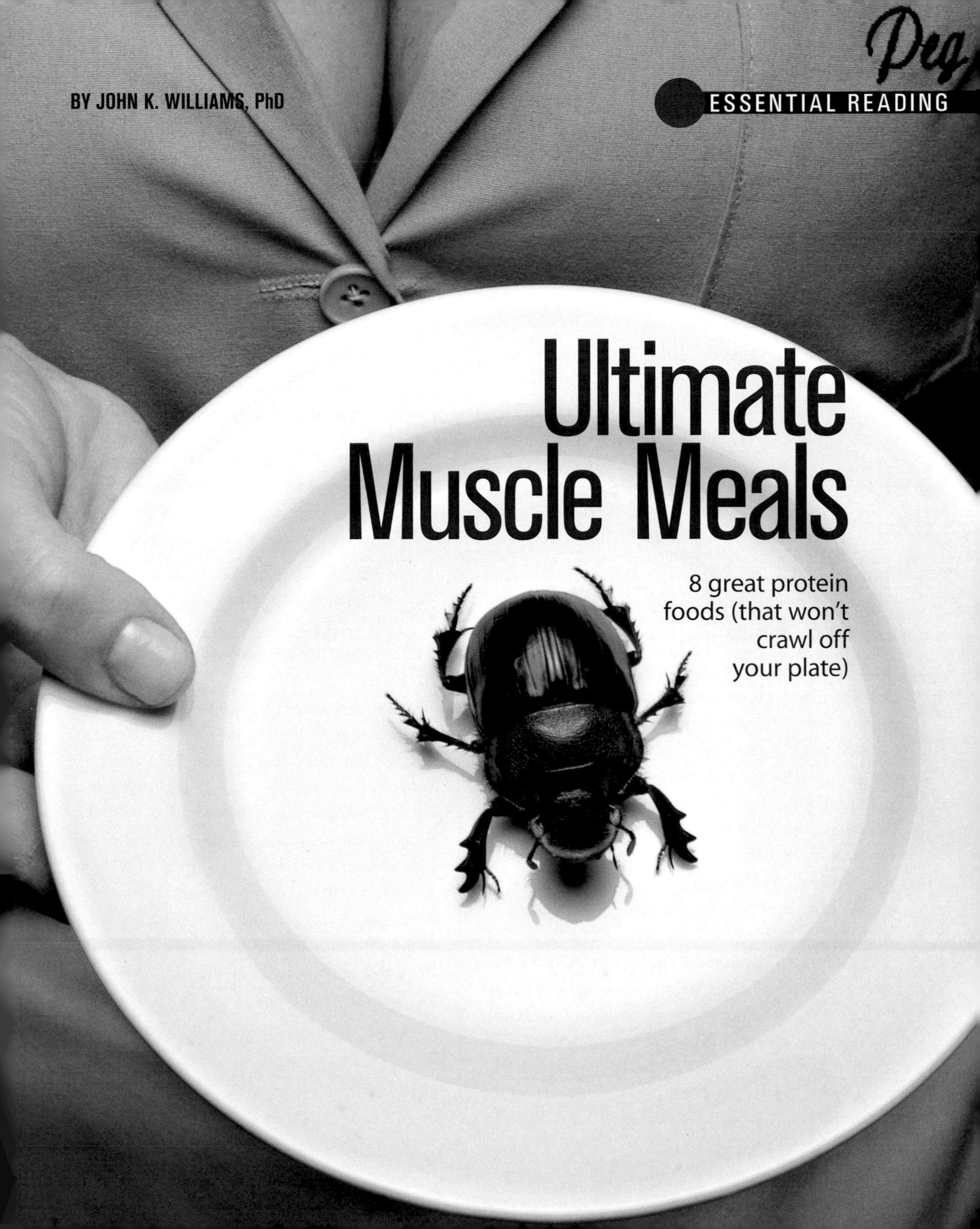

**D**id you know there's an all-natural, muscle-building snack that's free? It's called *Onthophagus gazella Fabricius* and a big handful contains 17 g (grams) of protein, just 4 g fat, and almost no carbs. The downside: You know it better by its common name—the dung beetle.

But don't be disappointed. We've found eight better-tasting ways to help you boost your protein intake. And, specifically, at the times when you need it the most: breakfast, lunch, and the snacks between meals. Why? Because most men consume two-thirds of their daily protein after 6 p.m., says Donald Layman, PhD, a professor of nutrition at the University of Illinois. In fact, Layman found that to optimally feed your muscles, you need 8 to 12 g of an amino acid called leucine spread evenly throughout the day. Trouble is, it takes 30 g of high-quality protein—such as that found in meat, eggs, and cheese—to provide a 2- to 3-g dose of this essential amino acid. And that's where most predinner meals fall short. Make sure yours don't, by using the following recipes.

## FRENCH TOAST WITH WHIPPED FRUIT TOPPING

1½ c low-fat cottage cheese

Splenda to taste

1 cup blueberries

2 eggs plus 2 egg whites, beaten

¾ cup low-fat milk

1 tsp ground cinnamon

½ tsp vanilla extract

6 slices whole-grain bread

To make the whipped topping, blend the cottage cheese, Splenda, and ½ cup of the blueberries on high for 30 seconds, or until smooth and creamy. Then set it aside. In a large bowl, mix together the eggs, milk, cinnamon, and vanilla extract. Soak the bread one slice at a time until it's saturated with liquid, then grill it over medium-high heat in a nonstick skillet coated with cooking spray until lightly browned on both sides. Serve with the whipped fruit topping and put the remaining blueberries on top.

Makes 2 servings

Per serving: 565 calories, 46 g protein (3.8 g leucine), 66 g carbohydrates, 13 g fat, 9 g fiber

## Protein Power: 3 Ways to Supplement Your Diet

**Optimum Nutrition 100% Whey Protein Powder.** Use it to make protein-packed shakes or cheesecake (see the recipe on page 163), or add it to your morning bowl of oatmeal. ($50 for a 5-pound container; www.optimumnutrition.com)

**Calorie Countdown 2% chocolate dairy beverage.** This low-sugar chocolate-milk substitute is essentially an inexpensive protein supplement. A big 16-ounce glass contains 16 grams (g) of protein and just 6 g sugar—compared with 60 g sugar in regular chocolate milk.

**Everyday Nutrition meal replacement.** At $5 for each 11-ounce carton, it's not cheap. But this is the healthiest ready-to-drink protein shake we've found. Each serving contains 20 g protein, 6 g fiber, 700 milligrams (mg) fish oil, 400 mg calcium, and just 1 g sugar. ($115 for a 24-pack; janaklauermd.com)

## BREAKFAST BURRITO

2 Tbsp salsa

¼ cup shredded low-fat Cheddar cheese

¼ cup fresh cilantro

1 large egg plus 4 large egg whites, beaten

½ cup chopped lean ham

1 large (8") whole-wheat tortilla

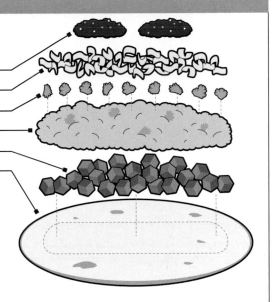

In a nonstick skillet coated with cooking spray, sauté the ham over medium-high heat, just until the surface starts to brown. Place the cooked ham in the tortilla, then add more cooking spray to the skillet and scramble the eggs together with the cilantro. Add the eggs to the tortilla, top with the cheese and salsa, and fold.

Makes 1 serving

Per serving: 410 calories, 48 g protein (2.4 g leucine), 33 g carbohydrates, 11 g fat, 3 g fiber

## YOGRANOLA

1 cup low-fat plain yogurt

½ cup low-fat granola

For this snack, simply put the yogurt in a bowl and stir in the granola. If desired, the plain yogurt can be sweetened with Splenda.

Makes 1 serving

Per serving: 349 calories, 19 g protein (1.8 g leucine), 63 g carbohydrates, 3 g fat, 3 g fiber

## OATMEAL AND WHEY

1 cup rolled oats

1 cup low-fat milk

½ cup berries (fresh or frozen, your choice of berries)

Dash of salt

Dash of ground cinnamon

Splenda to taste

1 scoop (28 g) vanilla whey-protein powder (see "Protein Power," at left)

Combine the oats and milk in a large bowl. Microwave for 1 minute, stir, then microwave for an additional minute. Mix in the berries, salt, cinnamon, and Splenda. Let the oatmeal cool slightly, then stir in the protein powder. (Very hot oatmeal can damage protein powder, causing it to lump and sour.)

Makes 1 serving

Per serving: 580 calories, 45 g protein (4.5 g leucine), 83 g carbohydrates, 7 g fat, 14 g fiber

## PITA PIZZA

½ cup shredded low-fat mozzarella cheese

¼ cup chopped pineapple

4 oz lean ham

1 Tbsp Italian seasoning (or dried basil and oregano)

2 Tbsp marinara sauce

1 whole-wheat pita (6" diameter)

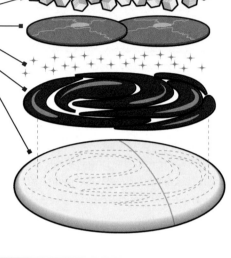

Preheat the oven to 425°F. Spread the marinara sauce over the pita, add the Italian seasoning, and top with the pineapple, ham, and cheese. Bake the pita for 8 minutes on a baking sheet on the center oven rack.

Makes 1 serving

Per serving: 650 calories, 55 g protein (3.5 g leucine), 62 g carbohydrates, 20 g fat, 8 g fiber

## CHOCOLATE PEANUT-BUTTER SHAKE

1 cup Hood Calorie Countdown chocolate 2% dairy beverage

½ cup low-fat cottage cheese

2 Tbsp peanut butter

1½ cup ice

Splenda to taste

Combine all the ingredients in a blender and blend on high for about 30 seconds, until the shake is smooth and creamy.

Makes 1 serving

Per serving: 400 calories, 35 g protein (2.8 g leucine), 17 g carbohydrates, 21 g fat, 2 g fiber

## NUKE-AND-EAT ASIAN STIR-FRY

*Make this recipe on Sunday, then freeze it in single-serving portions—you'll have a healthy fast-food meal ready anytime you want it.*

1 large egg, beaten

½ tsp salt

4 Tbsp soy sauce

1 lb beef sirloin, sliced into 2" strips

1 Tbsp sesame oil

1 Tbsp cornstarch

½ tsp crushed red pepper

1 Tbsp chopped garlic

2 tsp grated fresh ginger

2 carrots, sliced into 2" strips

1 8-oz can sliced water chestnuts, drained

1 medium onion, sliced

1 bunch scallions, sliced into 2" strips

Rice Expressions Organic Brown Rice (This frozen rice is precooked and packaged in individual microwaveable pouches. You can find it at riceexpressions.com.)

In a bowl, combine the egg, salt, and 1 Tbsp of the soy sauce, and stir well. Then add the sirloin strips and set aside to marinate. Next, heat the oil in a large nonstick skillet while you mix the remaining soy sauce, cornstarch, and crushed red pepper in a bowl—this is your sauce, to be used later. Once the skillet is hot, stir-fry the garlic and ginger for about 30 seconds, stirring constantly. Then, at 30-second intervals, individually add the carrots, water chestnuts, onion, and scallions. Next, remove all the vegetables from the skillet and place them in a bowl. Put the beef-marinade mixture in the skillet, cook for 2 to 3 minutes, then pour in the sauce, stirring and cooking until it's thick and bubbly. Finally, add the vegetables back to the skillet, and cook everything together for a couple of minutes, or until hot.

Let it cool, then place individual portions in plastic containers and freeze. When you're ready for a quick lunch, microwave the stir-fry for 3 minutes or until hot and serve with one pouch of the brown rice.

Makes 3 servings

Per serving: 486 calories, 42 g protein (2.2 g leucine), 45 g carbohydrates, 16 g fat, 7 g fiber

## STRAWBERRY CHEESECAKE
### Crust

1 cup graham-cracker crumbs

¼ cup milled flaxseeds

¼ cup raw oat bran

1 oz fat-free cream cheese, warmed in the microwave

⅓ cup water

### Filling

2 cups low-fat cottage cheese

1 package (28 g) powdered Jell-O Sugar Free, Fat Free Instant Pudding, cheesecake flavor

3 oz fat-free cream cheese

3 scoops strawberry or vanilla whey or casein Protein powder

### Topping

1 cup sliced strawberries

4 Tbsp sugar-free strawberry jam

To make the crust, mix the crust ingredients in a large bowl. Stir this mixture until it's all the same consistency, then press it into a 9-inch pie pan coated with cooking spray, easing the crust up the sides of the pan. For the cheesecake filling, blend the ingredients in a blender on high until smooth and creamy. Pour the blended mixture into the crust and refrigerate for 1 hour. Top with the strawberries and jam.

Makes 6 slices

Per slice: 240 calories, 27 g protein (2.8 g leucine), 27 g carbohydrates, 3 g fiber

BY TIM FOLGER

# Harness the Olympics Advantage

With the power of Olympic weight lifting, you'll experience the greatest workout known to man—and the best gains of your life

My introduction to the best-kept secret in fitness begins with a video that both inspires and intimidates me. I'm watching Pyrros Dimas, a three-time Olympic gold medalist from Greece, prepare for an Olympic weight-lifting competition. Pound for ripped pound, he's one of the strongest men on the planet.

Dimas is hoisting a bar so loaded with plates that it looks like a truck axle with the tires attached. Again and again, he tosses the weight from the floor over his head in one quick, graceful motion, almost casually. And that's just his warmup. In competition, Dimas once lifted 474 pounds over his head—considerably more than twice his body weight of 187.

"That move's called a snatch," says my trainer, Shane Miller, as he rewinds the video. Miller is the head trainer at Carl and Sandra's Physical Conditioning Center, a gym in Santa Fe, New Mexico, where I've come for a 2-hour beginner lesson in Olympic-style weight lifting. It's not that I have any Olympian aspirations; I'm here because the Olympic lifts, as they're called, have no equal for developing speed; flexibility; and coordinated, total-body strength and muscle.

Interestingly, there are only two official Olympic lifts: the aforementioned snatch and the clean and jerk. For a visual, think of the snatch as a deadlift, barbell shrug, jump squat, and overhead squat performed consecutively in one fluid motion. The clean and jerk? A combination deadlift, upright row, front squat, and push press.

To underscore the effectiveness of these movements, consider that in the most basic measure of raw athletic ability—the vertical jump—Olympic weight lifters excel above all others. "When I worked at the Olympic Training Center in Colorado Springs, we measured vertical jumps of athletes in nearly every sport," says Michael Stone, PhD, a professor of exercise science at Eastern Tennessee State University. "And Olympic weight lifters had higher average jumps than all other groups—basketball players, gymnasts, sprinters, everybody."

Even the bulkiest Olympic heavyweights make astonishing leaps. Shane Hamman, the top American lifter in the history of the sport, weighs in at 350 pounds but boasts a

*(continued on page 168)*

## PAINkiller

**I feel a lot of pain directly under my right kneecap, especially after sitting for a while or when I climb stairs. Should I see a doctor?**

First, try this test at the gym or at home: Lie facedown on the floor, and have someone grab your right leg and bend it toward your right buttock (don't resist or assist). If you don't have any pain when your foot is moved all the way to your butt, see the doctor. You might have ligament damage.

But if you feel extreme tightness in your quad muscle or you can't bend your leg anywhere near your butt, your quad is too short, and that could be causing patella alta (an abnormally elevated position of the patella tendon). This condition is common in people who don't exercise regularly, and the older you get, the more likely it is to occur. To alleviate the pain, stretch your quad using the movement described above. (On your own, loop a piece of rope or a towel around your ankle.) Over the next few weeks, do three 30-second stretches every day and work the muscle just short of feeling pain—no harder. If pain persists, see your doctor.

# The Olympic Workout

Twice a week, insert these two mini-routines into your current workout, performing them before you do any other exercises. Alternate between themRoutine 1 and Routine 2 so that you do only two of the modified Olympic lifts each session. (Or, for a complete training plan, see "Go Inside the NFL's Secret Training Camp" on page 124.) A couple of pointers: The high pull and the jump shrug are speed exercises, so use a weight that requires a strong effort to lift it quickly but isn't so heavy that you can't control the bar. For the front squat and push press, use the heaviest weight that allows you to do all the pre-scribed reps.

## Routine 1

### High Pull

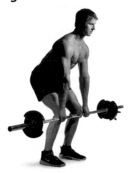

Hold a barbell just below your knees with a shoulder-width, overhand grip. With your back flat and arms straight, pull the bar upward as fast as you can by thrusting your hips forward and explosively standing up.

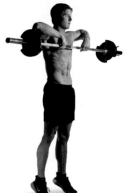

As the bar passes your thighs, continue moving upward onto your toes and pull the bar as high as possible by bending your elbows and raising your upper arms. Return to the starting position and repeat for three sets of three to five repetitions, resting 90 seconds after each set.

### Front Squat

Grab a bar with an overhand grip that's just beyond shoulder width and hold it on the tops of your shoulders. Raise your upper arms so they're parallel to the floor and let the bar roll back so it's resting on your fingers, not your palms. Stand with your feet shoulder-width apart and your back straight.

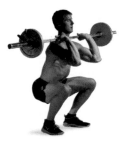

Without changing the position of your arms, lower your body until your thighs are at least parallel to the floor. Then push back up to the starting position. Do three sets of six to eight repetitions, resting 90 seconds after each set.

## Routine 2

### Snatch-Grip Jump Shrug

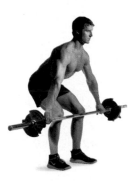

Hold a bar just below your knees with an overhand grip that's twice shoulder width.

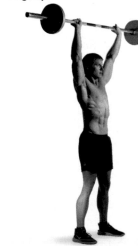

Keeping your back flat and arms straight, simultaneously thrust your hips forward, shrug your shoulders, and jump straight up. Land on the balls of your feet and repeat. Do three sets of three to five repetitions, resting 90 seconds after each set.

### Push Press

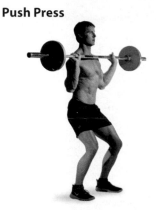

Grab a barbell with a shoulder-width, overhand grip. Stand holding the barbell at shoulder level, your feet shoulder-width apart. Dip your knees slightly.

Push up with your legs as you press the bar over your head. Then lower the bar to the starting position. Do three sets of eight repetitions, resting 90 seconds after each set.

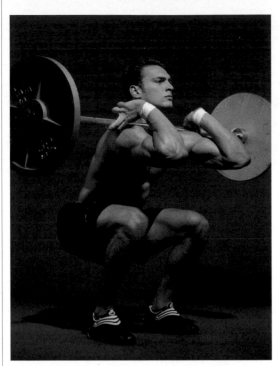

**When doing a front squat, keep your elbows high. This helps your torso stay more upright, reducing stress on your back.**

vertical jump of 36 inches. Most NBA players top out at 34 inches. Not only can Hamman dunk (he's 5'9"), he can also drive a golf ball 350 yards.

Then there's the pure vanity aspect. The Olympic lifters who aren't heavyweights are among the leanest—they're certainly the strongest—athletes in the world. One study of elite athletes found that Olympic weight lifters burn almost as many calories per day as marathoners do, and another reported that, on average, the lifters have as little as 5 percent body fat. Granted, these men are moving more than 175,000 pounds in a typical training week, but they also eat 6,000 to 8,000 calories a day.

So what is it about the Olympic lifts that works such magic on the human body? Most simply, they engage nearly all of your muscles to move weights farther and faster than conventional exercises. In fact, each repetition takes only a second or two from start to finish, which allows you to target your fast-twitch muscle fibers. These are the muscles with the greatest potential for size and strength—and the ones that are typically ignored in most men's weight workouts.

At this point, you might be wondering why, if these Olympic lifts are so great, you seldom see them practiced in gyms. The main reason is that they're technically difficult to perform, says Miller. Unlike a biceps curl, which requires little or no instruction to perform safely, these maneuvers call for a qualified instructor to teach you the nuances of each movement. Otherwise, you'll put yourself at risk of injury or, at the very least, perform them incorrectly—which is, of course, why I've come to Miller's gym in the first place.

But while anyone can find an instructor at the USA Weightlifting Web site (www.usaweightlifting.org), it turns out there's also a shortcut to experiencing the Olympic advantage. You see, the unique aspects of the Olympic lifts consist of two distinct parts: the "pull" phase and the "catch" phase. During the pull, you explode upward, yanking the barbell off the floor and in front of your thighs, as if you were trying to jump out of the gym. In the catch, you quickly move your body under the bar and catch the weight on your shoulders or above your head.

"In my experience, 95 percent of the benefits of Olympic lifts come from the pull phase, which is the simplest part of the movement," says Alwyn Cosgrove, CSCS, a certified USA Weightlifting coach in Santa Clarita, California. "And almost all of the technical difficulties occur during the catch phase." That's why Cosgrove has eliminated the catch portion of the movement from nearly all of his programs and why you can forget about it, too. "Most men need to worry about the catch only if they're interested in competing in the sport," he says.

To enable lifters at any level to benefit from these exercises, Cosgrove has broken down the Olympic lifts into their four most effective movements. (See "The Olympic Workout" on page 166.) Incorporate them into your routine and you'll build muscle and strength, burn fat, and boost sports performance faster than ever before. In fact, consider whatever you've been doing up till now preparation for your real workout.

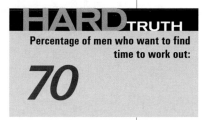

**HARD** TRUTH

**Percentage of men who want to find time to work out:**

*70*

# Simplify Your Lifting Plan, Supersize Your Strength

This four-step plan will transform your workout—and your body

**BY BILL HARTMAN**

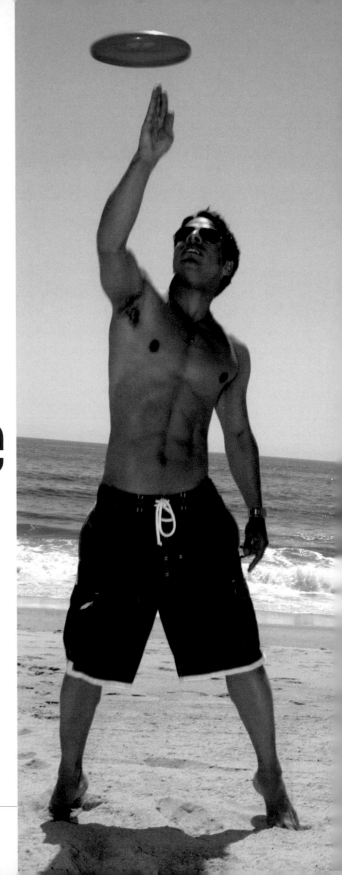

ummer presents a fitness paradox: You aspire to make your body look its best, but you want to invest the least possible gym time to get it that way. After all, what good are beach muscles if you never have the chance to show them off?

The solution, of course, is efficiency—the ability to work your muscles only as much as they need, so you can achieve maximum results in minimal time. Turns out, it's as simple as knowing when to hit the weights a little harder and when to finish early. All you have to do is let your body guide you.

It's important to know first that all of life's stressors, both physical and psychological, directly affect your performance in the gym—and they change from day to day. For instance, suppose you lift weights intensely on Monday after work, and then on Tuesday night you get only 5 hours of sleep instead of your usual 7. Wednesday morning, your "check engine" light comes on as you pull in to work, and 5 minutes later, your boss assigns you a high-priority project. When it's time for your evening workout, you aren't physically or mentally prepared to give your best effort. And that means your strength and endurance will fade faster than in your previous workout. When this happens, it's a signal from your body that your muscles have had enough—that doing more repetitions won't lead to greater growth but will only increase the stress on your body, slowing recovery time.

There's a flip side, too: If your life has gone perfectly over the past couple of days, you may feel like you can lift the world. This is the time to take advantage of your increased ability—by upping weights, sets, and repetitions—in order to accelerate your muscle gains.

You see, your body provides the best indicator of how long your workout should last. And, chances are you're doing more than you need—even on your best days. But use the four-step plan that follows, and you'll never waste another repetition...or a minute in the gym that could be spent in the sun.

## Step 1: Streamline Your Workout

Although most men perform three or four exercises for each muscle group, it's better to choose just one. Fact is, you obtain almost all the size-boosting benefits of weight lifting from the first exercise you do, when your muscles are fresh. For example, let's say

## Work Out at Warp Speed

When researchers at the University of Sydney had two groups of men perform biceps curls at either a slow tempo (3 seconds up, 3 seconds down) or a fast tempo (1 second up, 1 second down), they found that lifting fast builds 11 percent more strength than training at slow speeds. "Changing the speed of reps either from workout to workout or from set to set can build muscle," says Matthew Rhea, PhD. Try it: For the next 4 weeks, add a set of six to eight biceps curls to your workout 3 days a week. Use the heaviest weight that allows you to complete the reps fast without having to "cheat"— that is, without leaning forward or back.

you complete three sets of each of these three chest exercises: flat bench press, incline bench press, and dumbbell fly. By the time you do the last exercise, the amount of weight you can handle is so low that it's no longer challenging enough to stimulate muscle growth.

Don't believe it? Try doing the exercises in reverse order. Not surprisingly, you'll be able to lift far less than usual for the flat bench press—a weight you'd normally consider too light. That means there's no reason to think it's benefiting your muscles.

**How to do it:** You can apply this rule to your current workout—eliminating exercises that target the same muscle group—or use the 3-day-a-week plan below. It works your entire body with just four exercises each session—a perfect fit for your summer schedule.

Alternate between Workout A and Workout B every other day, doing the

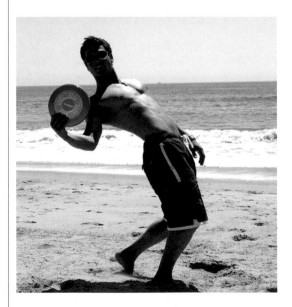

exercises in the order shown, and use this repetition strategy: The first time you perform Workout A, do 6 repetitions of each exercise; the next time, do 6 repetitions. In Workout B, do the opposite: 12 repetitions in the first session, 6 in the next. Continue to alternate for each workout. This ensures that you train your muscles for both muscular strength and muscular endurance, a method that leads to the fastest gains. As for the number of sets you'll perform, keep reading.

| WORKOUT A | WORKOUT B |
|-----------|-----------|
| Squat | Deadlift |
| Bench press | Chinup |
| Bent-over row | Lateral raise |
| Reverse crunch | Side bridge |

## Step 2: Rev Up Your Engine

Like Tiger Woods after blowing a third-round lead, your muscles perform better when they're fired up. So prime them for action by using a technique called the "ramp-up" method. By exciting the nerve pathways between your brain and muscles—without causing fatigue—it allows you to activate a greater number of muscle fibers than if you didn't warm up. The result: You'll be able to lift heavier weights and do more repetitions. And that means faster gains in both size and strength.

**How to do it:** For each exercise, estimate the weight you plan to use in your regular sets. (It doesn't have to be exact; just go with your best guess.) That's your base weight. Then perform the 2-minute warmup that follows. There's no need to rest between sets; just change the weight and repeat. Once you've finished all three warmup sets, you're ready to start your regular sets.

Set 1: five repetitions with 60 percent of your base weight

Set 2: three repetitions with 80 percent of your base weight

Set 3: one repetition with 110 percent of your base weight. By using a slightly heavier weight than your base on your last warmup set, you'll trick your brain into engaging even more muscle fibers during your regular sets.

## Step 3: Determine the Best Weight

Here's where it gets fun: After you warm up (step 2), you'll test your strength to determine the ideal weight to use for your regular sets, using the benchmark of technical failure. Technical failure is the point at which performance starts to decline, and it can be identified in two ways.

1. You can't maintain perfect form. The easiest gauge is when your posture changes—for instance, you have to arch your back to complete a bench press, or you need to lean your torso backward to complete an arm curl.

2. You aren't in total control of the weight. In this case, the speed at which you lift a weight slows down as you pass your "sticking point." The other yardstick:

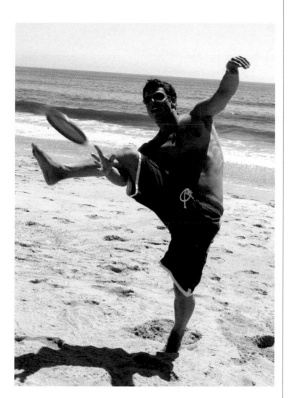

You aren't able to lower a weight back to the starting position at the same rate from top to bottom; that is, it feels as though the weight overtakes you.

When either of these conditions occurs, you've reached technical failure. Unlike in absolute failure, in which you can't perform even one more repetition, you'll probably feel as if you could pump out a couple more.

**How to do it:** For each exercise, start by estimating the amount of weight you think will allow you to complete your planned number of repetitions for that day. Don't worry if you're not sure; that's what the test is for. (Keep in mind this isn't a onetime assessment; you'll repeat the test for each exercise, every single workout.) Now do as

## Superior Squats

The classic barbell back squat develops all the muscles of your lower body, making it a must-have move in any workout plan. It develops strength and power in the quadriceps, hamstrings, and glutes, all in one basic movement.

Here, you'll find two upgrades that strengthen the same muscles while also engaging your core. An added bonus: You'll build an athletic body by improving the flexibility and stability of your lats, lower back, hips, and abs. As a result, you'll lift more weight when you return to the traditional back squat. (For more on that move, visit www.mens health.com/body.) Remember: Focus on staying upright and maintaining a natural arc in your back.

## Overhead Squat

This move forces you to control your center of gravity at a much higher point than in a back squat, so you'll strengthen your core. You'll also be able to press more weight overhead (for rock-hard shoulders), since the overhead squat conditions your back to stay straight.

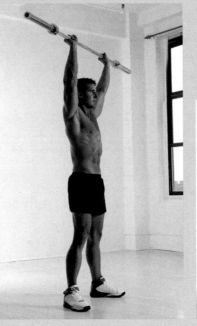

Stand holding a bar overhead with an overhand grip, hands wider than shoulder width.

Pull your shoulder blades together to keep the bar in line with or behind your ears throughout the move. As you lower your body into a squat, imagine pulling the bar apart and pushing up on it. Pause when your thighs are parallel to the floor.

Then push yourself back to a standing position. Do two sets of 12 repetitions. Make it harder: Trade the bar for a pair of dumbbells.

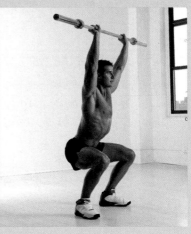

many repetitions as you can, ending the set when you reach technical failure.

If you're able to complete all your planned repetitions—but no more—without achieving technical failure, you've chosen the correct weight. For example, if your goal was six repetitions, you would have achieved technical failure on repetition seven.

However, if you reach technical failure before you complete all your intended repetitions, the weight is too heavy. And if you're able to complete more reps than you planned, the weight is too light. In either case, rest for a minute or so, adjust the weight accordingly (up or down), then repeat the test. It may take you a couple of tries to

### Triceps Plate Squat

This full-body exercise combines a squat, press, and triceps extension for a great cardiovascular and muscle-building workout. Perform 12 repetitions with the triceps extension in step 3, followed by 12 without it. Focus on keeping your movements slow and smooth. Grab a weight plate and hold it overhead with your arms straight and your palms facing each other.

Keeping your eyes forward and chest up, squat while bringing your arms down in front of you until the weight is beneath your butt and your thighs are parallel to the floor.

Reverse the move to position 1. Lower the plate toward your back and raise it overhead again. That's one rep. Make it harder: As you stand back up in each rep, rise onto your toes.

—Carter Hays, CSCS

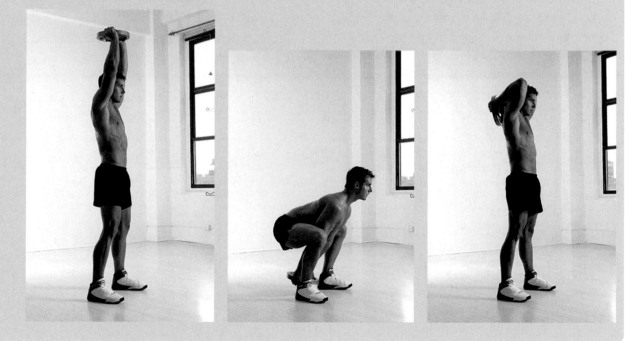

find the ideal weight, but that's okay; you're not wasting time because you're still challenging your muscles.

## Step 4: Lift Till You Drop

The rest is simple: Once you've used technical failure to determine the ideal weight to use for an exercise, you'll simply perform as many sets with that weight as you can—stopping when your performance drops off significantly. This is your cue that you've worked the target muscles maximally.

**How to do it:** Using the ideal weight (step 3), perform one set to technical failure. Next, rest as long as it takes for your breathing rate to return to normal (but no longer than 2

## Drink Up

University of West Florida scientists recently discovered that downing a sports drink with amino acids before you lift may make your workout easier. The researchers compared two sports drinks: one containing branched-chain amino acids (BCAA)—the proteins that are a major part of muscle tissue—and one without the added nutrients. The result: When the study subjects drank 16 ounces of the BCAA-infused drink before doing a set of bench presses, their perceived exertion declined by 16 percent, compared with that of men who consumed a regular sports drink. In the study, the scientists were testing a product called Amino Vital; you can find it at www.amino-vital.com or your local health-food store.

minutes). Then repeat the process as many times as you can, stopping when the number of repetitions you can complete is three lower than the number you planned. This is known as your performance drop-off. Consider this a signal from your body that it's time to move on to the next exercise in your workout (or to the locker room). So if your goal is six repetitions, you'll have performed your last set of that movement when you can't complete four repetitions without achieving technical failure. If your goal is 12 reps, the critical number is 10. You may be able to perform eight sets, six sets, or perhaps only one or two. Regardless, you can be sure that it's precisely the number your muscles need.

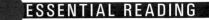
# Straighten Up

Poor posture may be
ruining your workout.
Here's how to get it
straight—and build a
better body

BY LORENZO GONZALEX, DPT

Consider this fact: The average human head weighs 8 pounds. And if your chin moves forward just 3 inches—as it tends to when you work at a computer—the muscles of your neck, shoulders, and upper back must support the equivalent of 11 pounds. That's a weight-bearing increase of 38 percent—often for hours at a time. Left untreated, the effect of chronic desk slump results in a postural dysfunction that physical therapists call upper-cross syndrome; you know it as rounded shoulders.

The consequences aren't simply a vanity concern; this little-known condition is a common cause of weight-lifting plateaus, as well as pain and injuries. Chances are, if you work a desk job or lift weights, you already suffer—or soon will—from this sinister syndrome. Your risk is even higher if you do both.

Use the self-test that follows to determine whether you're an upper-cross victim. Then reevaluate your workout and your job posture with our problem-solving guide. It'll show you how to repair the damage if you've already fallen prey and provide you with a preemptive battle plan for fending it off in the future. The bonus: Your shoulders will be bigger, stronger, and healthier than ever.

## The Self-Test: Are You Crossed Up?

Place two fingers at the top of your right shoulder and feel for a bony notch that protrudes from it. That's your acromion. Now grab a ruler and lie on your back on the floor, your right arm resting alongside your body. With your left hand, measure the distance from your right acromion to the floor, being careful not to raise or lower your right shoulder. If the distance is more than 1 inch, you have upper-cross syndrome.

Want a second opinion? Ask a friend to take a digital picture of you—shirtless—from the side. Stand tall but relaxed, the way you would if you weren't thinking about your posture. Check to see if the middle of your ear is in line with the middle of your shoulder, hip, and ankle. If you can't draw a straight line through these points, then you've just been diagnosed—again.

## Problem #1: Your Workout

The shoulder is the most complex and unstable joint in the human body. For it to function properly, you need to train all the muscles that help stabilize it. Trouble is, to the average guy, the shoulder muscles are the deltoids, the rounded muscles that cap the upper arms. Period. "Men suffer from an 'If I can't see it, why train it?' mentality," says Micheal Clark, DPT, president of the National Academy of Sports Medicine. And that means they'll do plenty of overhead presses and lateral raises— exercises that target the front and middle portions of the deltoid—but neglect the smaller, less-visible muscles at the back of the shoulder joint. The result: a strength imbalance, which makes the shoulder less stable. Poor stability not only increases your risk of injury—think dislocations and rotator-cuff tears—but also reduces your strength in almost every upper-body lift. That's because you can lift only as much weight as your shoulders can support. In fact, weak shoulder joints are the most common cause of longtime lifting plateaus.

Another workout issue: bench presses and lat pulldowns, two of the most popular exercises in any gym (except Curves). The first move emphasizes your pectoralis major—the primary muscle of your chest—and the second targets your latissimus dorsi, the largest muscle of your back. Both of these powerful muscles attach to the inside of the upper arm, which means they rotate it inward. If you perform these exercises more than you do moves that rotate your upper arms outward—such as bent-over and seated rows—your pectoralis major and lats will pull your arms inward, causing your shoulders to round forward.

This primer shows you how to train your "other" shoulder muscles. As a general rule, count the total number of sets of bench presses, shoulder presses, pullups, and lat pulldowns that you do in a week, and make sure you do an equal number of sets of exercises that work the following muscle groups.

## REAR DELTOIDS

The deltoid consists of three separate heads: the anterior head, or front deltoid; the medial head, or middle deltoid; and the posterior head, or rear deltoid. Though the shoulder press and lateral raise train the front and middle deltoids, they ignore the rear deltoid.

**Exercise R$_x$:** Try bent-over dumbbell raises and barbell bent-over rows using a wide grip. Do seated rows by pulling the rope handle to your neck instead of to your lower chest.

## ROTATOR-CUFF MUSCLES

These four tiny muscles—the teres minor, supraspinatus, infraspinatus, and subscapularis—stabilize your upper-arm bone (the humerus) in your shoulder socket, allowing you to rotate your arm in every direction.

**Exercise R$_x$:** Bolster your rotator cuffs by working them at least twice a week with external-rotation exercises and a move called PNF. (See "The Perfect Posture Plan" on page 180.)

## SCAPULAR MUSCLES

These muscles—the trapezius, serratus anterior, pectoralis minor, rhomboid major, and rhomboid minor—allow you to move and stabilize the shoulder blades, or scapulae. According to a study, 100 percent of people with shoulder-joint problems have unstable scapulae.

**Exercise R$_x$:** Focus on rowing movements, such as the bent-over row and seated row. Initiate rows and pulldowns by squeezing your shoulder blades together.

*(continued on page 182)*

**HARD**TRUTH

Percentage of gym weight-lifting equipment tested that was infected with viruses:

**73**

## The Perfect Posture Plan

### Fix your shoulders for good

If you have upper-cross syndrome, scrap your entire upper-body workout and perform the routine below 3 days a week for 4 weeks. Do two sets of 12 repetitions of each exercise. Continue to incorporate these moves into your workouts even after you've completed the program. If you have chronic shoulder pain, see an orthopedist or physical therapist who specializes in sports. Go to www.aaos.org to find a doctor near you.

### Shoulder-Adductor Stretch

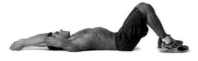

Lie on the floor with your knees bent and your arms straight up in the air. With your back flat, slowly move your arms back and down toward the floor, keeping them straight and close to the sides of your head. Hold for 20 to 30 seconds.

### Peel

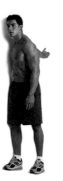

Stand facing a wall and place your right arm against it, fingers pointing to 3 o'clock. Keeping your shoulder and arm flush against the wall, rotate your body to the left by moving your feet. When you feel a stretch along your chest, hold for 20 to 30 seconds. Progression: After you've gained enough flexibility to perform the stretch with your body perpendicular to the wall, move your arm up to 2 o'clock, then progress to 1 o'clock.

### Kneeling Lat Stretch

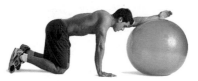

Kneel in front of a Swiss ball with your left arm on the ball and the other hand on the floor. Move your left arm forward until you feel slight tension. Hold for 20 to 30 seconds and repeat with your right arm. Progression: At the end of the stretch, when your arm is straight, slowly move it inward across your body until you feel tension.

### Swiss-Ball T

Grab a pair of 2- or 5-pound dumbbells and lie facedown on a Swiss ball. Start with your back flat, your chest off the ball, and your arms hanging down, palms forward.

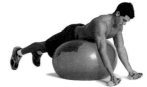

Squeeze your shoulder blades down and together as you extend your arms to the sides, creating a T with your torso. Pause, then return to the starting position.

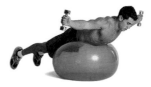

### Incline Dumbbell V Raise

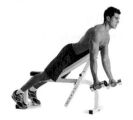

Lie facedown on an incline bench and hold dumbbells below your shoulders, thumbs pointing forward.

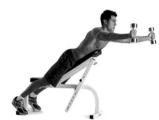

Raise the weights in front of you at 45-degree angles, forming a V with your arms, until your arms are almost parallel to the floor. Pause, then lower the weights.

### Kneeling External Rotation

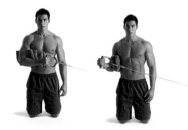

Kneel with a cable station to your left and a small folded towel under your right armpit. With your right hand, grab the low pulley handle.

Starting with the handle at your navel, rotate your arm away from your body to a 10 o'clock position. Pause, then return to the starting position. Finish the set, then repeat with the other arm.

### Single-Leg PNF

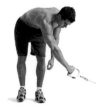

Stand with a cable station to your left. Lift your right foot off the floor and reach across your body with your right hand to grab the handle.

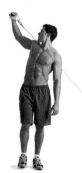

Pull the cable up and across your body while rotating your thumb to the right so that at the top of the move, your arm is straight and to the right of your shoulder. Reverse the move to the starting position and finish a set before repeating with your other arm.

### Standing Cable Reverse Fly

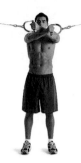

Grab the left handle of a cable-crossover system with your right hand and the right handle with your left.

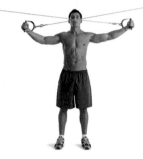

Lean back and pull the handles down and across your body while squeezing your shoulder blades down and together. Pause, then return to the starting position.

## Problem #2: Your Job

If you suffer from poor desk posture, changing your lifting habits isn't guaranteed to correct your problem. After all, the 30 minutes a day you spend exercising is only a fraction of the time you spend sitting in one position. If your shoulders are slumped forward for long periods of time, your chest muscles become shortened. That is, since these muscles attach to your upper arms, the distance they need to extend when you slouch is less than when your shoulders are drawn back. Over time, the chest muscles adapt to this position as their natural length, pulling your shoulders forward. As a result, many of the shoulder's stabilizers are overstretched, which makes them weaker.

**Exercise R$_x$:** Use the stretches shown in "The Perfect Posture Plan" on page 180 daily. They force your chest muscles to extend, which prevents them from becoming permanently shortened. At work, do 10 standing shoulder retractions every hour when working at a computer. Stand and pull your shoulders back as you squeeze your shoulder blades together. Hold each repetition for 3 seconds. And focus on keeping your head and shoulders directly above your pelvis at all times. It's an easy way to ensure that your body is in proper alignment.

# Double Your Bench

Learn from a master how to press twice as much
as you do now, in only 2 months

Joe Mazza looks like somebody, but you can't quite put your finger on who.

In recognition of his Hollywood tan and his black hair that would be undisturbed by a hurricane, Joe's buddies—a crew of 400-pound, ink-covered strongmen sporting shaved heads or Mohawks that descend into mullets—settle for calling him Mr. GQ.

Or Mazz. A full-time New Jersey cop with 19 years of experience under his belt and 19 inches of muscle under his sleeves, he ranks, pound for pound, as America's best practitioner of the bench press. You haven't heard of him because, while big money flows into bass fishing and poker, his sport remains beyond the fringe, with lightweights like him receiving even less publicity than heavyweights. That doesn't make his stats any less eye-popping, though. Weighing just 165 pounds, he has benched more than 400 pounds "raw" and has managed 625 pounds—for four reps—when encased in one of the straitjacket-like lifting shirts all world-class benchers use for meets. "My ultimate goal is to bench 700," says Mazza, who's been competing since 2001.

When Mazza lifts his fork at a Ruby Tuesday, his arm inflates like a balloon under his short sleeve. Yet unlike bodybuilders, he is concerned with a muscle's performance, not its appearance. Nor does he care how much he can squat and deadlift, as powerlifters do. Mazza simply wants to drive more weight off his chest than any man his size ever has before. During this primal challenge to gravity, the pectoral muscles of the chest push through the bottom half of the lift, and the shoulders and triceps take over from there. The key to doubling your own bench is strengthening those muscles and your back, all while honing your technique.

As Mazza and his compadres cinch one another into their lifting shirts and then bench amid rubber bands, boards, flying chalk dust, clanging metal, and screams, the vibe suggests exorcism as much as exercise. But method governs this madness. The shirt is most effective from the chest to the sticking point—the hardest moment of the lift—and the board and bands focus on the move from the sticking point on up, allowing lifters to nail the press by locking out, or fully extending, their arms.

We've figured out a way to take these principles and recast them in ways you can use at the gym tonight. In 2 months, you may not be benching three or four times your body weight like Mazza does, but you'll be benching twice what you do now.

## The Shirt

**How it works for pros like Mazza:** In competitive bench-pressing, it's all about the shirt, although you won't see these hanging on a rack at Brooks Brothers. Made of industrial-strength denim or polyester, this equipment (it's not really apparel) offers lifters the same kind of drive golfers seek with, say, the Nike SasQuatch. Among other advantages, the shirt gives a lifter more recoil when moving the bar off his chest. World-class competitors claim almost unanimously that it adds 200 or even 300 pounds to their bench presses, which explains why the very best heavyweights, such as Gene Rychlak, have now arrived at the 1,000-pound mark.

**How it can work for you:** No need to wear a lifting shirt like competitors do. Those artificially inflated gains would evaporate the moment you removed it, and you'd receive some really strange stares at the gym. But when you start benching two to three times your body weight, there's an incredible amount of force trying to pull your shoulders apart, and the shirt protects the delicate architecture of the joints. "I can train with my shirt and not have any problems," says Mazza.

This protective effect is something you should seek to duplicate through other means—namely, by strengthening your back, which Mazza does with heavy lat pulldowns and other back moves. (See "The Raise-the-Roof Workout" on page 186.) "Your back doesn't push the weight, but it gives your shoulders a more stable base," says Sean Waxman, CSCS, a former national-level Olympic lifter and the owner of Pure Strength in Southern California. Also, form is key: Pull your upper arms close to your torso when you bench, instead of flaring them out to the sides. This allows your latissimus dorsi (a.k.a. lats)—your largest back muscle—to help stabilize your shoulders, providing you with a better foundation

## Psych Yourself Up

It really is all in your head: U.K. researchers found that men bench press 12 percent more weight when they psych themselves up before a lift than when they're distracted. In the study, the scientists either gave experienced weight lifters 20 seconds to prepare mentally for three sets of five repetitions of a strength exercise or asked them to count backward from 1,000 in increments of seven before the sets. The take-home message: Before you approach the bench, skip the small talk and focus on the task at hand.

from which to press. For a visual cue, your upper arms should create roughly a 45-degree angle with your torso when the weight is lowered to your chest.

### The Bands

**How it works for pros like Mazza:** Bench pressers can hold more weight in the top position than in the bottom, but attaching giant rubber bands to the bar reverses this strength curve. At the top, where the lift is easiest, the bands are stretched, making it harder to push the bar. The benefit: "Your muscles have to generate more force than usual throughout the entire range of motion," says Waxman. A study published in the *Journal of Strength and Conditioning Research* found that training with bands significantly increased force and power in the squat, an effect Waxman predicts would carry over to the bench.

*(continued on page 188)*

# The Raise-the-Roof Workout

Follow this routine for 2 months, during which you can continue training your biceps, abs, and other muscle groups. As you become stronger, go heavier, so that the weights fully challenge your muscles in the rep ranges given. One final note: Always use a spotter, even if you don't think you need one.

## Monday: Heavy Bench Day

**Barbell Bench Press**

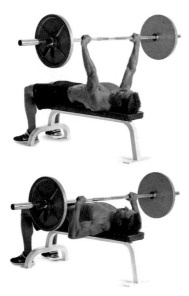

Lie on a bench and grab a barbell with an overhand grip, your hands slightly more than shoulder-width apart. Pull your shoulder blades down and together—which helps stabilize your shoulders—then unrack the bar. Slowly lower the weight to your chest, keeping your elbows tucked close to your body. Instead of just pushing the bar straight up, push it back slightly toward the rack. "That allows the weight to kind of do the work for you," says Mike Miller, a champion powerlifter.

### THE DRILL

1. After you warm up, set the bench at a 45-degree incline for three sets of four or five reps. (Start off using the heaviest weight you can for that rep range, and then drop as needed.) Rest for 2 to 3 minutes between sets.
2. Do two sets of six reps at the same incline. Rest for 2 to 3 minutes between sets.
3. Set the bench flat and repeat the same sequence.
4. Set the bench at a decline and do three sets of six reps. Rest for 2 to 3 minutes between sets.
5. Finish with a method called flushing, in which you use higher reps to increase the flow of nutrient-rich blood to your muscles. Do two sets, 8 to 10 reps apiece, of cable crossovers, in which you bring the handles of opposing cable stacks together in front of your chest. Rest for 1½ minutes between sets.

## Thursday: Close-Grip Bench Day

**Close-Grip Bench Press**
Lie on a bench in a power rack and grab a barbell with an overhand grip, your hands slightly less than shoulder-width apart. "Stops" should be set 5 inches above chest level.

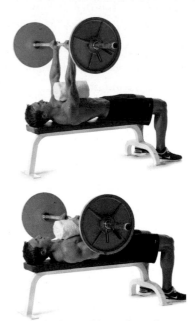

Unrack the bar and lower it to the stops, slowly and with control. Press the bar back up as quickly as possible. (If you have access to bands, attach those to the ends of the barbell and press at a normal pace. If you have a board, use that instead of the stops on the rack.)

### THE DRILL

1. Regardless of the apparatus, start out using a weight that's slightly more than you'd normally be able to lift for the prescribed rep range. (For example, if you usually do close-grip bench presses with 135 pounds, add an extra 10 to each side of the bar.)
2. Unrack the bar, then lower it until it touches the stopping point.
3. Press the bar up and repeat for the prescribed number of reps.
4. Complete three sets of four or five reps, and then three more sets of six

reps, resting for 2 to 3 minutes between sets.

5. A week or two later, lower either your board or the stops on the power rack by 1 inch, so the weight comes down closer to your chest. Now complete the same workout.

6. Continue removing blocks or lowering the stops every other week until the bar comes all the way down to your chest.

## Lying Triceps Extension

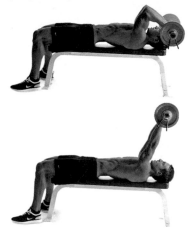

Lie on your back holding a bar at arm's length above you. Bend your elbows to lower the bar to your forehead. Press it back up to the starting position.

### THE DRILL

Do three or four sets of 6 to 10 reps.

## Saturday: Heavy Back Day

### Dumbbell Pullover

Lie on a bench with your feet flat on the floor and hold a dumbbell over your chest with both hands.

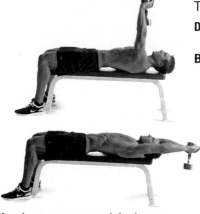

Keeping your arms straight, lower the dumbbell until your arms are in line with your body. Return to the starting position.

### THE DRILL

Do three or four sets of 6 to 10 reps.

### Lat Pulldown

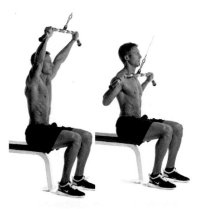

Sit on the seat and grab the handle so that your arms are fully extended and your torso is straight.
Pull the handle straight down to the top of your chest. Return to the starting position.

### THE DRILL

Do three or four sets of 6 to 10 reps.

### Barbell Shrug

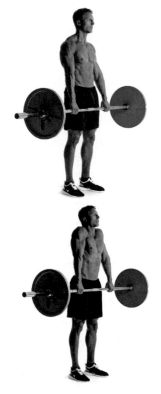

Stand holding a barbell at arm's length with a shoulder-width grip. Without moving your arms, raise your shoulders as high as you can. Return to the starting position. (To lift more weight, keep your elbows close to your torso as you lower and raise the bar.)

### THE DRILL

Do three or four sets of 6 to 10 reps.

**How it can work for you:** If you can, try lifting with a pair of Jump Stretch Mini Bands, which can be picked up at www.elitefts.com for about $10 apiece. Attach one to each end of the barbell, then to the base of a power rack, or even to heavy dumbbells anchored on the floor, and then double them up again on the bar. They'll provide an extra 70 to 90 pounds of resistance at the top of your bench.

If that's not feasible, mimic the effect of bands without actually using them, through a technique called compensatory acceleration training. "Bring the bar down slowly, but then rapidly accelerate it through the full range of motion," says Waxman.

## The Boards

**How it works for pros like Mazza:** Bench pressers place small wooden boards, ranging from 1 to 5 inches high, on their chests to reduce their range of motion and focus on the lockout portion of the lift. That's important, since the shirt has helped them push a ton of weight through the first half of the rep. "When you're using the boards, you would normally be using more weight than you could for a full repetition," says Jeffrey M. McBride, PhD, CSCS, a biomechanics expert at Appalachian State University. Reducing the range of motion also allows you to train hard for the bench press, with minimal strain on your shoulders.

**How it can work for you:** If you have access to boards, place one on your chest just like the big boys do. (If you don't, they can be purchased at www.elitefts.com; try the 3 Board Press for $20 and the 4 Board Press for $22.) If you don't want to carry around different-size boards in your gym bag to vary your range of motion, as Mazza does, McBride recommends benching in a power rack and gradually lowering the stops to achieve the same progressive effect. If you're really in a pinch, rolled-up towels can substitute for both. Adding lying triceps extensions to this workout will further develop your lockout.

# Build Strength and Size Where You Want It

The muscles in your chest increase your presence in the boardroom, win her over in the bedroom, and intimidate your opponents on the playing field. Build a powerful chest with this innovative plan

BY MYATT MURPHY AND ALYWN **COSGROVE**, CSCS

**W**e'll bet there are three things you don't know about your chest. First, you're most likely to rupture your chest muscles in your twenties and thirties. Chalk it up to ego. Tears in the pectoralis major—your largest chest muscle—typically occur in men trying to bench press more weight than they can handle, report Boston University researchers. The take-home advice: Always use a spotter.

Second, your chest can sabotage your posture. When your chest muscles are tight, they pull your shoulders forward, making you appear hunched instead of tall and straight. Use this doorway chest stretch twice a day to loosen up: Bend your right arm 90 degrees and place your forearm against a door frame. Then push your right shoulder forward until you feel slight tension in your chest. Hold for 30 seconds, then repeat on the other side.

Third, your chest is one of the first muscle groups to atrophy when you stop lifting weights. That's because you rarely stress your chest muscles in daily activities. Think about it: How often do you have to push heavy weight away from your chest? Keep in mind that losing muscle slows your metabolism, which means that regularly training your chest also benefits your abs.

All that said, here are the best exercises for your chest.

## Hard Move, Harder Muscle

Try this exercise at the start of your workout. Do as many repetitions as you can, then rest for 60 seconds and repeat. Continue until you're able to do only half the number of reps performed in your first set.

**TIP:** *Center your forearm on the Swiss ball.*

### SWISS-BALL FLY

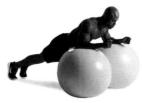

Place a pair of Swiss balls side by side and position a forearm on each, your elbows bent about 90 degrees.

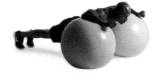

Without changing the bend in your elbows, lower your torso and upper arms downward, rolling the balls away from each other. Pull your upper arms toward each other to return to the start.

## BARBELL BENCH PRESS

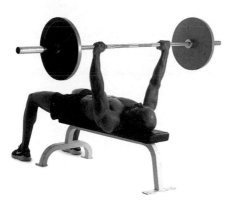

Lie on a bench with your feet flat on the floor. Grab the bar with your hands slightly more than shoulder-width apart and hold it over your chest.

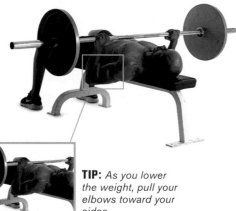

**TIP:** *As you lower the weight, pull your elbows toward your sides.*

Pull your shoulder blades down and together, then lower the bar to your chest. (Keep your elbows tucked in.) Pause, then push the weight back up.

## BARBELL INCLINE BENCH PRESS

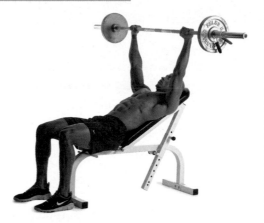

Lie faceup on an incline bench with your feet flat on the floor. Grab the bar with your hands slightly more than shoulder-width apart and hold it with your arms extended over your chest.

**TIP:** *Keep your wrists straight, instead of allowing them to bend backward.*

Slowly lower the bar until it touches your chest just above your nipples, then press the bar back up.

# Pick Your Plan

Choose one of these three routines for the results you want.

## The Chest-Chiseling Complex

The premise behind this workout is simple: Don't allow your muscles time to fully recover, and they'll learn to withstand fatigue better. As a result, over time you'll improve your ability to churn out more repetitions of any chest exercise. And that means more muscle.

**How it works.** Perform eight parallel-bar dips (see page 194) and eight pushups (see page 194) without pausing between exercises. Continue alternating between moves, reducing the number of repetitions you do by one each time. So you'll do seven dips and seven pushups next, then six and six, and so on, until you're down to one rep of each exercise. Rest for 90 seconds, then try to repeat the complex. As your strength improves, add one repetition to your starting number of reps. Do this workout once every 5 days, maximum.

## The Super-Strength Workout

Research shows that men who vary their repetition ranges in a wavelike fashion—known by scientists as "undulating periodization"—gain twice as much strength as men who do the same routine every workout.

**How it works.** Do three workouts a week, resting at least a day between sessions.

Monday—Workout 1: Perform four sets of the barbell bench press (see page 191), followed by four sets of the barbell incline bench press (see page 191). Do four to six repetitions of each exercise, resting for 90 seconds between sets.

Wednesday—Workout 2: Do three sets of the cable single-arm chest press (see opposite page), followed by three sets of the dumbbell incline bench press (see opposite page); perform 10 to 12 repetitions of each exercise, resting for 60 seconds between sets.

Friday—Workout 3: Do two sets of parallel-bar dips (see page 194), followed by two sets of pushups (see page 194). Perform 15 to 20 repetitions of each exercise, resting for 45 seconds between sets.

## The Time-Saving Trifecta

Sure, performing three consecutive chest exercises without resting saves you time. But organizing your workout this way also keeps your muscles under tension longer, which is an effective means of stimulating growth.

**How it works:** Perform one set each of three different exercises in succession, without resting—a routine known as a triset. Mix and match the movements, using these guidelines: Start your triset with four to six repetitions of either the barbell bench press (see page 191) or the barbell incline bench press (see page 191). Next, do 10 to 12 reps of either the cable single-arm chest press (see opposite page) or the dumbbell incline bench press (see opposite page), and finish with 15 to 20 reps of parallel-bar dips (see page 194) or push-ups (see page 194). Rest for 60 seconds after each triset and repeat for a total of four rounds. Perform this workout 2 days a week, resting at least 3 days between sessions.

## CABLE SINGLE-ARM CHEST PRESS

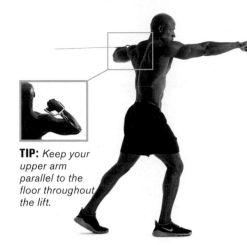

**TIP:** *Keep your upper arm parallel to the floor throughout the lift.*

With your left hand, grab the high-pulley handle at a cable station and face away from the weight stack. Place your right foot in front of your left and hold the handle next to your shoulder.

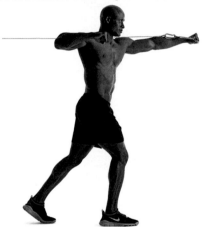

Without dropping your elbow, straighten your left arm. Do all the reps, then switch arms and legs, and repeat.

## DUMBBELL INCLINE BENCH PRESS

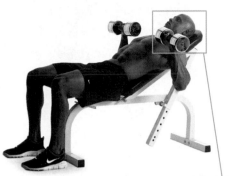

**TIP:** *To lift your best, push your head against the bench as you press the weight.*

Lie faceup on an incline bench and hold a pair of dumbbells along the outsides of your chest with an overhand grip (palms facing forward).

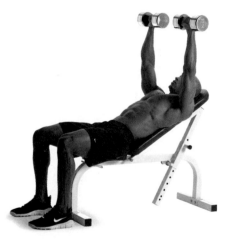

Press the weights straight above your chest. Pause, then lower them to the starting position.

## PARALLEL-BAR DIP

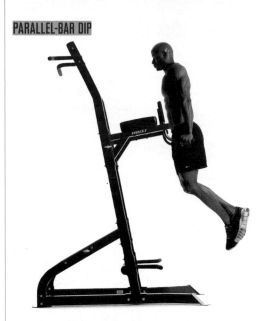

Grab parallel dip bars and lift yourself so your arms are straight.

**TIP:** *To prevent excess stress on your shoulder joints, don't allow your upper arms to move below the level of your elbows.*

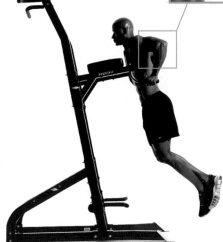

Keeping your elbows tucked close to your body, slowly lower yourself by bending your elbows until your upper arms are parallel to the floor. Pause, then push back up to the starting position.

## PUSHUP

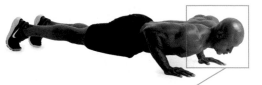

Get into the standard pushup position with your hands beneath your shoulders, slightly more than shoulder-width apart. Straighten your legs so your body forms a straight line from head to heels.

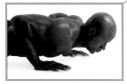

**TIP:** *For best results, pause for 1 second in the bottom position.*

Lower your torso until your chest is just off the floor. Push yourself back to the starting position.

# Lift Your Best

BY MIKE MEJIA, MS, CSCS

**P**ush past your sticking points in classic muscle-building exercises with this 3-day-a-week routine. You'll move the weight from a standstill every repetition, which ensures that every rep is equally challenging. What's more, you'll strengthen the weakest parts of your lifts—so when you return to your standard exercises, you'll see a big improvement. Complete the sets of one exercise before proceeding to the next. Do three sets of four or five repetitions, and rest 90 seconds between sets.

**Deadlift:** Stand with your feet shoulder-width apart and a loaded barbell on the floor in front of you. Bend at the knees and grab the bar with an overhand grip, just outside your legs.

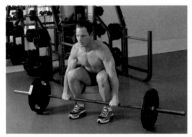

Keeping your back straight, stand up with the bar, driving your hips and glutes forward. Now lower the bar to the floor and stand up without it. Then repeat the move so that for each rep, you start with the bar on the floor.

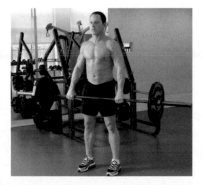

**Bench press off supports:** Position a bench between the uprights of a squat rack, and set the bar on the supports at a height level with your chin when you're lying on the bench. Use an overhand grip. (Your elbows should be bent and the bar just over your chest.)

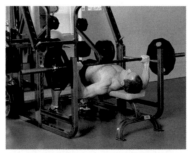

Press the bar up until your arms are straight, then lower it and rest it on the supports for 1 or 2 seconds before repeating.

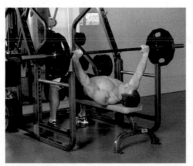

**Squat off supports:** Place a barbell on the supports of a squat rack, at the level where your shoulders will be when you're squatting with your thighs parallel to the floor. Lower your body under the bar with your back slightly arched and your chest up, and grab the bar.

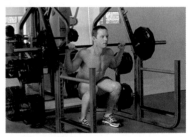

Drive the weight up until you're in a standing position, then lower it back onto the supports. Pause for at least 2 seconds before repeating.

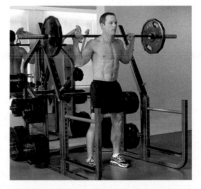

# Training

# Tips

## How can I maximize my body's muscle growth?

Start by suppressing hormones that break down lean muscle tissue. In one study, college football players who took a supplement called beta-hydroxy-beta-methylbutyrate, or HMB, lowered their levels of the stress hormone cortisol and creatine kinase, which is a marker of muscle damage. Another study shows that taking 3 grams of HMB daily builds muscle and strength in beginning weight lifters, although it has less effect in more experienced athletes. EAS makes a preworkout supplement called Muscle Armor that contains amino acids and HMB. It may stunt cortisol before your workout and help you recover faster afterward, keeping you in a constant anabolic, or muscle-building, state.

Another way to boost your body's natural growth hormones is by cycling your workouts according to the following plan. Alternate between these two phases to unleash a flood of hormones for a leaner and more muscular body.

**Phase 1 (weeks 1 through 4):** Do three to five sets of 10 to 15 repetitions of all your upper- and lower-body exercises. Training at a high volume can push your lactate threshold higher, improving your natural production of growth hormone.

**Phase 2 (weeks 5 through 8):** Reduce your volume but increase your intensity—complete four to six sets of three to six reps of all your major exercises. Lifting heavier weights for fewer repetitions triggers more testosterone release.

## Can I cut my gym time and still pack on serious muscle?

Sure—the key is boosting "workout density," a fancy term for the work you do in a given length of time. Here's a program for big gains, sans burnout.

**Rule 1: Fill your tank.** High-octane workouts stall if you don't gas up properly. A half hour before your workout, drink a glass of juice with a scoop of whey-protein powder mixed in, or eat a small cup of fruit, granola, and yogurt.

**Rule 2: Recover while you work.** Perform pushing and pulling exercises one after another in superset fashion, letting one muscle group recover while the other works. Follow with a core exercise (such as a side bridge or hip crossover).

**Rule 3: Work your whole body.** Exercising major muscle groups releases growth hormone and testosterone to build muscle and burn fat. Hit them all, whether you work out three times a week (with a day of rest between workouts) or four times a week (with a day of rest after your second session and 2 days' rest after your last session).

**Rule 4: Watch the clock.** After each pushing-pulling-core sequence, rest for 2 minutes, reducing this time by 15 seconds every week until you're down to 60-second rest periods. Here's one way to arrange your circuits.

**The ultimate total-body workout:** Do each circuit once or twice, depending on time, before moving on. Rest at least 1 minute after each exercise.

**Circuit 1:** Do an upper-body pushing movement (e.g., bench press, dumbbell military press), then a lower-body pulling movement (Romanian deadlift, Swiss-ball leg curl) and a flexion core exercise (Swiss-ball crunch, plank).

**Circuit 2:** Perform an upper-body pulling movement (e.g., pullup, row), followed by a lower-body pushing movement (squat, lunge) and a rotational core exercise (Russian twist).

**Circuit 3:** Finish with a vanity move for your shoulders, biceps, or triceps, such as a biceps curl to press—or an injury-prevention move for your hips or shoulders, such as a woodchopper or Swiss-ball T.

**Does it matter whether I lift the same weight for three sets of 10 reps or six sets of five reps? I'm satisfied with my size, but I'd like to focus on getting stronger, pound for pound. What should I do?**

Both questions get at the same idea: All sets are not created equal. The first question leads into the second: Though the total number of repetitions is the same for both schemes (sets × reps = 30), the two approaches will yield very different results. Assuming

the same tempo of reps, three sets of 10 should produce greater muscle size and endurance, while six sets of five will improve "relative strength," giving you more power per pound. That's what you're looking for in the end.

Use heavy weights and lower the weight slowly, lifting explosively. Add weight with each set and maintain perfect form. Finish with a down set of dynamic reps: Lighten the load to about half of your maximum, and do 10 or more fast-paced reps to fatigue—1 second down, no pause, explosive up. This formula can build strength without sacrificing size.

## How can I bench at home without a spotter?

We've all heard horror stories of men being pinned under more weight than they could handle. One solution is to do a variation on the "rest pause" principle, says *Men's Health* contributing editor Mike Mejia, CSCS. With rest pause, you end up handling more weight than you ordinarily could, by taking short breaks during a set. Here's how it works.

Select a weight that normally allows you to perform only four or five repetitions (without going to

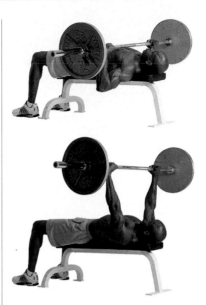

absolute failure). After doing four or five reps, pause and rack the weight for 10 seconds.

Next, grab the bar and crank out whatever you can safely do (usually about another one or two reps) before racking the weight again. This time, rest for 15 to 20 seconds, and then try for another couple of repetitions.

Rack the weight one last time and rest for 20 to 30 seconds before grinding out one or two more. By the time you're finished, you should have amassed anywhere from 8 to 12 repetitions with a weight that ordinarily allows you to do only four or five. The end result is more size and strength and a windpipe that remains intact.

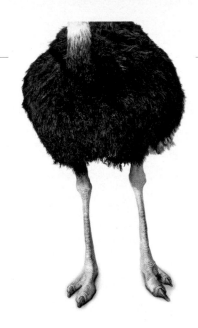

## I have long, skinny legs. How can I put some meat on my calves?

You've probably already tried calf raises with weights, but they seldom do the trick because they simply mimic the motions that calf muscles perform all the time—walking, running, climbing. To build muscle, you need to shock your calves with something new. Try an eccentric exercise, which emphasizes the lowering phase rather than the lifting part of a movement.

1. Stand on a 4-inch-high platform (a step also will work), position your right foot on the platform, and lift your heel as high as possible. Wrap your left foot behind your right ankle so your right leg supports all your weight.

2. During a slow five- count, lower your heel to the platform, then raise it. Repeat nine times.

3. Without resting, step off the platform and hop in place on your right foot 10 times without letting your heel or left foot touch the floor.

4. Repeat both parts of this exercise, this time with your left foot.

## Will I lose strength if I take a week or two off from weights?

If you've been lifting regularly, a week off might be good for you. Muscle needs time to heal. When you resume, don't be surprised if you achieve a new personal best in one or more of your lifts.

## I hit the gym at lunchtime 4 days a week to run and lift. What should I eat for breakfast?

You need a well-balanced meal that provides a total of about 500 calories: 200 in protein, 150 in carbs, and 150 in fat. Start with a smoothie or another drink that's high in protein; it will help your muscles recover faster from your workouts. Carb Countdown, a reduced-fat chocolate beverage, is a good-tasting choice; a 12-ounce serving has only 135 calories. The rest of the meal should include two servings of protein (two scrambled eggs or two links of lean turkey sausage), one serving of fruit (a cup of berries or melon, an orange, or an apple), and one to two servings of whole grains (a bowl of oatmeal, two slices of multigrain bread, or half a whole-wheat bagel).

## Should I do a specific number of repetitions or just crank out as many as I can?

High-rep phases build lean mass, and capping your reps by increasing weights adds strength. It takes both approaches to become well-rounded. Here's one way to get the best of both worlds—we call it the strength and size workout. This program features three 3-week phases for balanced growth.

**Lean-mass phase:** Perform two or three sets of 8 to 12 repetitions of each exercise. For your final set, use a lighter weight and do as many repetitions as you can. We call this "max reps" because it indicates the maximum amount of work your muscles can perform at a given weight. Each week, leave the weight constant during your max-rep test to track your success.

**Strength phase:** Aim for three or four sets of three to five repetitions with heavier loads. The goal is to hit the wall not because of a burning in your muscles or depleted energy stores but because the resistance is very high. Stopping short of failure actually makes your muscles smarter because the heavy resistance causes more motor units to fire within each muscle. This can stimulate the oft-ignored type 2a and 2b muscle fibers, which will make you both stronger and bigger.

**Combo phase:** Perform three sets of six repetitions with a heavy weight. Follow with two sets of 12 to 15 repetitions with 60 seconds of rest between sets.

### What's better: total-body training or split training?

First, a clarification: In total-body training, you work all major muscle groups every time you work out; in split training, you focus on different ones each session (e.g., chest and triceps one day; legs and abs another). I prefer the total-body approach. It virtually guarantees that you'll work each muscle group regularly. And the more muscles you work, the more calories you'll burn. Don't be thrown by the lack of pump you feel in individual muscles. Slow and steady wins the race, and your reward will be more lean muscle and accelerated fat loss.

### Does it matter if I lift weights in running shoes?

Does it matter if you run a marathon in Timberlands, Ted? "If you're doing standing exercises or anything with lateral movements [such as side

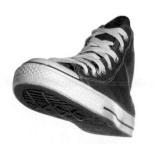
**A flat-soled sneaker gives weight lifters the stability they need.**

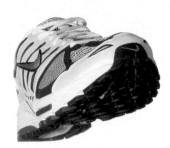
**The elevated heel makes a running shoe ill-suited for a weight-lifting session.**

lunges], running shoes can make you susceptible to injury," says Stephen Pribut, DPM, immediate past-president of the American Academy of Podiatric Sports Medicine. That's because they have extra cushioning, which can affect your balance. It's like standing on a foam cushion versus a hard floor, says Dr. Pribut. And that foam is like an angled platform, designed for forward motion—not good for power cleans or squats. "Cross-trainers and tennis shoes have flatter soles," says Dr. Pribut, "and provide better support for lifting." Conversely, never wear lifting shoes on a run. "You're more likely to injure yourself when running in the wrong shoes than when lifting," says Dr. Pribut.

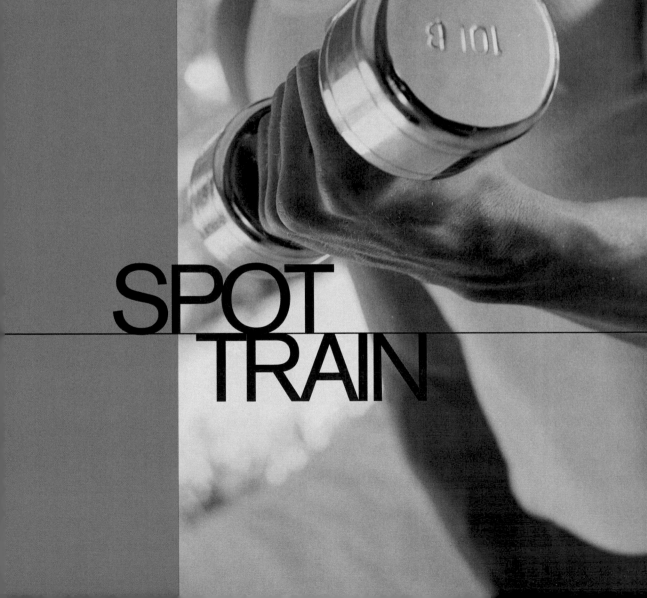

# SPOT TRAIN

## PART FOUR

Pick a part. Every man has a part of his body he yearns to improve; some of us have more than one. When we asked men which famous body part they would most like to have, 41 percent said Michelangelo's David's abs, 28 percent said Albert Einstein's brain, 17 percent said Dirk Diggler's unit, 7 percent said Hulk Hogan's arms, and 6 percent said Lance Armstrong's legs. Your brain and your unit are topics for whole other books entirely. But this one book holds the key to changing your other parts.

That's why we dedicated this section of the book to spot training. First, we offer the greatest abs workout ever. Chisel them in just 24 minutes a day. Then you'll build a bigger, stronger back with our workout that delivers the ultimate upper body. Next, you'll sculpt a powerful chest. With another, you can add 2 inches to your arms in just 24 minutes a workout. Then you'll strengthen your shoulders to build the rock-solid shoulders you want—in the time that you have. And more.

Turn the page to change your body one part at a time.

BY MYATT MURPHY

# Chisel Your Abs

The greatest abs workout ever—in just 24 minutes

ome beliefs are painfully slow to perish, like the one that declares intense aerobic exercise is the best method for burning fat. "This misconception could be what's keeping you from a lean physique," says Michael Mejia, CSCS, a *Men's Health* exercise advisor. The reason is simple: "Most men invest their energy in exercise that boosts their caloric expenditure only while they're working out," says Mejia—for example, a 45-minute spin on a stationary bike or a moderate jog through a park. Resistance training, on the other hand, elevates your metabolism for up to 48 hours afterward, so it pays fat-loss dividends long after your workout ends. Turns out lifting weights is highly underrated for burning calories during your session, too. A study from the University of Southern Maine found that an intense weight-training session burns as many as 71 percent more calories than previously thought—putting it on a par with aerobic exercise.

## The Payoff

**Faster fat loss!** The traveling deadlift and Turkish getup, featured here, force your body to engage more muscles than typical bodybuilding exercises do. And that means you'll burn more calories than ever before.

**Greater stamina!** The fast pace of this routine not only melts fat but also improves your overall endurance. As you progress, you'll be able to go harder and longer in each subsequent workout. The end result: You'll get leaner faster.

## Benchmark of Success

### How do you measure up?

Most men judge weight-loss success by their waistlines. And that's fine, but it doesn't measure your ability to burn fat. In this test, you'll sprint as fast and as far as you can. The farther you can run at your fastest pace, the better prepared your body is to last through high-intensity fat-burning workouts like this one.

Lace up your running shoes and head to an open stretch of road or track. After a 2- to 3-minute warmup jog, sprint at your top speed for as long as possible. Stop as soon as you feel yourself slowing down, and record either your time or your distance—whichever is more convenient.

### Track Your Progress

Record your time or distance on this chart. Then follow the plan, and retest yourself every 2 weeks.

Start (maximum time or distance) _____

Week 2 (maximum time or distance) _____

Finish (maximum time or distance) _____

**Extra muscle!** Because this plan incorporates power exercises—such as the hang clean and jump squat—it targets your fast-twitch muscle fibers. Since these fibers have the greatest potential for size and strength, that leads to bigger, stronger muscles.

## The Workout

Mejia's workout plan creates an enormous metabolic demand on your body by blending explosive exercises and combination lifts in a fast-paced circuit. Alternate between Workouts A and B, performing three

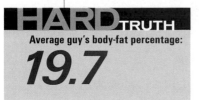
workouts a week and resting a day between sessions. In the first 2 weeks, do three sets of each exercise, resting 60 seconds between sets. In weeks 3 and 4, perform each routine as a circuit; that is, do one set of each exercise without resting between moves, then rest 90 seconds between circuits. Complete a total of three circuits.

## WORKOUT A

### HANG CLEAN TO FRONT SQUAT TO PUSH PRESS

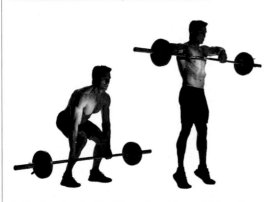

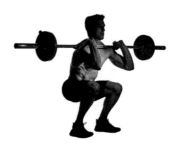

**1. Grab a barbell with a shoulder-width grip and dip your knees, as if you were about to jump.**

Quickly reverse the motion and shrug your shoulders as you pull the bar straight up and rise onto your toes. As the bar approaches chest height, bend your knees and swing your elbows forward to "catch" the bar in the crooks of your fingers.

**2. Now lower your body until your thighs are parallel to the floor.**

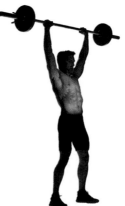

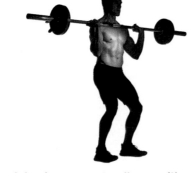

**3. Push back up to a standing position.**

**4. Then press the bar overhead. Lower the bar to the starting position. That's one repetition.**

**The plan:** Do six repetitions with a weight you would typically use to push-press six times. Perform three sets in weeks 1 and 2; do the move as part of a circuit in weeks 3 and 4.

### DUMBBELL DOUBLE WOOD CHOP

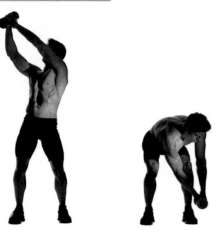

### PISTON BENT-OVER ROW

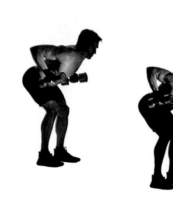

Hold a light dumbbell with a hand-over-hand grip, your arms extended above your right shoulder.

Keeping your arms straight but not locked, bend at the knees and forcefully rotate your torso to the left as you draw your arms down and across your body.

When your hands reach the outside of your left ankle, pause, then quickly reverse the movement with the same intensity, pausing at the top. That's one repetition. Do eight, then hold the weight over your left shoulder and repeat the move, this time chopping to your right.

**The plan:** Complete eight repetitions on each side. Perform three sets in weeks 1 and 2; do the move as part of a circuit in weeks 3 and 4.

Holding dumbbells, stand with your feet shoulder-width apart. Bend forward until your torso is almost parallel to the floor and your arms hang straight down, palms facing each other. Pull the weights to the sides of your chest. This is the starting position.

Keeping your right arm as still as possible, lower the weight in your left hand until your arm is straight. Lift the dumbbell back up to the side of your chest, then lower your right hand. Continue alternating.

**The plan:** Complete eight repetitions with each arm. Perform three sets in weeks 1 and 2; do the move as part of a circuit in weeks 3 and 4.

## WORKOUT A

**TURKISH GETUP**

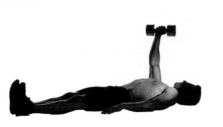 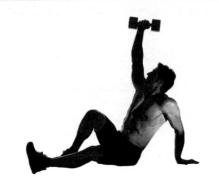

Lie on your back with your legs straight. Hold a dumbbell in your right hand with your arm straight above you.

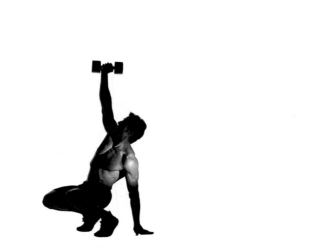

Keeping your elbow locked and the weight above you at all times, stand up. (Move your legs and left arm underneath you to push yourself up.) Still keeping your right arm straight and the weight above you, reverse the motion to return to the starting position.

**The plan:** Complete eight repetitions on each side. Perform three sets in weeks 1 and 2; do the move as part of a circuit in weeks 3 and 4.

**HARD**TRUTH
Percentage of men and women who want toned abs more than any other muscular trait:

## 60

## WORKOUT B

### PUSHUP/PULLUP LADDER

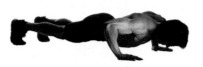

1. Stand next to a pullup bar and get into pushup position.

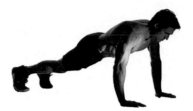

2. Do two pushups.

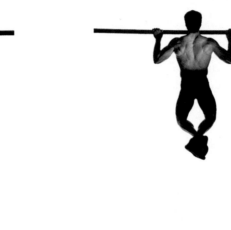

3. Then stand up and grasp the bar with your hands slightly more than shoulder-width apart.

4. Pull yourself up until the bar is at shoulder height, then lower yourself.

**The plan:** Add two pushups and one pullup each time you repeat the pair. So you'll start by doing two pushups and one pullup. Next, you'll do four and two, then six and three, and so on. Stop when you can do 10 pushups and five pullups or when you reach technical failure—that is, when your form falters or you can no longer control the speed of your repetitions. Perform three ladders in weeks 1 and 2; do the ladder as part of a circuit in weeks 3 and 4.

**HARD**TRUTH

Body-fat percentage needed for cover-model abs:

*Below 10*

## DUMBBELL JUMP SQUAT TO SQUAT THRUST

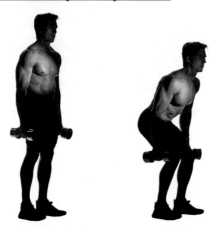

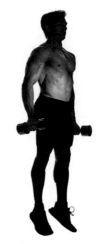

1. Stand with your feet shoulder-width apart and hold a pair of dumbbells at your sides.

Lower your body about 6 inches.

2. Then jump as high as you can.

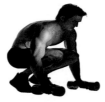

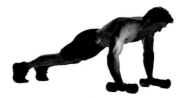

3. Land softly on the balls of your feet and immediately sink into a squat, lowering your body until you touch the dumbbells to the floor.

4. Kick your legs out behind you so you're in pushup position, with your hands on top of the dumbbells. Reverse the motion, bringing your legs forward so your feet are under your shoulders, then push back up to a standing position. That's one repetition.

**The plan:** Do eight repetitions. Perform three sets in weeks 1 and 2; do the move as part of a circuit in weeks 3 and 4.

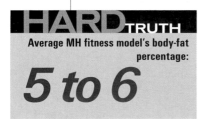

**HARD**TRUTH
Average MH fitness model's body-fat percentage:

## 5 to 6

## TRAVELING DEADLIFT

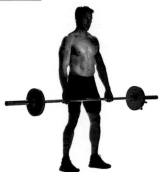

Stand with a light barbell on the floor in front of you, your feet shoulder-width apart and the bar directly over your toes. Bend your knees and grasp the bar with an overhand grip with your hands just outside your knees. Keeping your head and back straight and the bar close to your body, stand up.

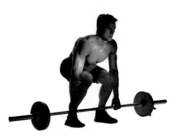

Next, step forward with your left foot and then with your right so your feet come together. Lower the bar to the floor and repeat the move, this time stepping forward with your right foot.

**The plan:** Do 8 to 10 repetitions. Perform three sets in weeks 1 and 2; do the move as part of a circuit in weeks 3 and 4.

## MEDICINE-BALL BICYCLE MANEUVER

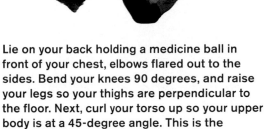

Lie on your back holding a medicine ball in front of your chest, elbows flared out to the sides. Bend your knees 90 degrees, and raise your legs so your thighs are perpendicular to the floor. Next, curl your torso up so your upper body is at a 45-degree angle. This is the starting position.

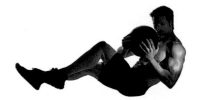

Bring your left knee toward your chest as you straighten your right leg, and simultaneously twist your upper body to the left until your right elbow meets your left knee. Reverse the move, drawing your right knee to your left elbow.

**The plan:** Do 10 repetitions on each side. Perform three sets in weeks 1 and 2; do the move as part of a circuit in weeks 3 and 4.

BY DAVID ZINCZENKO

# The Greatest Abs Workout Ever

Unleash your abs with this exclusive plan from *Get Fit, Stay Fit*, the sequel to the best-selling *Abs Diet*

## Live longer!

A 13-year Canadian study of more than 8,000 people found that those with the weakest abdominal muscles had a death rate more than twice that of the people with the strongest midsections.

## Lift more!

A stronger core supports your spine, so you can lift more weight in every exercise. Case in point: Canadian researchers found that men bench-pressed 40 percent more on a stable surface—which best supported their spines—than on an unstable surface.

## Prevent injuries!

Research shows that men with the best-conditioned abdominal muscles—guys who can perform at least 73 situps in 2 minutes—are five times less likely to suffer a lower-body injury than those who can knock out only 50.

## Improve your posture!

Tight lower-back muscles from excessive running pull your spine out of natural alignment. Strengthening your abs can correct this muscular imbalance, improving your body's posture to allow it to function properly.

### Men With Flat Stomachs Are . . .

50% less likely to develop heart disease.

16% less likely to die of a first heart attack.

50% less likely to have erectile dysfunction.

70% less likely to develop high blood pressure.

35% less likely to develop kidney cancer.

90% less likely to suffer from gallstones.

14% less likely to develop osteoarthritis.

19% less likely to die in a car crash.

## The Ultimate Abs Exercise Plan

Having worked at *Men's Health* magazine for more than 10 years, I've seen all the trends. (Uh, electrodes on my abs? No, thanks.) I've talked to trainers. I've tried just about every exercise ever concocted. In a lot of ways, my workout is my work. But I'm also busy with calls, meetings, and all the stresses that go with any job. So I know you want an exercise plan that fits into your life—not one that is your life. This routine is short and simple. In addition to performing this workout three times a week, train your largest muscle groups with classic moves like squats, bench presses, deadlifts, and rows. And add the 12 Abs Diet powerfoods to your diet. (See menshealth.com for a meal plan to go.) The end result: You'll lose fat, build muscle, flatten your stomach—and change your body forever.

### THE WORKOUT

This routine attacks your midsection from every angle, so your abs are constantly challenged. Choose one exercise from each section, for a total of five. Perform one move immediately after the other for the specified number of repetitions, then repeat the circuit. After 4 weeks, choose the exercise in each group that you didn't perform in your previous workouts. This ensures that your muscles are always adapting to new stress.

**Burn off your belly.** This interval routine is designed to strip away the excess flab that's hiding your six-pack. Do it 3 days a week, after your weight session or on the days in between. Use your mode of choice—a treadmill, stationary bike, or rowing machine.

## SECTION 1

### STANDING CABLE CRUNCH

Attach a rope to a high-pulley cable. Stand with your back to the weight stack and hold one end of the rope on the left side of your head and the other end on the right. Crunch your torso down. Pause, then return to the starting position. Do 10 to 15 repetitions.

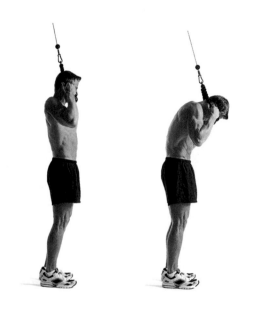

## SECTION 2

### PULSE-UP

Lie with your hands under your tailbone and your legs extended straight up toward the ceiling, perpendicular to your torso. Lift your hips off the floor in a straight line. Pause, then lower your hips. Do 10 to 15 repetitions.

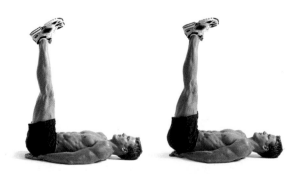

**Step 1:** Warm up for 3 to 5 minutes at an easy pace, about 30 to 40 percent of your best effort.

**Step 2:** Run, cycle, or row at 95 percent of your highest effort for 30 seconds.

**Step 3:** Perform active rest, slowing back down to your warmup speed for 90 seconds.

**Step 4:** Repeat five to seven times.

**Step 5:** Once you can complete eight intervals, reduce the length of your active rest periods by 5 to 10 seconds each workout, until they're only 30 seconds long.

## WEIGHTED CRUNCH

Lie on your back with your knees bent, and hold a weight plate or dumbbell on your chest. (If that's too hard, just do a traditional crunch.) Slowly crunch up, bringing your shoulder blades off the floor. Pause, then lower yourself to the starting position. Do 10 to 15 repetitions.

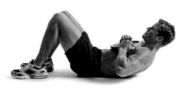

## FIGURE-8 CRUNCH

Lie on your back with your knees bent at a 90-degree angle, squeezing a light medicine ball tightly between them, and place your feet flat on the floor. Place your fingers behind your ears, then slowly raise your head, shoulders, and feet off the floor. Keeping your torso up, move your knees in a figure-8 motion. Each figure-8 is one repetition. Do 10 to 15 repetitions.

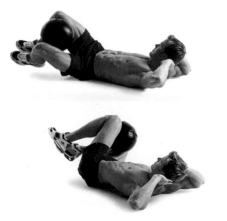

## SECTION 3

### MEDICINE-BALL TORSO ROTATION

Hold a medicine ball or basketball in front of
you as you kneel and sit back on your heels.
Quickly twist to your left and set the ball down
behind your back. Twist to the right and pick up
the ball, then bring it around to your left and
set it down again. That's one repetition. Do 10
to 15 repetitions.

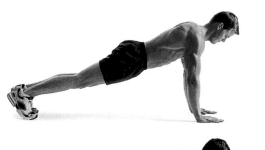

## SECTION 4

### TWO-POINT BRIDGE

Assume the standard pushup position. Lift
your right arm and left leg off the floor at the
same time. Hold for 3 to 5 seconds, then lower
them. That's one repetition. Return to the
starting position, then repeat, lifting your left
arm and right leg this time. Do 10 to 15
repetitions.

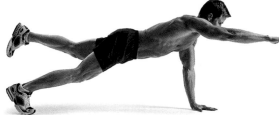

## SIDE JACKKNIFE

Lie on your left side, with your legs nearly straight. Also, lift your torso off the floor, with your left forearm on the floor for balance. Hold your other hand behind your right ear, with your elbow pointed toward your feet. Lift your legs toward your torso while keeping your torso stationary. Pause to feel the contraction on the right side of your waist. Then slowly lower your legs and repeat. Finish the set, then switch sides. Do 10 to 15 repetitions.

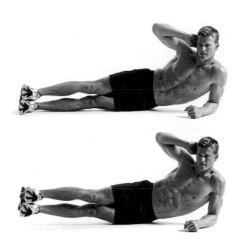

## NEGATIVE CRUNCH

Sit with your knees bent and your feet flat on the floor, shoulder-width apart. (Tuck your feet under weights to maintain balance.) Extend your arms in front of you with your fingers interlaced. Begin with your upper body at slightly less than a 90-degree angle to the floor. Lower your upper body toward the floor, curling your torso forward, rounding your lower back, and keeping your abs contracted. When your upper body reaches a 45-degree angle to the floor, return to the starting position. Do 10 to 15 repetitions.

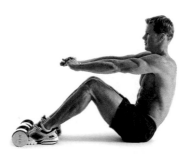

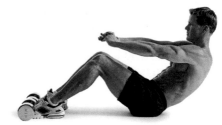

## BACK EXTENSION

Position yourself in a back-extension station, and hook your feet under the leg anchor. Hold your arms straight out beyond your head. Lower your torso, allowing your lower back to round slightly, until it's just short of perpendicular to the floor. Pause, then raise your upper body until it's slightly above parallel to the floor. At this point, you should have a slight arch in your back, and your shoulder blades should be pulled together. Do 10 to 15 repetitions.

## TWISTING BACK EXTENSION

Position yourself in a back-extension station, and hook your feet under the leg anchor. Lace your hands behind your head. Lower your torso, allowing your lower back to round slightly, until it's just short of perpendicular to the floor. Raise and twist your upper body until it's in line with your hips and facing right. That's one repetition. Repeat the move, this time twisting to your left. Do 10 to 15 repetitions.

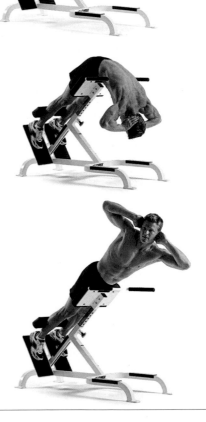

BY MYATT MURPHY

# Build a Bigger, Stronger Back

In just 25 minutes, this workout
delivers the ultimate upper body

When it comes to back exercises, most men favor pullups and lat pulldowns, since these movements primarily target the latissimus dorsi (a.k.a. lats), your largest back muscle. And the average guy's back workout rarely consists of anything else. Trouble is, "largest" doesn't mean "only." Focusing solely on your lats is sort of like working your chest but skipping your abs; and you'd never treat your "front" that way.

## Benchmark of Success

### How do you measure up?

The inverted row tests the strength of your back and rear shoulders and also requires a solid grip—a key factor in upper-body pulling movements. See Workout 2 (on page 220) for an exercise description and photos. Do as many reps as you can in 30 seconds, but don't sacrifice technique for speed. If at any time your form falters (for example, if your butt sags, your back arches, your chest doesn't touch the bar, or your arms fail to straighten fully), stop and record the number of reps you were able to complete with good form.

### Track Your Progress

Record the number of repetitions you performed in the inverted-row test. Then follow this workout and retest yourself every week.

Start (repetitions) _____
Week 1(repetitions) _____
Week 2 [repetitions]_____
Week 3 [repetitions]_____
Finish (repetitions) _____

## The Payoff

**Bigger muscle!** This workout trains your rear deltoids, rhomboids, and trapezius—all commonly neglected muscles of your upper body. By shoring up these weak spots, you'll pack on muscle and build a more symmetrical physique.

**A wider upper back!** The pullup and lat pulldown in this workout are slightly different from standard versions. You'll initiate each move by sliding your shoulder blades down. This allows your lats to contract through a larger range of motion, so they develop fully.

**Total-body strength!** The deadlift is more than just a muscle builder for your lower back and hamstrings. It strengthens your back from top to bottom and conditions your "posterior chain"—all the muscles on the back of your body—to work in coordination.

## The Workout

"Training the muscles surrounding your lats, particularly your rhomboid and trapezius muscles, will quickly add strength and size to your upper body," says C.J. Murphy, owner of Total Performance Sports in Everett, Massachusetts. Your rhomboids and trapezius stabilize your shoulder blades, which allow your shoulder joints to move your arms in every direction. By developing these muscles, you'll add mass to your upper back and rear shoulders and see improvements in every upper-body lift. Complete Murphy's routine once a week.

**DEADLIFT**

**PULLUP**

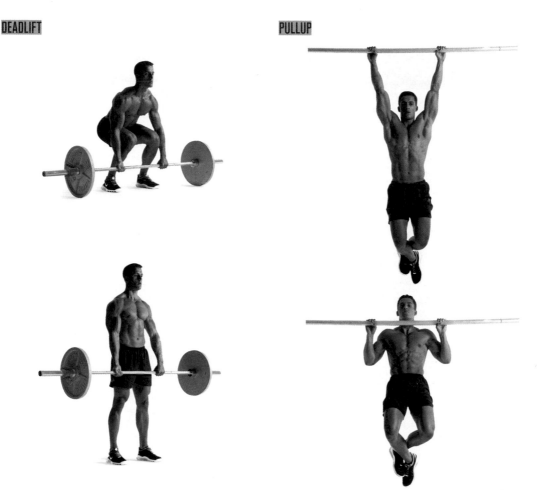

Stand with a barbell on the floor in front of you, with the bar over your toes. Bend your knees and grasp the bar with an alternating grip (one palm toward you, the other facing away), your hands just outside your knees. Keeping your head and back straight, stand up. Keep the bar close to your body as you lift it. Slowly lower the bar.

**The plan:** Do three sets of three reps using the heaviest weight that allows for perfect form. Rest for 60 seconds between sets.

Grab a chinup bar with an overhand grip (palms forward), your hands slightly more than shoulder-width apart. Hang with your arms straight, then pull your shoulder blades down. Pull your chest to the bar. Pause, then lower yourself to the starting position.

**The plan:** Do six to eight reps. Perform this move and the next as a superset; that is, move from one exercise to the other without rest.

## WORKOUT 1

### BACK RAISE

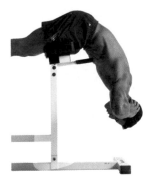

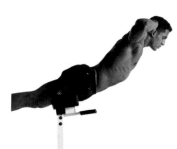

Position yourself in a back-extension station, and hook your feet under the leg anchor. With your upper thighs resting on the pad, lock your hands behind your head and bend forward at the hips until your upper body is just short of perpendicular to the floor. Slowly raise your torso until it's in line with your lower body, then lower it.

**The plan:** Do six to eight repetitions, then rest for 60 seconds. Repeat the superset two more times for a total of three sets.

## WORKOUT 2 (WEEK 2)

### DEADLIFT

**See the deadlift in Workout 1 for an exercise description and photos.**

The plan: **Do three sets of five repetitions using the heaviest weight that allows you to maintain perfect form. Rest for 60 seconds between sets.**

### INVERTED ROW

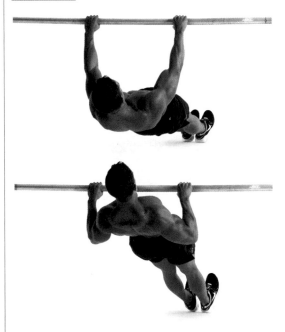

Sit under a Smith machine or squat rack with your legs straight and a bar set a few inches higher than arm's length. Grab the bar overhand, hands shoulder-width apart. Keeping your body straight, pull your chest to the bar. Pause, then lower yourself.

**The plan:** Perform this exercise and the next (the lat pulldown) as a superset. Do 10 repetitions of each.

## LAT PULLDOWN

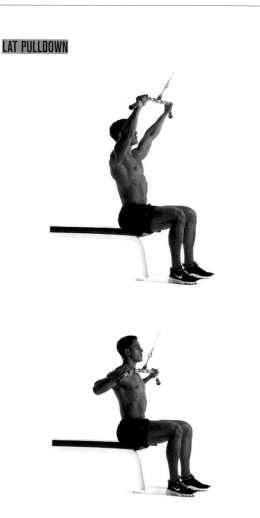

Sit at a lat-pulldown station and grab the bar with an overhand grip, your hands slightly more than shoulder-width apart. Keeping your head and back straight, pull your shoulder blades down, then pull the bar to your chest. Slowly let the bar rise.

**The plan:** Do 10 to 12 reps, then rest for 60 seconds. Repeat the superset two more times for a total of three sets.

## WORKOUT 3 (WEEK 3)

### SCAPULA PULLDOWN

Sit at a lat-pulldown station and grab the bar overhead. Keeping your arms straight, squeeze your shoulder blades together, then down. This movement is very slight. Pause, then allow your shoulder blades to rise to return the bar to the starting position.

**The plan:** Do 10 reps. Move to the next exercise without resting.

*(continued on page 224)*

## The 10-chinup challenge

Stop hiding at the lat-pulldown machine. You know the chinup is the best exercise for your back. Practically every fitness book and article proclaims it the granddaddy of back moves. Yet men avoid it for one reason: It's hard. Athletes in Winchester, Massachusetts, think chinups are tough, too. But there, nearly all the men and women can do a chinup with more weight than they can bench press. (They attach weight plates to a dip belt to add pounds.) Okay, not all athletes in town can do it—only those coached by Michael Boyle, MA, ATC. "It's amazing what a lost art the chinup is, when you see how well it works," says Boyle. Here's his plan for raising body to bar, over and over again.

This workout will help you build a broader back. Why? Because chinups primarily target your latissimus dorsi—the fan-shaped muscles of your back. Another benefit is if you go big on the bench, shoring up your back muscles will help realign your joints. And last, it will help build your arms. Chinups require more effort from your biceps and place less strain on your shoulders than pullups do.

### STEP 1: TEST YOUR PULLING POWER

Do as many chinups as you can. Start from a full hang, hands shoulder-width apart, palms toward you. Pull yourself up until your chin is over the bar and lower yourself to the starting position.

### STEP 2: SET THE BAR HIGH

If you can't do one chinup, then that's your initial goal. Aim for one more chinup every week. If you did five, strive for 10 by the fifth week.

### HOW TO DO THE WORKOUTS

These exercises develop the back and arm strength necessary to lift your body weight. Rest 3 minutes between sets. Do each workout once a week, resting 2 days between sessions.

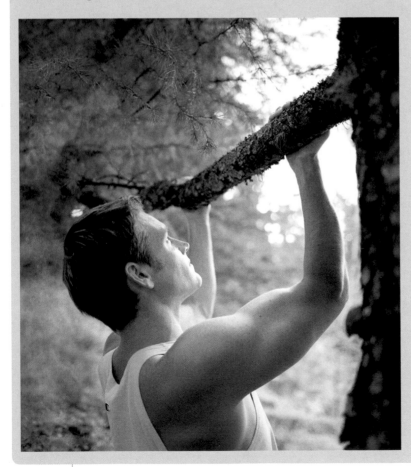

## WORKOUT 1

### Chinup

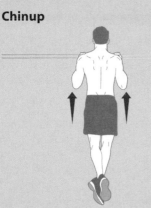

Perform your maximum number of chinups, which you determined in step 1. Rest, then do another set of one less than your max. Perform a third set of two less than your max.

### Dumbbell Row

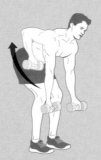

Grab a pair of heavy dumbbells with an underhand grip, knees slightly bent. With your torso almost parallel to the floor, pull one weight up until your elbow is higher than your torso, then lower it. Do three sets of six reps per arm.

### Biceps Curl

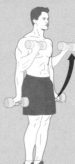

Hold dumbbells at arm's length, palms forward. Keeping your upper arms against your sides, curl the weights toward your shoulders. Squeeze your biceps at the top, then lower the weights. Do three sets of six reps.

## WORKOUT 2

### Parallel-Grip Pullup

Grab the parallel bars of a pullup bar so your hands face each other. Do one set of as many pullups as you can. Perform a second set of one less than your maximum from set one. Then do a third set of two repetitions less than your max.

### Inverted Row

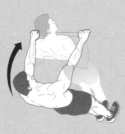

At a Smith machine, grab the bar overhand. Keeping your body straight, pull your chest to the bar, then lower yourself. Do one set of as many reps as you can. Do one rep less than your max for the second set and two less for the third.

### Hammer Curl

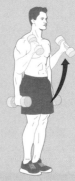

This is the same as the biceps curl, but hold the dumbbells with a neutral grip (palms facing each other). Do three sets of six repetitions using the heaviest weight you can handle with perfect form.

## BARBELL SHRUG

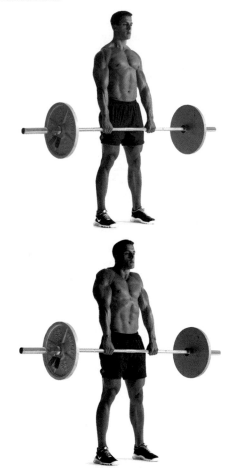

Stand holding a loaded barbell with an overhand grip in front of your thighs. Keeping your arms straight, raise your shoulders toward your ears. Pause when your shoulders are as high as they can go, then push them down as far as possible. That's one repetition.

**The plan:** Do 12 reps. Move to the next exercise without resting.

## BACK RAISE

See Workout 1 for an exercise description and photos.

**The plan:** Do 12 repetitions, then rest for 90 seconds.

Repeat this circuit (scapula pulldown, barbell shrug, back raise) three more times, for a total of four circuits, resting for 90 seconds after each circuit.

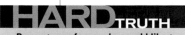

**HARD**TRUTH

Percentage of men who would like to double their upper-body muscle mass:

## 16

## FACE PULL

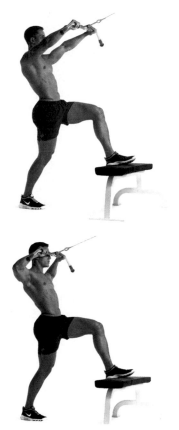

Stand facing a lat-pulldown machine and grasp the bar above with an overhand grip. Stagger your feet and place your front foot on the seat in front of you. Lean back as far as you can without arching your back. Pull your shoulders back, then pull the bar toward you until it's in front of your nose. Allow your arms to straighten slowly to return to the starting position.

**The plan:** This is the first move in a circuit. Do six reps, then move on.

Do eight reps when you repeat the circuit. Do 10 reps the third time around.

## LAT PULLDOWN

See Workout 2 for an exercise description and photos.

**The plan:** Do eight repetitions, then move to the next exercise in the circuit (the back raise). When you repeat this move, do 10 reps. In the third circuit, do 15.

## BACK RAISE

See Workout 1 for technique.

**The plan:** Do 10 reps, then rest for 90 seconds. Repeat the series two more times, resting 90 seconds after each circuit. When you repeat this exercise, do 12 reps. Do 15 reps for your final set.

## PAINkiller

**I sprained my knee more than 2 months ago, and I still have pain. Do I need to go back to the doctor to have it checked out?**

Probably. Unless you also have arthritis, which can slow your recovery, most knee sprains should heal within 8 weeks, depending on your age. If you can't run or move laterally without pain, you should see an orthopedic specialist. It could be a sign of something more serious, such as a torn meniscus or ligament.

BY MYATT MURPHY

# Sculpt a Powerful Chest

You're just 18 minutes away
from the perfect upper body

**T**his routine attacks the primary cause of puniness. "The mistake most men make when looking for more chest size and strength is always sticking to the traditional 8-to-12-repetition principle," says Jason Ferruggia, owner of Renegade Strength and Conditioning in Warren, New Jersey. Ferruggia's first rule: Diversify your repetition schemes and emphasize heavier-weight, lower-repetition sets. This allows you to target your body's fast-twitch muscle fibers, the ones with the greatest potential for growth.

## The Payoff

**A stronger upper body!** The heavy weights you'll use in this workout develop muscle fibers that produce strength and power. And because your chest is one of your largest muscle groups, this added strength improves performance in many upper-body and total-body lifts.

**Extra muscle!** This routine uses several body-weight moves that train stabilizing muscles, in addition to your largest muscles, so you end up working more muscle overall while improving your sense of balance.

**Fewer crunches!** The pushups and dumbbell single-arm bench press challenge your core stabilization while building your chest. The result: Your entire midsection works just as hard as in any ab exercise.

## The Workout

At times, this workout calls for you to lift only your body weight while in a suspended position. Think gymnasts, who build rock-hard bodies without ever picking up a weight. "Moving your body through space is more taxing to your central nervous system than regular weight training," says Ferruggia. This means you'll improve your brain-to-muscle connection, which will train your body to recruit more muscle in every exercise.

Do Phase 1 for 4 weeks, working your chest twice a week with two separate routines (day 1 and day 2). (Do the exercises shown here as the chest portion of your upper- or total-body routine.) Rest at least 2 days between workouts. Complete Phase 2 workouts in the next 4 weeks.

## Benchmark of Success

### How do you measure up?

The best barometer of chest strength is your maximum bench press—the most weight you can lift in a single repetition. To determine your max, you'll need a spotter.

Perform 10 repetitions of the barbell bench press. (See page 232 for a description.) Rest for 30 to 90 seconds, then add 20 to 40 pounds and repeat. Continue this process until the weight feels difficult. Then do only one repetition per set until you work up to the heaviest weight you can lift once—your one-repetition maximum (1RM), or one-rep max.

### Track Your Progress

Record your 1RM on this chart. Then follow the plan and retest yourself every 4 weeks.

Start (weight in pounds) _____

Week 4 (weight in pounds) _____

Finish (weight in pounds)_____

# PEAK
## performance

## We're with the Band

Try this chest and core workout from Juan Carlos Santana, owner of the Institute of Human Performance in Boca Raton, Florida. Move from one exercise to the next without rest, and try to perform the routine in the recommended 65 seconds. We like JC Bands from www.performbetter.com.

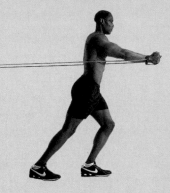

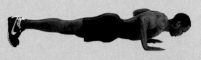

### Pushup

Assume the standard pushup position, with your hands beneath your shoulders and your body in a straight line. Bend your elbows to lower yourself toward the floor, then push yourself back up. Try to perform 20 repetitions in 15 seconds.

### Staggered-Stance Fly

Same setup as for the press, but begin with your arms at chest height and extended out to your sides, palms forward. Pull the handles together in an arc, then allow them to return. Do 10 in 10 seconds; do 10 more with your other foot forward.

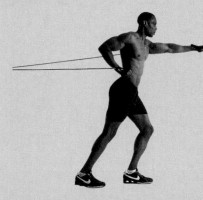

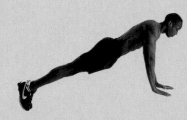

### Staggered-Stance Press

Secure a band and walk forward for tension. Hold the handles at your ribs with one foot forward. Extend one arm, return to the starting position, and then repeat with the other arm. Do 10 in 10 seconds; do 10 more with your other foot forward.

### Explosive Pushup

Same technique as for the pushup, but push yourself up with enough force that your hands come off the floor at the top of the move. Land and immediately lower yourself into the next pushup. Aim for 10 reps in 10 seconds.

## DAY 1

### DUMBBELL SINGLE-ARM BENCH PRESS

### DUMBBELL INCLINE BENCH PRESS

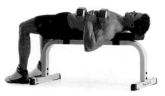

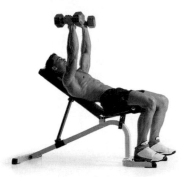

Lie on your back on a bench with a heavy dumbbell in one hand along the side of your chest, palm facing in. Hold your opposite arm straight out to the side for balance.

Lie faceup on an incline bench and hold a pair of heavy dumbbells along the outsides of your chest with a neutral grip (palms facing in). Slowly press the weights straight above your chest.

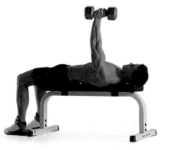

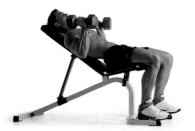

Push the weight up so your arm is straight above your chest. Pause, then slowly lower the weight to the starting position.

**The plan:** Do five to seven repetitions with each hand. Complete four sets, resting 2 minutes after each set.

Pause, then lower them to the starting position.

**The plan:** Perform six to eight repetitions. Do three sets, and rest 2 minutes after each set.

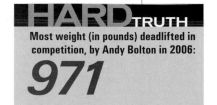

HARD TRUTH
Most weight (in pounds) deadlifted in competition, by Andy Bolton in 2006:

*971*

## DAY 2

### SUSPENDED PUSHUP

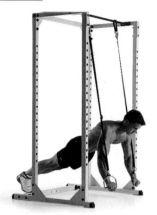

If your gym has Blast Straps (www.elitefts. com, $57) or chains, try this pushup variation. (Otherwise, do the weighted pushup on page 232.) Loop the straps or chains around the bar so the handles hang a few inches off the floor.

Now assume the standard pushup position with your hands grasping the handles, so only your feet touch the floor.

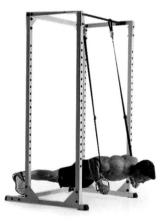

Bend at the elbows to lower your body until your upper arms are parallel to the floor, then push yourself up.

**The plan:** Do as many pushups as you can, then rest for 1½ minutes. Do a total of three sets.

### DUMBBELL INCLINE FLY

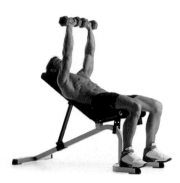

Lie on an incline bench and hold a pair of dumbbells over your chest with your arms straight, palms facing forward.

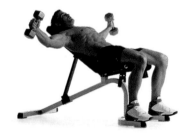

Keeping your palms forward, slowly sweep your arms down and out to your sides in an arc until the weights are level with your chest.

Pause, then reverse the motion until the weights are once again above you.

**The plan:** Perform this exercise as a superset with the next move; that is, do 8 to 12 repetitions of the dumbbell incline fly, then immediately move to the parallel-bar dip.

## PARALLEL-BAR DIP

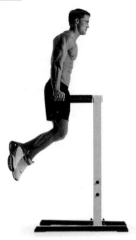

Grab parallel dip bars and lift yourself so your arms are straight.

Keeping your elbows tucked close to your body, slowly lower yourself by bending your elbows until your upper arms are parallel to the floor.

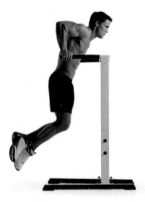

Pause, then push yourself up to the starting position.

**The plan:** Do as many reps as you can, then rest for 3 minutes and repeat the superset one time, performing a total of two sets of each exercise.

## SIDE-LYING SINGLE-ARM EXTERNAL ROTATION

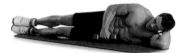

Lie on your left side with your left arm bent and your head resting on your left hand. Holding a light dumbbell in your right hand, bend your right arm 90 degrees and tuck your upper arm against your right side. Let the weight hang in front of your midsection.

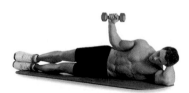

Keeping your upper arm stationary, slowly rotate your forearm until it points toward the ceiling. Then rotate your forearm back to the starting position.

**The plan**: Perform 12 to 15 repetitions, then rest for 1 minute. Do two sets.

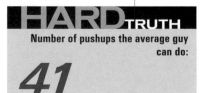

HARD TRUTH

Number of pushups the average guy can do:

*41*

## DAY 1

### BARBELL BENCH PRESS

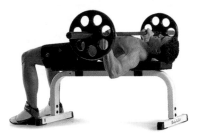

Lie on a bench with your feet flat on the floor. Grab the bar with your hands slightly more than shoulder-width apart, and hold the weight over your chest. Pull your shoulder blades back and together, then lower the bar to your chest. (Tuck your elbows in at 45 degrees; don't let them flare out to the sides.)

Pause, then push the weight back up.

**The plan:** Do five sets of four repetitions using 80 percent of your 1RM. In week 6, do six sets of three reps with 85 percent of your 1RM. In week 7, do five sets of two reps with 90 percent of your 1RM. In week 8, repeat the max bench press test described in "Benchmark of Success" on page 227, then do four sets of one repetition with approximately 90 percent of your new 1RM.

## DAY 2

### WEIGHTED PUSHUP

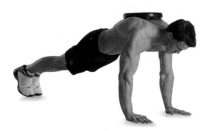

Assume the standard pushup position with your hands beneath your shoulders. Ask your workout partner to place a weight plate on your back between your shoulder blades.

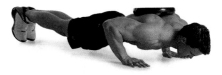

Keeping your body straight, lower yourself by bending your elbows until your chest touches the floor. Pause, then push yourself back up.

**The plan:** Perform this exercise as a superset with the next move: Do 8 to 12 repetitions, then immediately move on to the cable lying fly.

## CABLE LYING FLY

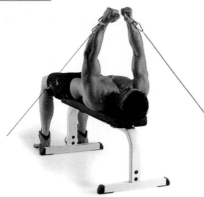

Place an exercise bench between the stacks of a cable crossover station and attach stirrup handles to the low-pulley cables. Grab a handle with each hand and lie faceup on the bench with your feet flat on the floor. Hold your arms straight above your chest, palms facing each other.

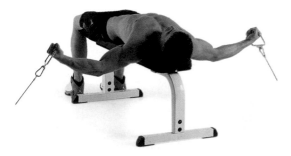

Keeping your elbows slightly bent, lower your hands out to your sides in an arc, then reverse the motion to return to the starting position.

**The plan:** Do 8 to 10 repetitions, rest 2½ minutes, then repeat the superset (pushup and cable lying fly) two times for a total of three sets.

## SEATED SINGLE-ARM EXTERNAL ROTATION

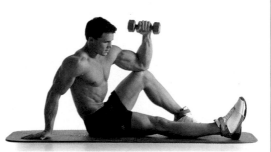

Sit on the floor with your left knee bent and your right leg flat on the floor. Hold a light dumbbell in your left hand and rest your left elbow on your left knee. Bend your left arm 90 degrees and allow the weight to hang down over your right leg.

Keeping your elbow in place, slowly rotate your left arm upward. Pause when your forearm points to the ceiling, then reverse the motion until the weight is again hanging over your right leg.

**The plan:** Do 10 to 12 repetitions with each hand, then rest 1 minute. Repeat one time for a total of two sets.

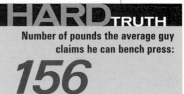

**HARD**TRUTH
Number of pounds the average guy claims he can bench press:
*156*

## Core Power to You

Have a basketball? Then you've got a piece of fitness equipment. You can strengthen your abs, back, and hips with this 5-minute routine from Alan Stein, CSCS, owner of www.eliteathletetraining.com. Perform each exercise for 1 minute in the order shown.

### Plank

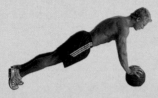

Assume the pushup position with your hands beneath your shoulders, on top of the ball. Keep your abs tight and hold your body in a straight line from heels to shoulders.

### Knee-to-Elbow Plank

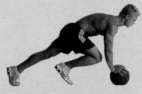

Use the same body position as in the plank, but allow your back to arch and attempt to touch your right knee to your right elbow. Hold for 30 seconds, then try to touch your left knee to your left elbow and hold for 30 seconds.

### Lying Woodchop

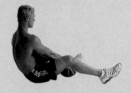

Lie on your back with your knees slightly bent. Hold the ball behind your head with your arms slightly bent. (Maintain this arm angle throughout the move.) As you do a situp, bring the ball to the floor, between your legs. Then return to the starting position.

### Side-to-Side Twist

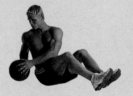

Sit and lean back slightly, with your knees bent and feet off the floor. Hold the ball in front of your chest with both hands. Now twist your shoulders from side to side, touching the ball to the floor next to each hip.

### Over and Under

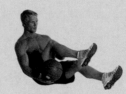

This is like the old figure-8 drill but seated, with your legs slightly bent and your upper back off the floor. Move the ball over and under your legs, from one hand to the other, while you alternate drawing your knees toward you and pushing them away from you.

BY MYATT MURPHY

# Pump Up Your Arms

With this simple workout,
you can add 2 inches to your
arms—in just 24 minutes

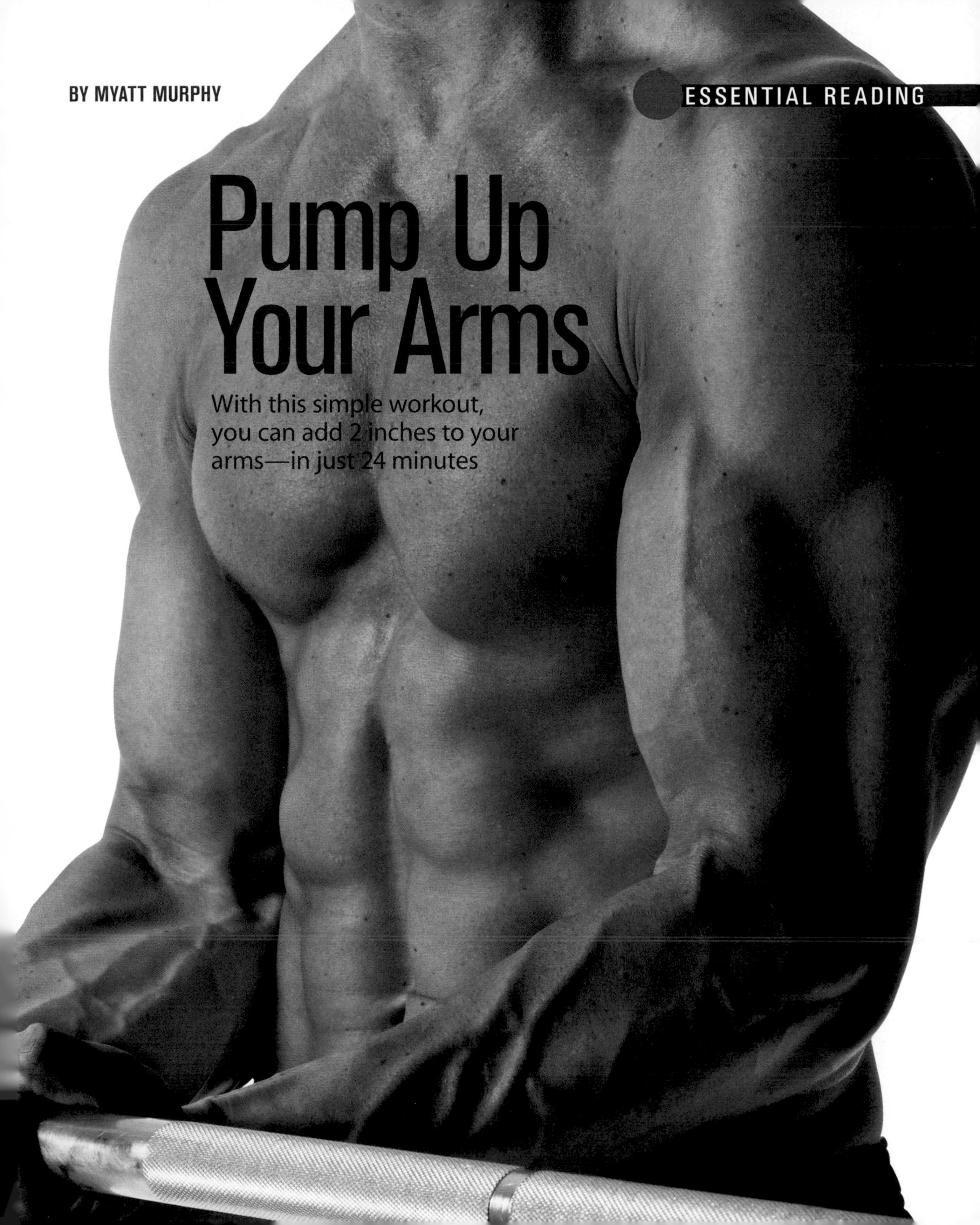

Unless you can complete a set of five chinups and eight dips, you should limit exercises that isolate your arms, such as biceps curls and triceps extensions. "Your arms will grow best when you focus on the basics," says Kelly Baggett, a certified personal trainer with the International Sports Sciences Association. The basics, he explains, are compound exercises—such as the chinup and dip—that force you to move at more than one joint. These movements allow you to use heavier weights than you would with single-joint isolation exercises, while also training either your chest or back. So don't worry: You'll fully engage the muscles of your arms with each repetition, and you'll also shore up any weaknesses in the larger muscles of your upper body.

## The Payoff

**Fuller biceps!** This routine places your arms in front of you during some arm curls and behind you or at your sides during others. Varying arm positions builds the biceps evenly. As a result, you'll raise your peak and build thickness throughout your arms.

**Stronger triceps!** Your triceps consist of three distinct muscles—the lateral head, on the outside of the arm; the long head, which provides bulk; and the medial head, which lies between the other two. This plan develops all three.

**A bigger upper body!** The chinup and bench press in this workout develop your arms with help from your back and chest, respectively. The benefit: You'll build a bigger and more balanced upper body to support larger—and stronger—arms.

## The Workout

If you can't yet perform five chinups and eight dips, do Workout A twice a week. When you're able to complete a full complement of both exercises, progress to Workout B, performing the routine once every 3 to 5 days for bigger arms—and a better total body.

## Benchmark of Success

### How big are your arms?

Since it requires only a tape measure, finding the circumference of your arms is an excellent way to gauge the effectiveness of your arm workout.

Your arms may look slightly larger after a workout or meal, when blood and water rush to your muscles. So, for the most accurate results, take all your measurements at the same time of day, such as before breakfast. Extend your arm in front of you (unflexed) and wrap a measuring tape around the largest portion of your upper arm. Record the circumference, then measure your other arm.

### Track Your Progress

Record the total circumference of both your arms in the chart below. Then follow this workout and remeasure every 2 weeks.

Start (total inches) _____

Week 2 (total inches) _____

Finish (total inches) _____

## WORKOUT A

Do this workout if you can't complete five chinups and eight dips.

**NEGATIVE CHINUP**

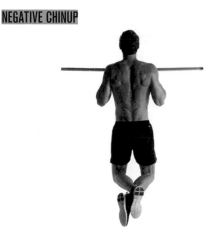

Set a bench under a chinup bar, then stand on the bench and grasp the bar with an underhand grip (palms facing you) and your hands about shoulder-width apart. Give yourself a boost from the bench so you don't have to use much effort to pull your chest up next to your hands.

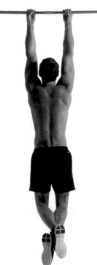

Slowly lower yourself for a count of 6 seconds. Then hop back up to the bar and repeat.

**The plan:** Perform five or six repetitions. Rest for 1½ minutes, then move to the next exercise.

**NEGATIVE DIP**

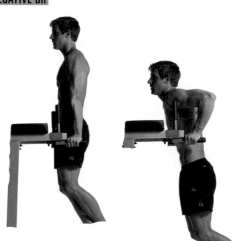

Grab parallel dip bars and use your legs to boost yourself up so your arms are straight and all your weight is resting on your hands.

Keeping your elbows tucked close to your body, slowly lower yourself by bending your elbows for a count of 6 seconds. Your upper arms should be parallel to the floor at the end of the move. Place your feet on the floor to boost yourself back up, and repeat.

**The plan:** Do five or six repetitions. Rest for 1½ minutes, then perform a second set of negative chinups (at left). Continue alternating between exercises for a total of four or five sets of each movement, resting for 1½ minutes between sets.

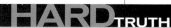

**HARD** TRUTH

Percentage greater chance of death for older men with small amounts of arm muscle compared with those with large amounts:

## 95

## CLOSE-GRIP BENCH PRESS

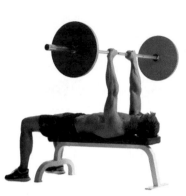

Lie faceup on a bench with your feet flat on the floor. Grab the bar with an overhand grip, your hands shoulder-width apart.

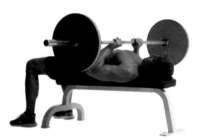

Keeping your elbows tucked at your sides, lower the bar to your chest, then press the weight overhead.

**The plan:** Perform six to eight repetitions. Rest for 1 minute, then move on to the next exercise.

## BARBELL CURL

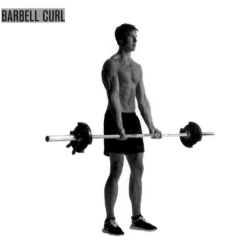

Stand holding a barbell in front of your thighs with an underhand grip, your hands shoulder-width apart.

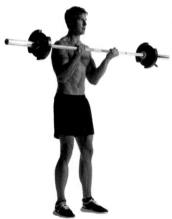

Keeping your back straight and your elbows at your sides, slowly curl the bar up in a semi-circular motion until your forearms touch your biceps. Pause, then slowly lower the bar to about an inch in front of your thighs before repeating the move.

**The plan:** Perform 8 to 10 repetitions. Rest for 1 minute, then do a second set of close-grip bench presses (at left). Alternate between exercises for a total of three or four sets of each move, resting for 1 minute between sets.

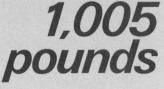

**HARD TRUTH**

World record for the bench press, held by Gene Rychlak Jr.:

## 1,005 pounds

## WORKOUT B

Perform this workout when you're able to complete five chinups and eight dips.

### CHINUP

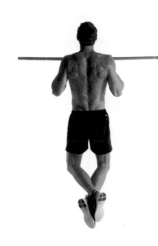

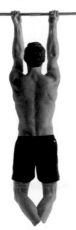

Grab a chinup bar with an underhand grip (palms toward you), your hands about shoulder-width apart. Pull yourself up until the bar is below your chin.

Squeeze your biceps at the top, then slowly lower yourself until your arms are almost straight; keeping a slight bend maintains tension on your biceps.

**The plan:** Do six to eight repetitions. (If you can do more, ask a workout partner to place a dumbbell between your feet.) Rest for 1½ minutes, then move to the close-grip bench press (see opposite page).

### DUMBBELL TRICEPS EXTENSION

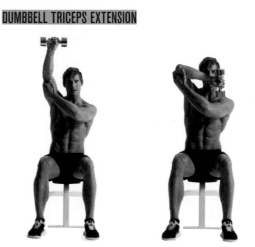

Sit on a bench holding a heavy dumbbell in your right hand. Extend your arm straight overhead with your palm facing forward, and place your left hand on your right elbow for support.

Without moving your upper arm, lower the weight down in front of your face until the end of the dumbbell touches the top of your chest. Finish the set before repeating with your other arm.

**The plan:** Do 8 to 10 repetitions with each arm. Rest for 1 minute, then move to the next exercise.

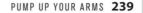

**HARD** TRUTH
Percentage of muscle in your upper arms made up of your triceps:

*67*

## WORKOUT B

### CABLE PREACHER CURL

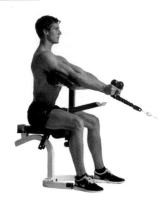

Place a preacher-curl bench in front of a low-pulley cable station. Attach a rope to the cable and grab an end with each hand. Rest your upper arms on the pad in front of you with your palms facing each other.

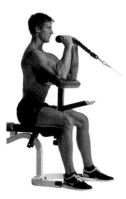

Keeping your back straight and your upper arms pressed against the pad, bend your elbows to curl the rope up toward your shoulders. Pause, then slowly lower your arms to the starting position.

**The plan:** Do 8 to 10 repetitions. Rest for 1 minute, then perform a second set of the dumbbell triceps extension (see page 239). Alternate between exercises for a total of three sets of each, resting for 1 minute between sets.

### CABLE INCLINE-BENCH PRESS TRICEPS EXTENSION

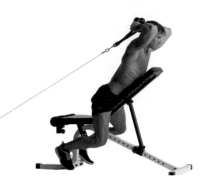

Attach a rope to a low-pulley cable and place an incline bench a couple of feet in front of the pulley. Grab the rope and lie facedown on the bench with your arms straight and beside your ears.

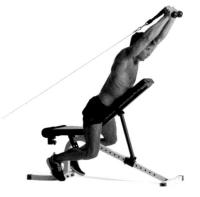

Without moving your upper arms, bend your elbows 90 degrees. Pause, then straighten your arms.

**The plan:** Do 12 to 15 reps. Rest 45 seconds, then go to the next exercise.

## CLOSE-GRIP BENCH PRESS

Lie faceup on a bench with your feet flat on the floor. Grab the bar with your hands shoulder-width apart. Keeping your elbows tucked at your sides, lower the bar to your chest, then press the weight overhead. (See the photos in Workout A on page 238.)

**The plan:** Perform six to eight repetitions. Rest for 1½ minutes, then do a second set of chinups (see page 239). Continue alternating between exercises for a total of four sets of each move. Rest for 1½ minutes after each set.

## CABLE SINGLE-ARM CURL

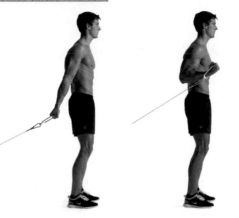

Stand with your back to the weight stack of a cable station and grab the low-pulley handle with your right hand. Step forward so your right hand is a few inches behind you and your arm is straight.

Keeping your elbow in place, curl the handle up until it reaches the side of your chest. Pause, then slowly lower your arm.

**The plan:** Do 12 to 15 reps with each arm. Rest for 45 seconds, then do a second set of the cable incline bench triceps extension. Rest for another 45 seconds, and do a second set of this cable curl.

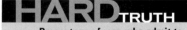

**HARD TRUTH**

Percentage of men who admit to overworking their biceps while ignoring their triceps:

*26*

BY MYATT MURPHY

# Strengthen Your Shoulders

Here's how to get the rock-solid shoulders you want—in the time that you have

The best way to build muscle isn't always the most obvious. For instance, conventional wisdom says that if your shoulders are weak, you're not working them hard enough. In fact, just the opposite is true, especially when it comes to the most obvious exercise. "Men do entirely too many shoulder presses," says Jon Crosby, CSCS, performance director for Velocity Sports Performance. "Excessive pressing exercises can destabilize your shoulders by overworking the front portions of the muscles, which eventually causes the shoulder joints to be pulled out of alignment." So instead of growing stronger, your shoulders—and all the muscles that attach to the shoulder joints, including those of your chest and arms—become weaker over time.

## The Payoff

**Greater strength!** The alternating shoulder press in this workout helps you look great all over. Because you work each arm separately, both sides of your body are trained evenly—helping you avoid muscle imbalances.

**A bulletproof upper body!** This workout emphasizes your rotator cuffs—the primary stabilizers of the shoulder joints. Since the shoulders are the most unstable joints in the body, shoring them up helps protect you from injury and allows you to lift more in every upper-body exercise.

**The ultimate pump!** This routine incor-

## Benchmark of Success

### How strong are your shoulders?

The classic military press builds the largest muscles of your shoulders, including your deltoids, rotator cuffs, and trapezius, making it a great exercise to measure shoulder strength.

Sit on a bench with your feet flat on the floor, and grab an empty bar with your hands slightly more than shoulder-width apart. (Use a spotter.) Keeping your back straight, press the bar overhead until your arms are straight, then lower it to the top of your chest. Do 10 repetitions, rest 1 minute, then add 10 to 20 pounds and repeat for a set of eight repetitions. Rest again, add another 10 pounds, and do a third set, this time of five repetitions. Continue adding weight in increments of 5 to 10 pounds—increase your rests to 2 to 3 minutes—until you work up to the heaviest weight you can lift five times. That's your five-repetition maximum (5RM), or five-rep max.

### Track Your Progress

Record your 5RM in the chart here. Then follow the plan and retest yourself every 2 weeks.

Start (weight in pounds) _____
Week 2 (weight in pounds) _____
Finish (weight in pounds)_____

porates a sequence called the Javorek complex, named after former Romanian Olympic weight-lifting coach Istvan Javorek. It works your shoulders from five angles, forcing a surge of blood that'll make your upper body appear larger right after your workout.

## The Workout

This workout, courtesy of Crosby, is designed to work the entire shoulder girdle—all the muscles that hold your upper-arm bone in its socket and allow the shoulder blade to move. This includes your deltoids, trapezius, rhomboids, and scapular stabilizers. Although logic might suggest that such a well-rounded approach would require extra time in the gym, Crosby took into account that most chest and back exercises involve your shoulders—so you need to use this workout only once a week. Perform Workout A in the first 2 weeks and Workout B in weeks 3 and 4. Do the exercises in the order shown, finishing all sets of an exercise before moving on to the next one.

### WORKOUT A (WEEKS 1 AND 2)

**ALTERNATING SHOULDER PRESS**

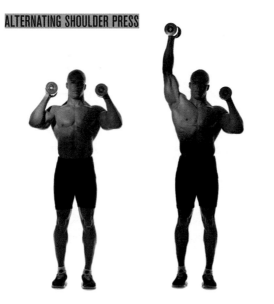

Stand holding a dumbbell in each hand just above your shoulders, with a neutral grip (palms facing each other).

Press the weight in your right hand straight above you until your arm is fully extended, then slowly lower the weight to the starting position. Now press the dumbbell in your left hand straight up and lower it. Continue to alternate arms throughout the set.

**The plan:** In week 1, do two sets of 10 repetitions with each arm; in week 2, do three sets of eight reps with each arm. Rest for 1–1½ minutes between sets.

**DUMBBELL UPRIGHT ROW**

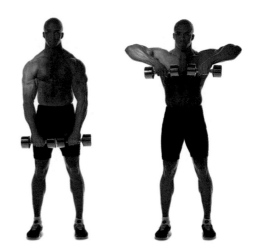

Stand holding a pair of dumbbells at arm's length in front of your thighs, your palms facing your body.

Keeping your forearms pointed down and the weights close to your body, lift your upper arms. Pause when the dumbbells are just below your chin, then slowly lower them.

**The plan:** Perform two sets of 10 repetitions in week 1 and three sets of eight in week 2. Rest for 1–1½ minutes between sets.

## STANDING SCAPTION

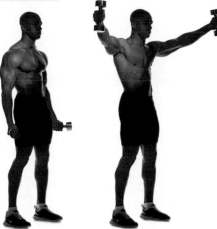

Stand holding a light pair of dumbbells in front of your thighs with a neutral grip (your palms facing each other).

Raise your arms forward and out at 45-degree angles until they're at eye level. The weights should point to 10 o'clock and 2 o'clock at the top of the move. Slowly lower your arms.

**The plan:** Perform two sets of 12 repetitions, resting for 45 to 60 seconds between sets.

## INCLINE ROW TO EXTERNAL ROTATION

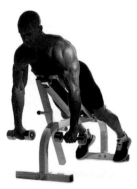

1. Lie facedown on a bench that's set at a 45-degree incline, and hold a light dumbbell in each hand with an overhand grip. Your arms should hang straight down with your palms facing your feet.

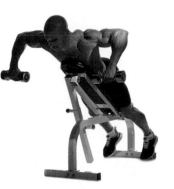

2. Keeping your head down, pull the weights up until your upper arms are parallel to the floor. Your elbows should point out to the sides and should be bent at 90-degree angles.

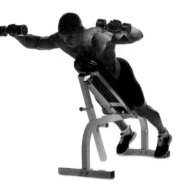

3. Keeping your upper arms stationary, rotate the weights forward until your palms face the floor. Pause, then reverse the movement to return to the starting position.

**The plan:** Perform two sets of 12 repetitions, resting for 45 to 60 seconds between sets.

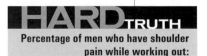

**HARD TRUTH**

Percentage of men who have shoulder pain while working out:

*28*

## WORKOUT B (WEEKS 3 AND 4)

### SWISS-BALL ALTERNATING SHOULDER PRESS

### DUMBBELL SHRUG

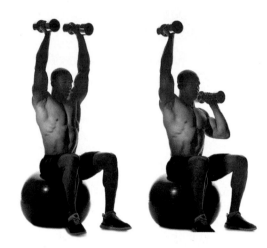

Sit on a Swiss ball with your feet flat on the floor. Hold a pair of dumbbells just above your shoulders with a neutral grip, your palms facing each other. Press the weights overhead until your arms are straight.

Keeping your right arm extended, slowly lower the weight in your left hand to its starting position, then press it back up. Next, keeping your left arm extended, lower the weight in your right hand and press it back up. Continue alternating arms.

**The plan:** Perform three sets of six repetitions with each arm, resting for 1–1½ minutes between sets.

Stand holding a heavy dumbbell in each hand at arm's length, with your palms facing the sides of your thighs.

Keeping your arms straight, shrug your shoulders up as if you were trying to touch them to your ears. Pause, then slowly lower your shoulders until your arms hang down as far as possible.

**The plan:** Do three sets of eight repetitions in week 3 and four sets of six reps in week 4. Rest for 1–1½ minutes between sets.

**HARD**TRUTH

Percentage of men who've continued to work out after feeling a pull or pain:

## 56

# PEAK
## performance

## Focus on Your Feet

When was the last time you worked your feet? Top trainers know that two secrets to big athletic gains are at the ends of your legs. By focusing part of your workout on your feet, you'll gain greater speed, agility, power, and balance. "And certainly, strong and flexible feet and ankles put you at less risk of sprains, strains, and other injuries," says Richard Cotton, PhD, chief exercise physiologist at myexerciseplan.com.

### Single-Leg Balance

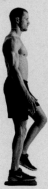

Fold a towel in half and roll it up. Step on the towel with your right foot, raise your left foot, and balance for 30 seconds. Do 10 on each foot.

### Toe Spreader

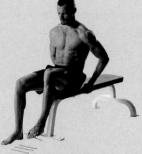

Scatter marbles, pebbles, pencils, or other small objects across the floor. While seated, start picking them up with your big toe and its neighbor.

### Single-Leg Hop

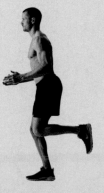

Stand with your feet together. Lower yourself into a quarter squat. Raise your right foot 2 inches off the ground, then take a small hop, keeping the quarter-squat position. Land back on your left foot. Do three sets of five jumps on each foot.

### Stork Jump

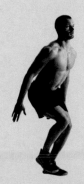

Stand with your feet hip-width apart, hop forward, and land on your right foot with your knee slightly bent. Stick the landing, holding yourself in a stork position (left foot off the ground, knee bent 90 degrees) for 10 seconds. Do 10 hops and holds on each foot.

## WORKOUT B (WEEKS 3 AND 4)

### LYING SWISS-BALL ROW TO EXTERNAL ROTATION

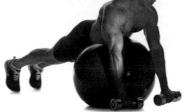

Holding a light dumbbell in each hand, lie facedown on a Swiss ball with your chest off the ball so your body is inclined. Your arms should hang down in front of the ball, palms facing your feet.

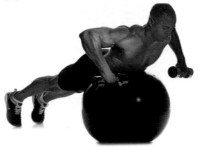

Keeping your neck straight, slowly pull the weights up until your upper arms are parallel to the floor.

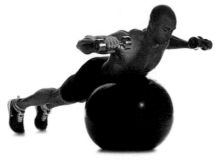

Then rotate your forearms forward until your palms face the floor. Pause, then reverse the motion to lower the weights to the starting position.

**The plan:** Perform two sets of 10 repetitions, resting for 45 to 60 seconds between sets.

### JAVOREK COMPLEX

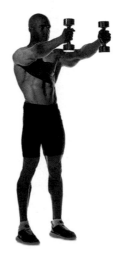

1. Stand holding a pair of dumbbells, arms at your sides, palms facing each other.

2. Raise your arms in front of you until they're parallel to the floor. Lower the weights and repeat for a total of six repetitions.

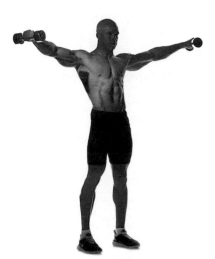

3. Now raise your arms out from your sides until they're parallel to the floor, and lower them. Again, complete six reps.

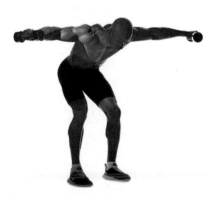

4. Next bend forward at the waist until your torso is almost parallel to the floor. Raise your arms out to your sides, lower them, and repeat for a total of six reps.

5. Stand up and place your hands in front of your thighs, palms toward you. Pull both weights up until they're just below your chin. Lower and repeat for six reps.

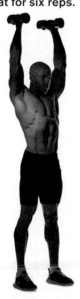

6. Finally, turn your palms so they face each other, curl the weights up to your shoulders, and press them overhead. Reverse the move and repeat for six reps.

**The plan:** Perform two sets, resting for 1½ minutes between sets.

BY MYATT MURPHY

# Sculpt a V-Shaped Torso

A bigger back, broader shoulders, and stronger abs

Even if you're unfamiliar with unilateral training, you practice it every day. Any movement in which your arms or legs function independently—even walking—is unilateral. Certain single-arm or single-leg exercises, such as the single-arm bench press, require a great deal of balance and thus limit the amount of weight you can lift. Others, like most of the moves in this workout, help you lift more by focusing your strength on one limb.

"Think of it this way: If you were to perform a row using two arms, you might grab a pair of 30-pound dumbbells. But use just one arm, and you could probably only handle a 50-pound weight," says Robert Dos Remedios, CSCS. This workout includes a mix of single-arm and traditional two-arm exercises to help you pack on muscle and eliminate imbalances. The benefit, says Dos Remedios, is that you'll build a more balanced body in strength and appearance. You'll train 3 days a week, resting at least a day between workouts and alternating between Workout A and Workout B. Rest for 60 to 90 seconds between sets.

## The Payoff

**Wider lats!** Performing the single-arm pullup demands nearly superhuman strength, which is why so few men attempt it. But you can still emphasize one side of your body at a time—and build bigger latissimus dorsi—with the side-to-side pullup in this workout.

**Bigger muscle!** Just because you can't see

## Benchmark of Success

### How do you measure up?

Don't be discouraged if your body shape initially looks more like the letter I than like a V—the average guy's back-to-waist ratio is 1:1.

To measure the width of your upper back and waist, stand up straight with your arms at your sides. Ask a friend or workout partner to wrap a tape measure completely around your body at the outer edges of your shoulder blades, just under your armpits. This measures your back width. Measure your waist by wrapping the tape around you so it rests at the top of each hip bone.

### Track Your Progress

Record your measurements in the chart below. Then follow this workout and remeasure yourself every 2 weeks.

Start (back/waist) _____

Week 2 (back/waist) _____

Finish (back/waist) _____

a muscle in the mirror doesn't mean you should ignore it in the gym, especially when your goal is building a V. The exercises in this plan develop your back while building your shoulders, abs, and arms.

**A harder core!** The corkscrew and side bridge reach in this workout condition the rectus abdominis—a.k.a., the six-pack muscle—and the obliques, located along the sides of your torso. The result: a powerful midsection that looks great from every angle.

### SIDE-TO-SIDE PULLUP

### DUMBBELL SINGLE-ARM ROW

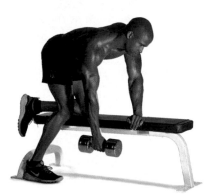

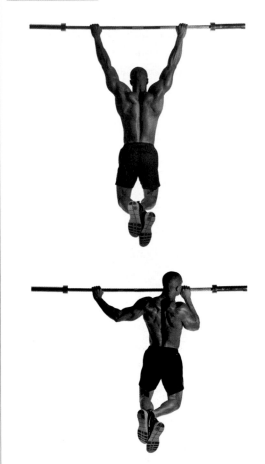

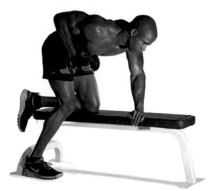

Grab a chinup bar with an overhand grip, your hands wider than shoulder width. Pull yourself up and to the right with the goal of bringing your chin to your right hand. Lower yourself. Next, pull yourself up and toward your left hand, then lower yourself.

**The plan:** Do four sets of five repetitions with each arm in weeks 1 and 3. In weeks 2 and 4, perform five sets of three reps with each arm. If you can't complete all the repetitions, place a step or bench under the bar so you can step up to the bar and complete the negative, or downward, portion of each rep.

Holding a dumbbell in your right hand, place your left hand and knee on a bench. Your right arm should be straight and hang just in front of your shoulder. Keeping your back flat and your right elbow close to your body, pull the dumbbell up and back toward your hip. Pause, then slowly lower the weight.

**The plan:** Perform four sets of 10 repetitions with each arm in weeks 1 and 3. Do four sets of five reps with each arm in weeks 2 and 4.

## PUSH PRESS

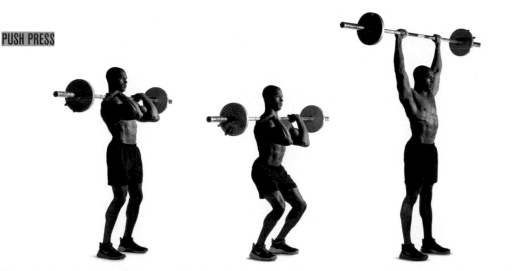

Stand with a light barbell across the front of your shoulders, your hands slightly wider than shoulder-width apart and your elbows pointed straight ahead. Bend at the hips and knees to descend about 6 inches, then quickly rise back up and explosively push the weight overhead until your arms are fully extended. Lower the weight to the starting position.

**The plan:** Do four sets of eight repetitions in weeks 1 and 3. Perform four sets of five reps in weeks 2 and 4.

## DUMBBELL CORKSCREW TO SINGLE-ARM CUBAN PRESS

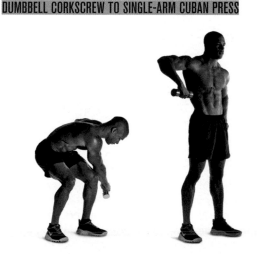
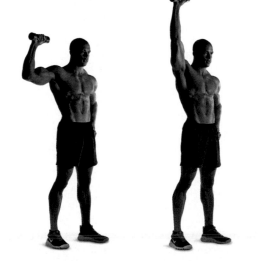

Stand holding a dumbbell in your right hand. As you squat, rotate your torso to the left and reach behind your left leg with your right hand. Push back up, twisting your torso to the right and bending your right arm 90 degrees. Leading with your elbow, lift your arm until you're standing and your elbow is in line with your shoulder. Now rotate the weight up until your forearm is vertical, then press the weight overhead. Return to the starting position.

**The plan:** Do four sets of eight reps with each arm in weeks 1 and 3. Perform four sets of six reps with each arm in weeks 2 and 4.

## CABLE SINGLE-ARM PULLDOWN

## SEATED ROW TO CHIN

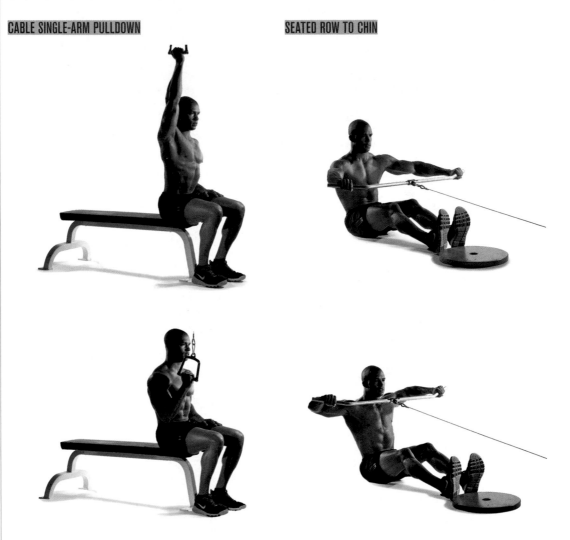

Attach a stirrup handle to the cable of a lat-pulldown machine. Grab the handle with your right hand so your palm faces left and sit on the seat. Keeping your back straight, pull the handle down to the right side of your chest. Resist the weight back to the starting position.

**The plan:** Perform four sets of 10 repetitions with each arm in weeks 1 and 3. Do four sets of six reps in weeks 2 and 4.

Attach a lat pulldown bar to the cable of a cable-row station. Sit on the bench and bend forward at the waist to grab the bar with a wide grip. Keeping your back straight, pull the bar inward and upward toward your chin. Resist the weight as it pulls your arms back out in front of you.

**The plan:** Do four sets of 10 repetitions in weeks 1 and 3. Perform four sets of six reps in weeks 2 and 4.

## SINGLE-ARM LEANING SHOULDER RAISE

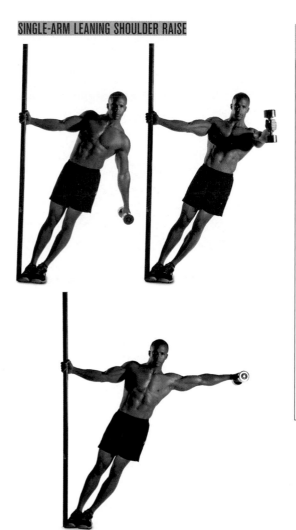

Stand with your right side toward a squat rack or a sturdy machine. Hold a light dumbbell in your left hand and grab the rack with your right hand. Lean to the left as far as you can. From here, raise your left arm in front of you. Pause when it's parallel to the floor, then lower your arm. Next, raise your arm out to your side until it's parallel to the floor, then lower it. That's one rep.

**The plan:** Do four sets of 10 reps with each arm in weeks 1 and 3. Perform four sets of six reps in weeks 2 and 4.

## SIDE BRIDGE REACH

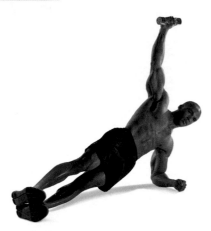

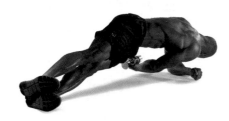

Holding a light weight in your right hand, lie on your left side with your feet stacked. Bend your left elbow 90 degrees and prop yourself up so that only your forearm and left shoe touch the floor and your body is straight. Extend your right arm. Now bring the weight down and under you, reaching with your arm until the weight is behind you and you face the floor. Reverse the motion to the starting position.

**The plan:** Do four sets of 10 repetitions in weeks 1 and 3. Perform four sets of five reps in weeks 2 and 4.

# Cut to the Core

**BY MIKE MEJIA, CSCS**

**E**very move in this workout strengthens the muscles of your abs, back, and hips. But this core routine also loosens your hamstrings, lower back, calves, hip flexors, and other areas, so you'll finish feeling stronger and stretched. Perform the workout as a circuit, moving from one exercise to the next without rest. Pause 60 to 90 seconds after each circuit, and do three circuits in all. Do the workout 3 days a week, taking at least a day off between workouts.

**Pike walk:** Stand with your legs straight and your hands flat on the floor. (You'll probably need to begin with your hands a couple of feet in front of you.)

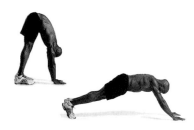

Keeping your legs straight, walk your hands forward as far as possible. Concentrate on keeping your stomach tight, with your navel pulled in toward your pelvis. Then take tiny steps to walk your feet forward to your hands, ending in the starting position. Repeat the movement for a set of five repetitions.

**Straight-arm side bridge:** Lie on your left hip with the outer side of your left leg flat on the floor and your upper body propped up on your left arm. (The arm should be straight, palm on the floor.)

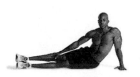

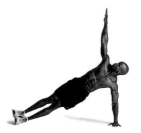

Pushing against the floor with your left arm, raise your hips and legs off the floor and simultaneously lift your right arm straight up in the air so your body forms a T. Hold for a second, then lower your hips and right arm. Do six repetitions per side.

**Glute bridge with abduction:** Lie on your back with your knees bent, feet flat on the floor. Raise your hips so your lower back is off the floor.

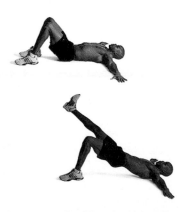

Then, holding this bridge position, straighten your right leg and move it out to the side as far as possible. (Don't let your hips drop.) Slowly bring the leg back in, lower your foot to its starting position, and slowly lower your hips to the floor. Repeat with your left leg. Do six repetitions to each side.

**Hindu pushup:** Start with your feet shoulder-width apart and your butt high in the air. Look back at your heels.

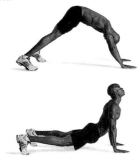

Bend your arms at the elbows, moving your head toward the floor while keeping your legs straight. Then lower your hips (but don't allow them to touch the floor) as you push up with your arms. Finish with your head up and your back arched. Then push yourself back up to the starting position. Do 8 to 10 repetitions.

# Training
# Tips

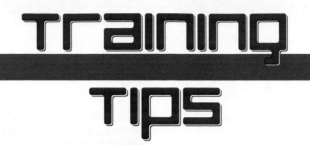

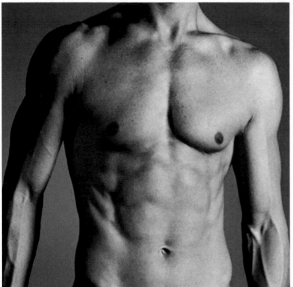

**If keeping my abs tight during exercise improves my posture and strength, should I do it even when I'm not working out, like when I'm at work?**

No. Just focus on feeling tall from the hips through the top of your head—whether you're sitting, standing, or working out. This naturally activates your body's postural muscles, including your abs. Most guys at the gym have terrible posture—their chins and shoulders slump, and they don't stand tall, so their guts slide down and out. Pay attention to these points—keep your abs braced, your shoulder blades hanging back and down, and your breastbone elevated during every exercise you do, and you'll notice improved posture outside of the gym as well.

**I'm bored with my abs routine. How can I shake it up?**

Use your Spidey sense. "The spider lift works on several planes of motion, especially the transverse, or diagonal, plane," says C.J. Murphy, MFS, owner of www.totalperformancesports.com. Most abdominal exercises crunch your torso forward or bring your legs up toward your chest, ignoring rotation and stabilization, Murphy says. The spider lift builds strength and stability throughout the torso and develops the quadratus lumborum, a muscle close to the spine that helps guard against back pain.

Grab a pair of dumbbells with a neutral grip (palms toward your thighs) and stand with your knees soft and your feet more than shoulder-width apart. Extend your left arm overhead, keeping your right arm at your side. Rotate your right hip back and your left hip forward, and look up at the dumbbell overhead.

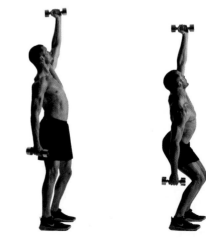

Lower the weight in your right hand straight down as far as you can. As you go, push your hips back and allow your knees to bend slightly. Perform 8 to 10 reps, then reverse the movement so your right hand is overhead and your right hip is forward. Do another 8 to 10 reps in this position.

### Do chinups work your biceps better than arm curls?

Pullups with a close, underhand grip (also called chinups) can challenge your biceps—and are a great upper-body muscle builder. But to answer your question of what "works" the biceps harder, we'll need to do some math. The effective load on your biceps and other pulling muscles would be determined by this formula:

body weight + external weight × reps × sets = cumulative load

Let's say you weigh 185 pounds, chain 15 pounds to your waist, and do three sets of eight repetitions: $(185 + 15) \times 8 = 1,600$ pounds $\times$ 3 sets $= 4,800$ total pounds

Contrast this with a biceps blaster from the Arnold era— straight-bar curls with 100 total pounds, an extreme weight for most men: $100 \times 8 \times 3 = 2,400$ total pounds

The workloads aren't identical: The 2,400 pounds of cumulative load from the bar curl has been applied in more of an isolated fashion, which is good for building strength and size. But if time is limited and you want your upper body to perform and look better, go with the weighted pull-ups—they're a more efficient all-around muscle builder.

### How can I strengthen my grip?

When it comes to grip strength, the rule of specificity applies; you need to train your gripping muscles to become stronger in the exercises in which they're weakest. Do this by altering your grip. If it fails quickly during chinups, for example, use a thumbless grip (grasp the bar with an overhand grip, but don't wrap your thumbs around it). Doing so will alter the angle of resistance and work different muscle fibers. The same goes for deadlifts or shrugs: Use a mixed grip (one hand palm up,

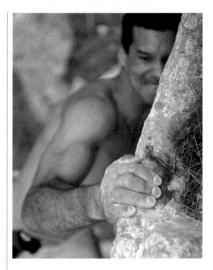

the other hand palm down) or a hook grip (in which you cover your thumb with your index and middle fingers). Your repetition count might decline initially while your muscles adapt to the new strain, but you'll know your grip is getting stronger when you can handle more weight in just a few weeks.

### Which grip attachment at the row machine should I use?

Depends on what you want. But before you worry about grips, master the fundamentals of the seated row. Sit upright with your knees bent, pushing your chest out and pulling your shoulders back while maintaining an upright torso throughout the move.

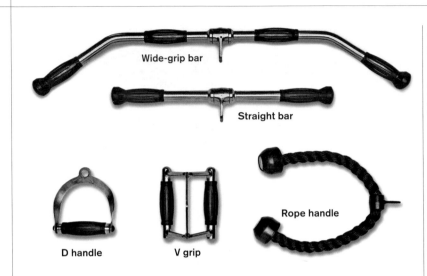

Wide-grip bar

Straight bar

Rope handle

D handle

V grip

"Rounding your lower back at any time during the exercise can cause injury," says Craig Ballantyne, CSCS, owner of www.turbulencetraining.com. The seated row trains your back (lats, rhomboids, and traps) and shoulders (deltoids), providing greater spine support. By changing the angle of your arms, these grip options target different areas of your back and shoulders.

*Wide-grip bar:* mid- and upper back, rear shoulders.

*Do it right:* The overhand wide grip is best for building the upper back. Cut the weight stack by 10 percent (compared with a straight bar) and pull toward your abdominals.

*Straight bar:* lower back, biceps.

*Do it right:* An overhand grip focuses the gains on your lower back. Narrow underhand (palms up) brings your biceps into play; add 10 to 20 percent more weight.

*D handle:* mid- and upper back, shoulders, biceps.

*Do it right:* Use it for single-arm seated rows. Sitting upright, grasp the handle with one hand. Without rotating your hips, row it toward your side at belly-button height.

*V grip:* midback.

*Do it right:* With your elbows in, draw your shoulder blades together and pull with your back. Bring the handle toward your belly, then slowly return to the starting position.

*Rope handle:* rear shoulders, upper back.

*Do it right:* The rope allows you to row the weight toward your upper chest without straining your shoulders. Do so as you pull your hands apart. Keep your elbows below shoulder height to avoid impingement.

### Is there a way to build my hamstrings without doing leg curls?

Try the keystone deadlift. It places the hamstrings in a slightly stretched position at the start and end of the move. "When a muscle is stretched, it can contract harder," says strongman C.J. Murphy, MFS, owner of www.totalperformancesports.com. It'll pay off in greater strength and flexibility throughout the entire posterior chain—that is, your hamstrings, glutes, and lower back. "If you do only leg curls, you get only one-third of the benefit; you neglect the other two muscle groups that contribute to speed, strength, and stability of the knee," says Murphy.

*Do it right:* Stand holding a barbell with an overhand grip, at arm's length in front of your thighs. Keep your knees slightly

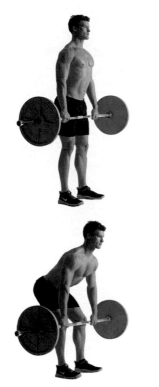

bent and your feet shoulder-width apart. Push your butt back and up by arching your back. This is the starting position. Without changing the angle of your knees, push your butt back as far as you can so the bar travels down your legs. (The bar should stay in contact with them throughout the move.)

As the bar reaches your knees, move your butt back as far as you can to stretch the hamstrings, then squeeze your glutes and drive your heels into the floor to reverse the move-ment back to the starting position. Do three sets of eight repetitions.

## Is there an exercise that will reduce the amount of time I need to spend training my legs?

Try the Bulgarian split deadlift. It develops all the major muscles of your lower body—so you don't need to bother with a clutter of leg exercises. The instability of the exercise (because it's done while standing on one leg) calls more muscle into play as you try to stay balanced, says Alwyn Cosgrove, CSCS, owner of Results Fitness, in Santa Clarita, California. Perform two or three sets of three to five repetitions to gain strength; do two sets of 8 to 12 reps to build muscle.

Place a loaded barbell on the

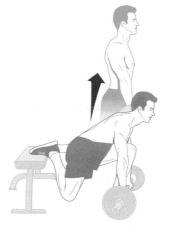

floor 2 to 3 feet in front of a bench. Facing away from the bench, place one foot on the floor so that your shin touches the barbell, and rest the instep of your other foot on the bench. Keeping most of your weight on your front leg, bend your front knee and lean forward to grab the bar with an overhand grip (palms down). This is the starting position. Lift the bar as you return to an upright stance, then return to the starting position. Complete your reps, then switch legs and repeat.

## Where should I look when I squat?

Look up. Look forward. Just don't look down. A recent study at Miami University in Ohio found that doing so can increase your forward lean by 4 to 5 degrees, increasing the likelihood of lower-back strain. Here's the best technique: Focus on a point directly in front of you, and hold that gaze as you lower your body (be sure to keep your back straight). When your thighs are parallel to the floor, pause; then return to the starting position. This will help you maintain proper form and get the most out of each rep.

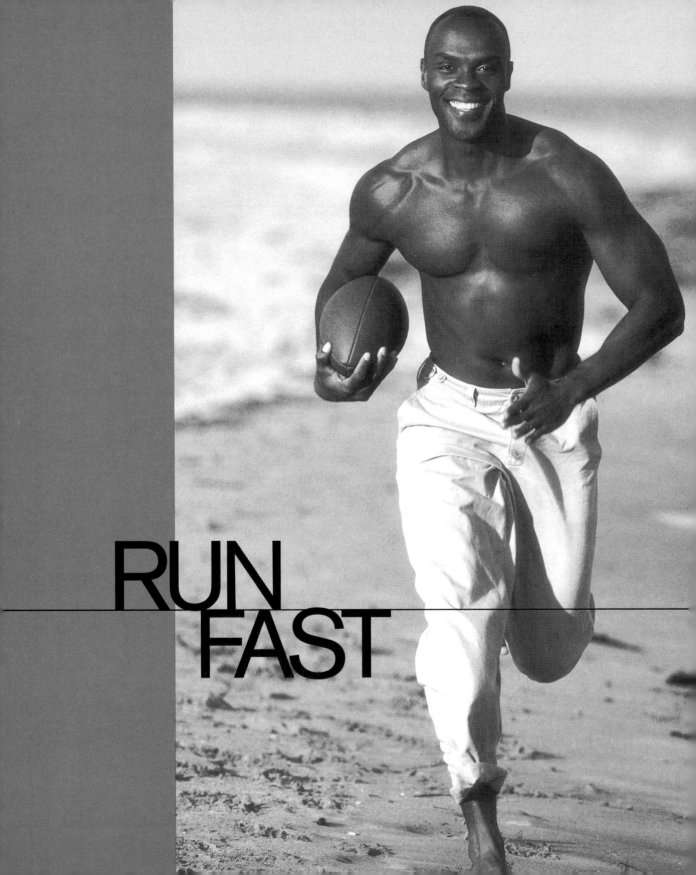

# RUN
## FAST

## PART FIVE

According to a survey by the National Sporting Goods Association, nearly 25 million Americans are active runners. That's a whole lot of feet pounding the pavement.

What gets you running? Perhaps you're running toward better health or after your kid or to stay ahead of the pit bull that lives next door. Whatever your purpose, running is one of the purest, simplest ways to work your body.

That's why we've dedicated this entire section to it. Here you'll read the story of one runner's quest to discover what really matters as he runs across the Sahara. You'll learn how to train for and run your first race—quite possibly slimming down, beating stress, and rewarding yourself with a huge dose of satisfaction in the process. Next, you'll find a troubleshooter's guide to the hazards of the road. You'll shore up your weak links by focusing on five form wreckers and the running rehab to fix them. Then, revolutionize your leg workout with the best exercise you're not doing. (It's the single-leg squat.)

With dozens of tips from running experts, we hope this section helps you to run wherever it is you're headed, faster than ever.

BY DONOVAN WEBSTER

# Transport Yourself

A portrait of one runner's quest
to discover what really matters

harlie Engle is 6 inches too short to have played North Carolina basketball alongside Michael Jordan. He's too honest and sincere to have become both America's top car salesman and a hit TV producer. He couldn't possibly have entered a 100-kilometer ultramarathon by accident—and won. And what's most unbelievable of all is the notion that this vital, accomplished 43-year-old used to spend weeks at a time holed up in cheap motels, burning through thousands of dollars in crack cocaine.

But every one of those things happened.

And on this morning in late 2005, with all of those lives trailing behind him, Charlie Engle is nothing more than a lonely speck on the horizon, the tiniest dot of dark clothing amid the rolling gold dunes and black, wind-scoured buttes of the Sahara in eastern Niger. Out here, in the belly of the world's largest desert—a barely habitable wasteland the size of the United States—Engle is busy exercising another of his gifts: his standing as one of the world's top endurance athletes. He's slowly and relentlessly trotting toward his support vehicles, getting used to the aridity and the gravelly sand beneath his feet.

And here's the strangest part. For Charlie Engle, this lope across the Sahara's dead zone isn't merely his next epic challenge; it's something he has to do to keep himself alive.

Seeing Charlie Engle today, with the Porsche Boxster, the Hermosa Beach bachelor pad, the pretty/smart/cool girlfriend, and the LA senior-producer title, it's

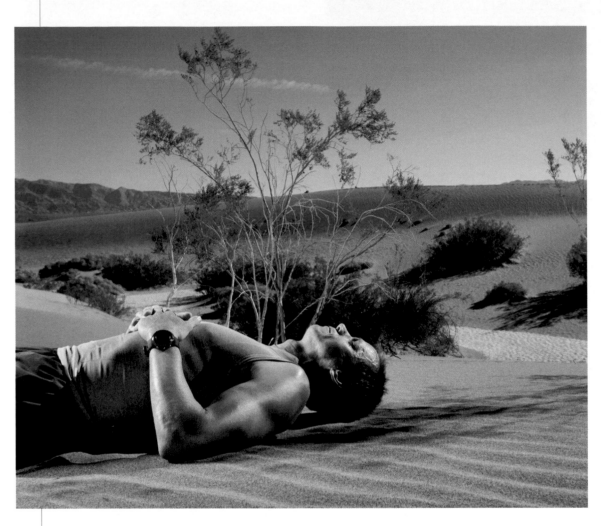

difficult to believe his life ever strayed very far from the golden-boy image he oozes. But there was a time, just over a decade ago, when Engle's idea of an endurance test was sitting alone in a crappy $14-a-night room at the edge of some blighted urban landscape, using beer as his sole food group and waiting for someone to bring him another crumbly pile of crack cocaine. Back then, the scope of his life had grown so small it could be cooked down in a glass bowl smaller than a thimble.

"It was all about smoking that rock; that's all I could think about," he says. "And what's amazing is, back at that time, I had no ability to see the thousands of little decisions that had put me there."

Like every golden boy, he had an advantageous start. He participated in North Carolina's Boys' State summer schools for exceptional students and captained his high-school football, track, and cross-country teams. By the time he arrived in Chapel Hill for college in 1980, Engle was playing junior-varsity basketball with Jordan under the tutelage of Dean Smith. "Charlie has always been really, really likable," says his father, Richard Engle. "Everybody's always wanted to help him, which, in his case, has proved both a blessing and a curse."

But after his sophomore year at North Carolina, Engle crashed. "After 2 years in JV, if you don't move up to varsity—which it was clear I wasn't going to do—that's all you get," he says. "I lost a connection to basketball, something I'd loved since I was a kid; it was then that my life began to unravel." Though he took up recreational running to fuel his exercise needs, he also began using copious amounts of drugs and alcohol and dealing on the side to support his habits. Alerted to the trouble by one of Charlie's frat brothers, Engle's father transplanted his son to Seattle, cleaned him up, and let him join the family business: buying and managing a series of Baskin-Robbins franchises along California's Monterey Peninsula. Soon, however, Engle was back to his old habits. Several times a week, he'd snatch $300 from his cash register, score a big pile of cocaine, sell some of the haul to defray his costs (replacing the original $300 in the till), and personally dispose of the rest of the drugs. "Eventually, I stopped selling a cut of the drugs to repay the money I'd taken, so the day soon came when I couldn't replace the $300," Engle says. "Then came a lot more days like that."

Within a couple of years, Engle was forced to sell his foundering franchise back to his father. "I gave it to my dad, really," he says. "Let's just say I left the ice-cream business ungracefully."

To prove himself after the ice-cream debacle, Engle took a job selling Toyotas in the peninsula town of Seaside. And, as in so many other corners of his life, it took no time at all for him to grow very good at it. "I had a unique sales technique," he says. "Naked honesty. Maybe I was trying to atone for my drug and alcohol behavior, but on the sales floor, I was so honest that my customers had no choice but to actually believe me. I'd ask, 'What do you need?' And they'd tell me. I'd say, 'No, you don't need that car, try this one, it's less expensive and just as good . . . ' The customers loved me for it."

In 1989, wielding his honesty shtick, Engle rocketed to the top of the salesman heap, ultimately snatching the company's national award for salesman of the year in Toyota's National Walk-Around competition.

But for the revived golden boy, darker clouds remained on the horizon. Although he had married and begun entering marathons, "I'd never really stopped using drugs," he says. "And really, this is the period when I started trying crack."

Soon after came a stint in rehab, but the cure didn't take for long. By the early 1990s, Engle had quit selling cars and gotten into the auto-dent-repair business, and it was booming. He was earning upward of $2,000 a day fixing dents at car dealerships while guiding a four- to eight-man work crew nonstop around the country: Denver, Orlando, Rapid City, Oklahoma City . . . you name it. In each place, he'd arrive, talk with

the owners of dealerships where he did most of his work, and casually ask, "What neighborhoods should I avoid?" Then, once he had sufficient cash in his pocket, he says, "those bad, drug-dealing neighborhoods would be my first stop. I was the boss, and when I'd disappear, my work crews kept the job going. They knew what I was doing, but they also knew a good thing when they saw it."

The whacked-out, crack-related stories start to spill out.

There was the time in Denver when, on a crack bender and out of cash, Engle offered his Toyota 4Runner to his drug dealer as collateral. When the dealer didn't return with the car after a few days, Engle—unable to pay the $14-a-day hotel tab—was forced onto the street. "So there I was. I'd been awake for about 6 days. There was a foot of

snow on the ground. I didn't even have a coat, and I was out of money for my room. So I just began walking around Denver."

After a few hours of aimlessly wandering the streets, Engle confronted a miracle. Up the street, sitting in the driveway of a house, with the keys in the ignition and the engine running, sat his Toyota. "I thought, 'Unbelievable,'" he says. "It's definitely my car; same license plates and everything. So I took it back. I just climbed in, backed it down the driveway, and drove off."

He'd gotten three blocks when he heard a baby crying behind him. Turning, Engle looked toward the backseat. Sure enough: an infant.

"So I turned the car around and drove back to the house where I'd found it. There was this black woman in the street—God, she looked terrified, distraught; her arms flying up and down—and she saw my car coming back. I stopped the car right in front of her. Without saying a word, she opened the back door, got the baby, and shut the door. It was a totally wordless exchange. And I drove away."

Finally, one night in Wichita, Kansas, Engle hit the end of his string. "I'd spent 6 days smoking about $4,000 in crack. I could no longer leave my hotel room. I was totally paranoid: watching the shadows out in the hallway by looking under the door, fearing somebody might be right outside. Once again, I'd given my car to the dealers, and they'd left with it—and they'd been gone for about 2 days."

Knowing on a subconscious level that he

had to change his life, Engle called the police. "I reported my car stolen," he says.

The police informed Engle that they'd found his car—with four bullet holes in it. "So I go there," he says, "and the police had found a crack pipe under the driver's seat. It was one of my crack pipes. At first, I thought: 'Hey, I hope there's some crack left in there,' but when the police asked, 'Is this yours?' I said, 'No, of course not.'"

That was when he realized how pointless his life had become. "I was sitting there, on the curb, waiting for the police to finish checking my car, and I knew it was now or never. I knew that, because of crack, I was going to die soon. And I said this prayer quietly but out loud: 'Please remove this craving; I'll do anything, just please remove this craving . . .' And it happened, just like that. I began going to AA meetings again. I was in Wichita, with nothing to prove to anybody except myself. But now I really wanted to be sober. And from that day to today, I've never had a craving again."

Engle had been sober about a year—and he and his wife, Pam, had had two sons in 20 months—when fate grabbed him again. He was prospering and now had his eight-man crew helping him undent cars worldwide, from the Midwest to Singapore. He was also training hard at running when, during a several-month stint in Australia, he saw a weekend race advertised and thought he might enter.

Unfortunately, he misread the advertisement. Instead of being a 10-kilometer race, it was 100 kilometers. "It was called the Nanango Rainforest Ultra," he says. "When I showed up for it and realized my mistake, I thought, 'Why not?' I decided to try doing the race . . . and I won!"

Engle had found his calling. In less than 2 years, he'd shifted from the blue-flamed heat of drug-and-alcohol addiction to a burning desire to be the best endurance athlete on the planet. He began competing in triathlons (he's since been in more than 100), as well as marathons and ultramarathons, clawing his way up the ladder of endurance-racing success and gaining commercial endorsements at each new rung.

"In some ways," he says, "drug addiction and endurance sports are similar; they both take you to this strange place, far outside usual reality. But it's more complex than that. Drug addiction and alcoholism take you in a very dark, confining direction; endurance sports always transport you to a new landscape, a new part of the world, where you embrace the outdoors with other people. You learn to go past what you thought your limits were . . . which is very different than being locked in some $14-a-night room, waiting for your next delivery of crack."

Over the past decade, Engle has competed in endurance races on four continents. He's won the Jungle Marathon of the Amazon in Brazil and the Gobi March in northern China, and he's finished among the top five in adventure races or ultramarathons in Costa Rica, New Zealand, and Chile.

Around the same time, with his athletic star on the rise (and his troubled marriage over), the CBS News program *48 Hours* came to Engle with a proposition: Would he consider carrying a small handheld video camera across the entire Eco-Challenge Borneo race, filming his ordeal for the program's viewers? Without hesitating, Engle said yes.

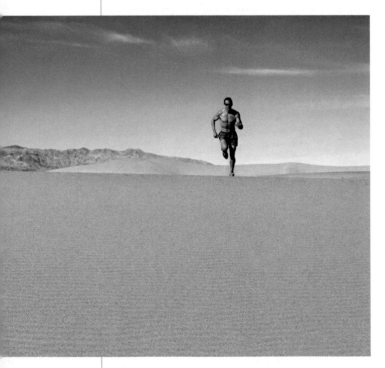

The race director was an up-and-coming TV producer named Mark Burnett, who scoffed at the idea of Engle carrying a camera. "He'll never finish the race with it," Burnett wagered. This was precisely the fire Engle needed. He arrived at the finish line 10 days later, his camera still running. Along the way, as he'd slogged through the jungle, slid down muddy hillsides, and paddled the sea off Borneo in withering sun and the clammy dark of night, a lonely and miserable Charlie Engle had told the camera the whole, agonizing story of his addiction and redemption.

Sensing they had something unique, CBS paid for Engle to visit New York City and watch the show with Dan Rather and the *48 Hours* crew on the night of its screening. "I'll never forget it," Engle says. "When I walked into the editing booth, I got a standing ovation from people I'd never met before. They'd all been watching, like, 30 hours of my tape for weeks, getting it ready for broadcast. And this one guy, Mike Malloy, who was the head of editing, said to me, 'You're crazy if you don't make a career out of this.'"

Engle did. He began traveling to California for extended stays, sleeping on couches and working the edges of the entertainment industry with his handheld-camera approach. By late 2003, Malloy and *48 Hours* producer Tom Forman had also decamped to join Endemol, one of the largest producers of reality-TV programming in Los Angeles, and they hired Engle for their new show: *Extreme Makeover:*

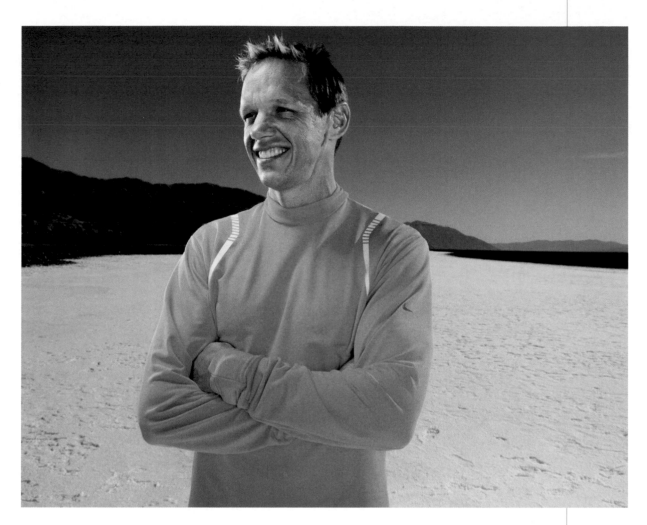

*Home Edition*. It quickly became a block-buster.

Engle often worked 18- to 20-hour days, catching naps in the production bus between events, and he rose from lowly camera guy to senior producer. "I was still training hard, though," he says. "I'd get done with an 18-hour day of shooting and, instead of going home and going to sleep, I'd put on my running stuff, still at the job site, and go off on a 2-hour run. Fact is, I needed to run more than I needed to sleep."

Out here in the middle of the Sahara, Charlie Engle is closing in on his life's dream. He's now only a half mile from where his expedition staff members sit in their air-conditioned Toyota Land Cruisers. His gray shirt is lined with sweat; he holds a water bottle in his left hand and a digital video camera in his right, filming as he goes. As he gets closer with every step, it's obvious he's thoroughly enjoying himself, letting the desert morning wash over him.

In the desert's quiet, Engle gives a whoop

across the sand, and one of the expedition crew members—a tall, blue-robed Tuareg tribesman named Adoua Mohamed—can't contain himself. Adoua stands and, with a strange pogolike gait, runs out to meet Engle. They trot toward and then past the vehicles, heading off into the still deeper desert while barely slowing to acknowledge the cars in the midst of this huge sand sea. Finally, as he sees Engle has no interest in stopping, Adoua slows to a walk while Engle continues alone.

"It just feels too good to stop right now," Engle says, turning and yelling back as he leaves the team behind. "Drive ahead of me another 10 miles or so, so I can follow your tire tracks . . . I'll just keep going until I get tired."

That could be a long, long time.

BY SARA WELLS

# Hit the Pavement

To slim down, beat stress, and reward yourself
with a huge dose of satisfaction, train for
and run your first race

**B**ill Bowerman had a name for anyone who laces up running shoes and hits the pavement: hamburger.

Bowerman was the famed University of Oregon running coach who transformed the Ducks into a distance powerhouse and is credited with igniting recreational running in America.

And he loved hamburgers.

"They are never going to run any record times," he said of the hamburgers on his team, "but they can fulfill their own potential."

And in that statement is the unequivocal appeal of this purest of individual sports. Every time you run, it's just you—body and mind—plus time and distance. Condiments optional.

How far do you go? It's up to you.

How fast do you go? Up to you.

Do you even go?

No one is chasing you. You have to want to run. You have to want to test your potential. But allow us to give you a little nudge by sharing some new research about the health and antiaging benefits of running.

**You'll live longer.** Danish researchers studying more than 4,000 men for 5 years found that regular joggers were 34 percent less likely than nonrunners to die of any cause.

**You'll reduce your risk of heart disease.** Results from the National Runners' Health Study of 8,290 men showed that participants' risk of a heart attack decreased dramatically with each 10-mile increment in weekly running distance.

**You'll be smarter.** A recent German study found that runners who jogged for 30 minutes at least twice a week improved their concentration and visual memory. The researchers compared the joggers' ability to recall images and complete visual tasks with that of the control group and found that the runners made far fewer mistakes than the nonjoggers.

**You'll stay harder.** Researchers at Harvard University looked at the sex lives of 31,742 men ages 50 and up. They found that men who ran at least 3 hours a week had a 30 percent lower risk of erectile dysfunction than those who got little or no exercise.

**You'll be happier.** Psychiatrists at Duke University studying the effects of exercise on mental illness concluded that rigorous exercise is even more effective at lifting mood than Zoloft and other antidepressants. But it has to be tough, push-yourself-hard exercise, not jogging a slow mile and calling it a day.

## PAINkiller

**Sometimes after an extremely difficult workout, my chest feels sore. Is my diaphragm just tired from working so hard?**

What you're probably feeling is the result of oxygen debt—your body isn't getting enough oxygen—which causes the already overworked muscles around the lungs, including the diaphragm, to become flush with lactic acid. Your lungs and diaphragm work closely together, but they're distinct parts of the body. The diaphragm, the muscle that separates your chest from your abdominal region and expands your lungs, can be trained. Keep exercising to develop your aerobic conditioning—running intervals will help—and the burn should disappear.

## Perfect Form

Run efficiently and you'll go farther before getting tired. "The key is to hold yourself together, maintain good posture, and not let yourself get sloppy," says exercise physiologist Greg McMillan. Practice perfect form, as detailed below, so it'll feel natural by the time you start training for the half marathon.

Your eyes should look straight ahead, not down at your feet. Run "tall" with your head over your shoulders, your shoulders over your hips, and your hips over your feet.

Keep your shoulders relaxed. Don't let them creep up toward your ears as you tire. If they do, shake them out to release tension.

Don't hunch, or your pelvis will tilt forward as well, which can put pressure on your lower back and throw the rest of your lower body out of alignment.

No tight fists. Keep your hands relaxed, as if you're cupping a tiny bird.

Don't lift your knees too high; it'll wear you out quickly. Instead, flex your knees slightly so they bend naturally upon impact. The proper stride length is one in which your feet land directly below your body.

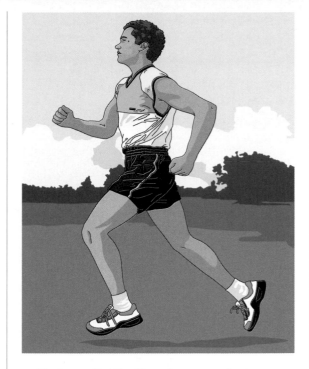

Try to run lightly. If you hear your feet slapping the pavement, you're overstriding. Shorten up.

Your arms should move forward and backward in line, not side to side. Your elbows should be bent at 90-degree angles.

**You'll win nice trophies.** Running is something you can get better at with age. When Yale University researchers compared the race times of masters runners with those in other age groups over a 16-year period, they found that the older runners improved their running times at a greater rate than the younger athletes did.

Have we convinced you that getting back into running can be pretty damn rewarding healthwise? Here's something more: It also delivers a sense of accomplishment, especially when you've crossed the finish line of your first race.

So sign up for a race. Now. Even before you start training. Studies have shown that exercisers who have measurable, deadline-oriented goals (like that 5-K in town next month) are more successful at sticking with a training program than guys who work out without putting their goals in writing.

Even if the last time you laced up running shoes was 20 years ago in gym class, you can become a runner. You can easily finish a 5-K (that's just 3.1 miles) or a 10-K after 4 weeks of training, and believe it or not, with just a little more effort, you can complete your first half marathon in just 12 weeks.

You heard right: a half marathon, 13 miles, 192$^1/_2$ yards. It's a challenging distance, sure, but it has serious health benefits, above and beyond those you get training for shorter races. Remember that study of 8,290 men? It found that those who ran 50 miles or more per week reduced their risk of hypertension by 50 percent and required less medication to control their blood pressure. It seems the greater benefits come from upping the intensity of the run. Train for the half marathon, and you will be pushing yourself enough to reap grand health rewards but won't be overdoing it and risking boredom, burnout, or injury. That's because you have to run only 3 days a week, leaving yourself plenty of time to

spend on the rest of your life. "This plan is for the guy who's not a runner yet and therefore needs to build up slowly, but who's likely to get bored if he has to run every day," says marathoner Matt Fitzgerald, author of *Performance Nutrition for Runners.*

## Getting Started

All you need are the right pair of shoes (see "Cinderella Story" on page 282) and some comfortable clothing. While it doesn't matter what you wear, always dress for a run as if it's 10°F warmer outside. This way you're dressed for how warm you'll feel at midrun, not the first mile, when your body is still heating up.

The key is to start slowly and gradually build endurance. Trying to do too much too fast is the number one mistake beginners make, says Greg McMillan, an exercise physiologist and certified track-and-field coach. (His Web site, www.mcmillanrunning.com, offers personalized training.) "Injuries occur when runners push themselves to increase their mileage or speed too quickly."

To avoid injury, first assess your fitness level. If regular exercise isn't part of your routine, you need to start with walking: 3 days a week for 20 to 30 minutes, with five 1-minute easy jogs scattered throughout. (Easy means you're not gasping for breath.) "This will get your legs used to the impact very, very gradually," says Fitzgerald. When you can comfortably complete this workout, increase the jogging intervals by half-minute increments and decrease the walking breaks until you're running the whole time.

The next step—or the first if you're in good aerobic shape—is to start increasing the duration of the runs. "The idea is to challenge yourself until you can run for 50 to 60 minutes," says McMillan.

Start running for 20 minutes 3 days a week at an easy pace. If you still need to take walking breaks, that's okay. "You don't want to get out of breath during these runs; if you do, you're going too fast," says McMillan. In fact, pushing the pace doesn't mean you're getting a better workout. Research shows that if you can carry on a conversation while training (known as the talk test), then your heart and breathing rates are within your target aerobic zone; if you're huffing and puffing, you're running too hard.

When you feel like you could continue running for another 10 to 20 minutes, lengthen two of the runs. For example, you might run 20 minutes on Monday, 25 minutes on Wednesday, and 30 minutes on Friday; the next week it could be 20, 30, and 35 minutes. Once you can run for about 50 minutes, you can start training in earnest.

## Preventing Injury

Following the guide above will ease you into running and help you avoid injuries, but there are other measures you should take to prevent aches and pains. Most important after getting properly fitted for shoes: Always warm up. This doesn't mean just a few stretches but, rather, a slow walk/easy run for 5 to 10 minutes, long enough to break a sweat. Be sure to cool down afterward, too.

Vary the terrain so you're not always pounding the hard pavement. This is especially crucial if you have back pain, in which case you should try to do most of your running on grass, trails, tracks, and treadmills to soften the force of impact. The half-marathon plan you're about to start incorporates cross-training and weight training, which will make you a stronger, healthier runner while giving your primary running muscles a rest, says Fitzgerald. In addition, our plan includes a weekly speed workout. A 2002 study shows that speed work can reduce risk of injury by almost 50 percent.

## The Plan, in Detail

Now that you're comfortable running about 5 miles, follow the training schedule outlined in the chart on page 279. Here's a detailed explanation.

**The long run:** This Sunday run is the most important of the three runs that you will do. The runs start at 4 miles, increasing in distance each week—with the exception of weeks 4, 7, and 10, which are recovery weeks—and work up to 12 miles right before race day. "Do this run at an honest pace—an intensity level of 6 or 7 on a scale of 1 to 10," says Fitzgerald. "But the most important thing is to make it through the prescribed distance."

Also, use the long runs to practice taking in fluids. Carry a water bottle or stash a few bottles along the course beforehand. "You should take a swig of water or sports drink every mile or every 10 minutes," Fitzgerald says. "Don't guzzle. Just listen to your body."

**The hard run:** This Wednesday interval workout is designed to make you a more efficient runner. Start with an easy 5- to 10-minute warmup. Then do four to six hard runs of 1 to $1^1/_2$ minutes each, separated by jogs of the same duration. Cool

down with another 5 minutes of light jogging. Try to run these at an effort level of about 8 with the recovery jogs at level 4 or 5. "This workout should be hard, but you want to stay relaxed. You should be able to finish the last interval at the same pace at which you started the first one. If you start out like a bat out of hell, you're not going to be able to maintain that pace," says Fitzgerald.

**The maintenance run:** This 4- to 6-mile run on Friday maintains your base level of fitness. Again, run at a steady effort level—6 to 7 on a scale of 1 to 10.

**The cardio workout:** Once a week, do some form of low- or nonimpact cardiovascular workout for at least 20 to 40 minutes. The elliptical trainer is the best cross-training option for a runner because it works many of the same muscles running does. Bicycling, deepwater running, swimming, and stair climbing are other good options.

**The strength workout:** "Most running injuries are caused by instability at key joints, like the hips, pelvis, and knees," says Fitzgerald. "You need to lift to strengthen your muscles to the point where they can stabilize your joints properly." Plus, powerful muscles allow you to take longer, quicker strides. You can do any exercises you want, but focus on those that strengthen the legs, abs, and back.

**The 5-K and 10-K:** Not only are these races interim goals that'll keep you running, but "these are also dress rehearsals for the half marathon," says McMillan. "Use them to practice your routine so nothing goes

## PAINkiller

### How do I get rid of side stitches?

Get your diaphragm under control. It's spasming, probably as a result of your taking short, shallow breaths, running too soon after you eat, or neglecting to build strong core muscles, says Lorenzo Gonzalez, a physical therapist in New York City and an athletic trainer for several NFL players.

If a stitch strikes midrun, slow your pace and focus on belly breathing, expanding your stomach as you inhale and contracting your abs as you exhale. If that doesn't work, apply pressure to the problem area while pursing your lips and exhaling forcefully. "That will stretch your diaphragm and ease the pressure," says Gonzalez. To prevent spasms, follow these tips.

**Run on empty.** Avoid eating foods that require heavy digestion (meats, fats, cheeses) for 2 to 3 hours before you run. "Otherwise, your body will send blood to your stomach and intestines rather than to your diaphragm and respiratory muscles," says Gonzalez. Do, however, drink plenty of fluids—6 to 8 ounces for every 20 minutes of exercise. Muscles spasm when they're dehydrated.

**Support your organs.** Stitches can also result from the jostling of internal organs, including your liver, pancreas, and intestines. Support them by strengthening your inner abdominal muscles with this exercise: Lie on your back with knees bent and feet flat on the floor. Place a Swiss ball between your knees, then tighten your abs and lift your pelvis until it's in line with your knees. Hold for 2 seconds, then lower the ball. Do three sets of 15 reps three times per week for a month.

# 12-Week Half-Marathon Training Plan

| WEEK | SUN | MON | TUES | WED | THURS | FRI | SAT |
|------|-----|-----|------|-----|-------|-----|-----|
| 1 | 4-mile run | Rest | Strength workout | Intervals (4 × 30 seconds) | Rest or strength workout | 4-mile run | Nonimpact cardio |
| 2 | 5-mile run | Rest | Strength workout | Intervals (5 × 30 seconds) | Rest or strength workout | 4-mile run | Nonimpact cardio |
| 3 | 6-mile run | Rest | Strength workout | Intervals (6 × 30 seconds) | Rest or strength workout | 4-mile run | Nonimpact cardio |
| 4 | 5-mile run | Rest | Strength workout | Intervals (4 × 30 seconds) | Rest or strength workout | 4-mile run | Nonimpact cardio |
| 5 | 7-mile run | Rest | Strength workout | Intervals (5 × 30 seconds) | Rest or strength workout | 5-mile run | Nonimpact cardio |
| 6 | 8-mile run | Rest | Strength workout | Intervals (5 × 30 seconds) | 5-mile run | Rest | 5-K race |
| 7 | 6-mile run | Rest | Strength workout | Intervals (4 × 30 seconds) | Rest or strength workout | 5-mile run | Nonimpact cardio |
| 8 | 9-mile run | Rest | Strength workout | Intervals (5 × 30 seconds) | Rest or strength workout | 5-mile run | Nonimpact cardio |
| 9 | 10-mile run | Rest | Strength workout | Intervals (6 × 30 seconds) | 6-mile run | Rest | 10-K race |
| 10 | 6-mile run | Rest | Strength workout | Intervals (5 × 30 seconds) | Rest or strength workout | 6-mile run | Nonimpact cardio |
| 11 | 11-mile run | Rest | Strength workout | Intervals (6 × 30 seconds) | Rest or strength workout | 6-mile run | Nonimpact cardio |
| 12 | 12-mile run | Rest | Strength workout | 4-mile run | Nonimpact cardio | Rest | Half-marathon race day |

wrong in the big race." They'll help you decide on the most appropriate clothing and the best foods to eat before the longer race. Shorter races also help you figure out your pace. "You need to learn to distribute your effort across a race," says McMillan. For instance, if you run the 10-K in 49:43—an 8-minute-mile pace—you should be able to finish the half in 1:49, or about an 8:22 pace per mile. "If you're motivated by numbers, having a goal pace will help you train better," says Fitzgerald.

BY SARA WELLS

# Beware!

## A troubleshooter's guide to the hazards of the road

I've been beaned in the head with a pack of cigarettes thrown from a car, forced off the road by a Ford Excursion that didn't see me, and flashed by a man wearing nothing but a ski mask. I've had to deal with ankle twists from potholes and glass in my Asics and have been chased by all manner of animals, from angry dogs to curious skunks and ground-hogs. The road can be a dangerous place for runners. But that's no excuse to miss a workout. Here's a troubleshooter's guide to the most common running hazards.

## SUV vs. YOU

**Rule #1:** Run against the flow of traffic, on the left side of the road, so you'll see cars coming at you.

**Rule #2:** Never assume a driver sees you. When you need to cross, make eye contact with the driver and wait to be waved on. Also, cross behind the first car at a crosswalk, rather than in front of it.

**Rule #3:** When running at night, wear a flashing light and shoes and clothes bearing reflective stripes. According to AAA tests, drivers can clearly see reflective strips from 700 feet, more than twice the length of a football field. In comparison, they can see fluorescent clothing only from 100 feet.

## Bad Dog

If a dog gives chase, the best thing to do is stop running, make a quarter turn, and walk away, says Dennis Fetko, PhD, an animal behaviorist and trainer. "By changing your body orientation slightly, you let the dog know in a nonthreatening way that you know he's there and that you're prepared to defend yourself if he attacks," 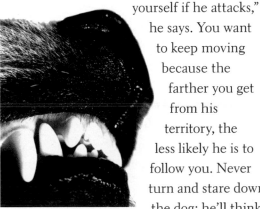 he says. You want to keep moving because the farther you get from his territory, the less likely he is to follow you. Never turn and stare down the dog; he'll think you want to attack him. For extra protection, carry a bottle of Spray Shield (formerly known as Direct Stop; about $10). When sprayed in a dog's face, it overwhelms him with the scent of citronella, disorienting him for 30 seconds or so.

## A Pain in the Knee

Switch to the other side of the road. Changing the angle of the road surface (most streets slope slightly) will relieve pressure on your knee. If that doesn't help, move to a more yielding surface, like a dirt path, which isn't as hard as asphalt, says Richard Braver, DPM, a sports podiatrist in New Jersey. Still feeling pain? Stop running and sit down with your legs straight in front of you. Tighten your quads for 2 seconds, then release. Repeat five times. "This helps squeeze out excess fluid around the knee-cap, which may be causing pain, and releases synovial fluid, which lubricates the knee to reduce pain," says Braver. If the knee still hurts, walk home. Consider seeing your doctor.

## A Blister

If you start to feel a hot spot, stop running and suss out the irritant. Is it a wrinkle in your sock? Is your shoe too tight? Fix it by adjusting your sock or removing the shoe's insole (it'll make the shoe feel roomier).

If you already have a blister, gently pop it and drain the fluid, but leave the skin intact as a protective covering, says Braver. Take off your other sock and wear it over the sock

## Cinderella Story

### How to find the perfect shoe and proper fit

Each foot strike during a run shocks your legs with pressure equal to four to five times your total body weight. For a 170-pound man, that's 680 to 850 pounds of pressure on each leg, every stride. Need a better reason to spend time choosing good running shoes?

To get the best shoe, you need to know your foot type. Identify yours with the "wet test." Pour just enough water to cover the bottom of a shallow pan. Step into the pan, then onto a blank piece of heavy paper. Step off and observe the shape of your foot.

If you can see about half of your arch imprinted on the paper, you can wear almost any shoe but will probably do best in a stability shoe, which provides moderate arch support.

If you can see most of your foot in that wet footprint, you probably overpronate: Your foot hits the ground, and your arch collapses inward too much, increasing your risk of shin splints and runner's knee. You'll do best in either a motion-control shoe, which provides firm support to limit your foot's range of motion, or a stability shoe.

If you see almost no arch, you most likely underpronate: Your arch doesn't collapse enough to absorb the pounding, and too much shock can travel up your legs. A neutral-cushioned shoe, which has a soft midsole and no added stability devices, is your best bet.

Once you've taken the wet test, head to a specialty running store, to be fitted for the right shoe.

"The best time to go is late afternoon, because your feet swell over the course of the day," says Warren Greene, special projects editor at our brother magazine *Runner's World*. Test several pairs of shoes—the store should have a treadmill for this purpose—before making your pick. Expect to pay at least $85 for a good pair of shoes, says Greene.

on the blistered foot for added protection. When you get home, apply an antibiotic cream. Minimize this problem in the future by wearing synthetic or Teflon-coated socks or using a skin lube to reduce friction.

### A Side Stitch

Continue running, but slow down. Contract your abs and rib muscles, then take a deep breath in and out through pursed lips. Repeat. This forces you to more fully activate your breathing muscles. "If that doesn't work, stop, bend over, and retie your shoes. This helps to relax the breathing muscles," says exercise physiologist Greg McMillan. "Then resume running at an easy pace, focusing on keeping your body relaxed." Next time out, avoid a stitch by making sure you're hydrated and not running on a full stomach.

### Neutral-Cushioned

**Brooks Radius 6 ($85):** The Radius is best suited for underpronators (guys with high arches) who need maximum midfoot cushioning with minimal arch support. Brooks increased the number of flex grooves in the forefoot and repositioned some of the grooves under the heel to better disperse impact shock.

### Motion Control

**Asics GEL-Evolution II ($110):** This shoe is recommended for runners with average to large builds (over 165 pounds) who are moderate to severe over-pronators and need a well-cushioned, supportive shoe. It provides maximum rear-foot control and extra support in the arch to help prevent injuries.

### Stability

**Saucony Grid Hurricane 8 ($125):** This is a great shoe for mild to moderate overpronators with normal to low arches who need a blend of cushioning and stability with moderate arch support. It features a substantial medial (inner) side for better stability and added cushioning foam in the heel and forefoot for a softer ride.

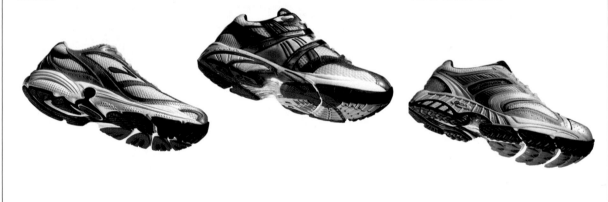

## Lightning

If you can't get inside a building, head for a car or other fully enclosed structure (partially open structures are no good), says Mary Ann Cooper, MD, head of the Lightning Injury Research Program at the University of Illinois at Chicago. Avoid open spots, because you could be the tallest thing in the area; stay away from water and tall objects, including trees.

To figure out how close lightning is (in miles), count the number of seconds between the lightning and the thunder, then divide by five. Right before lightning strikes, you may feel your hair stand on end or hear some staticky noise.

## Get a Leg Up

These variations on the classic Romanian deadlift, which range from the easy waiter's bow to the difficult core Romanian deadlift 2, from strength coach Carter Hays, CSCS, will improve hamstring strength and endurance and strengthen your core. Before the deadlifts, perform the waiter's bow to loosen your hamstrings and lower back—two areas often tight for men. Athlete's bonus: This stretch helps golfers, soccer and tennis players, and other athletes by building lower-back strength and increasing balance and single-leg stability.

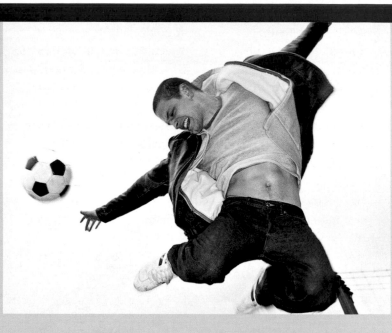

### Waiter's Bow

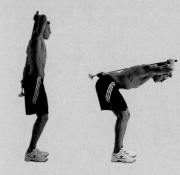

Hold a broomstick vertically against your back. Keep your knees slightly bent and your back arched naturally as you bend forward at the hips. The stick should stay in contact with your head, back, and butt. Pause just before the stick lifts off your butt. Hold the stretch for 20 seconds, then return to a standing position. Repeat the stretch two more times.

### Core Romanian Deadlift 1

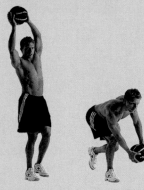

Stand on your right leg, holding a medicine ball over your right shoulder. Push your hips back and bring the ball down toward the inside of your right leg. Pause when your torso is as close to parallel to the floor as possible, making sure it's not too rounded or flattened. Then reverse the move. Do 12 repetitions, then repeat the move on the left side.

### Core Romanian Deadlift 2

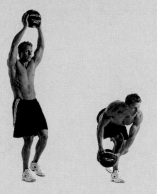

Perform this exercise exactly like the core Romanian deadlift 1 (described at left), but add this tweak to make it harder. Start with the ball over your left shoulder. Sweep down and across your body with the ball as you bend over. This will improve your balance, coordination, flexibility, and strength. Perform 12 repetitions on each side.

# Shore Up Your Weak Links

Good form can be difficult to achieve if certain muscles aren't strong enough. Five culprits and the running rehab to fix them

**H**ere's how five common weak points affect your body, plus the exercises to fix the problems.

## Weak Deltoids

**The effect:** shrugged shoulders. "These muscles are critical to maintaining a runner's arm mechanics and proper form," says Jonas Holdeman, track coach at McMillan Running Company.

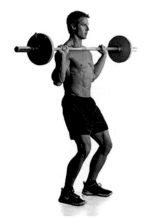

**The fix:** Activate your deltoids. Rest a barbell on the front of your shoulders, arms in. Lower yourself a few inches, then immediately drive up with your legs and thrust the weight toward the ceiling. Slowly return to the starting position. Do three or four sets of six to eight reps.

## Weak Midback

**The effect:** rounded shoulders. "Poor posture throws off lower-body alignment," says Scott Jurek, a seven-time Western States Endurance Run champion and coach. You waste energy and risk injury.

**The fix:** Target your middle and lower trapezius muscles. Hold a dumbbell at your

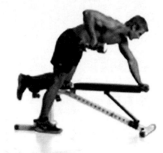

side with your arm hanging just in front of your shoulder. Keep your back flat, and use your back muscles to pull the weight up and toward your hip, elbow in. Pause, then return to the starting position. Do three or four sets of six to eight reps.

## Weak Buttocks

**The effect:** unstable legs. Your glutes "stabilize the hip and pelvis when you're driving forward on one leg," says Jurek.

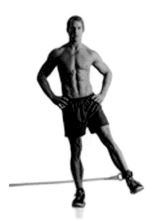

**The fix:** standing abductions. Stand sideways with your outside leg strapped to a low-pulley cable, slightly in front of your other leg. Pull it away from your body as far as you can without shifting your torso. Pause, then slowly return. Finish 15 reps with that leg, then repeat with the other leg.

## Adidas adiStar GCS Shoes

Sports like football, soccer, and lacrosse require quick lateral cuts, but most shoes aren't made to support side-to-side shuffling. This pair's insoles feature impact-dampening pods. Inside each pod, independently moving plates adjust with each step to absorb shock and support your ankles. $100. adidas.com

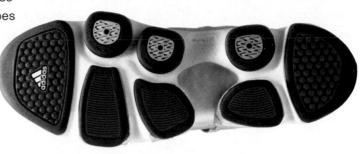

## Weak Hip Flexors

**The effect:** poor knee lift and leg drive. "Minimizing ground contact enhances speed," says Holdeman. "And strong hips help propel you forward against gravity."

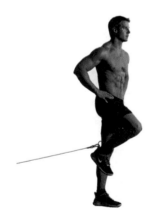

**The fix:** Mimic the upward drive of your knee. Strap one ankle to the low-pulley cable on a cable machine. Stand facing away from the weight stack about a foot behind you and slowly drive your weighted leg up to mimic a sprinting motion. Complete three or four sets of six to eight repetitions.

## PAINkiller

**My foot hurts under the arch when I'm out for a run. What's the problem here? Do I need to hang up my shoes for awhile?**

You might be suffering from plantar fasciitis, a repetitive-stress injury to the connective tissues of the foot. One telltale symptom: The pain sets in when you get out of bed in the morning but subsides as you go about your day.

Try thoroughly stretching the calf muscles before a run or rolling a golf ball with the underside of your foot to warm up the ligaments. A tweak to the basic standing calf stretch against a wall—move your back leg inward and point your toes toward the opposite heel—loosens the peroneal muscles of your lower leg, which pull on your foot when they're tight. The tighter they are, the more unevenly your foot will land on the ground, causing inflammation of the plantar fascia. After

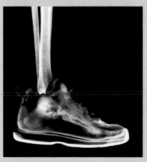

your run, take anti-inflammatories and ice the arch of the foot. You can also vary the stress by training in different shoes and on different surfaces. If the pain continues, you might need an x-ray to look for a hairline fracture. Remember, pain is the body's way of telling you to stop, so have it checked out before serious damage is done.

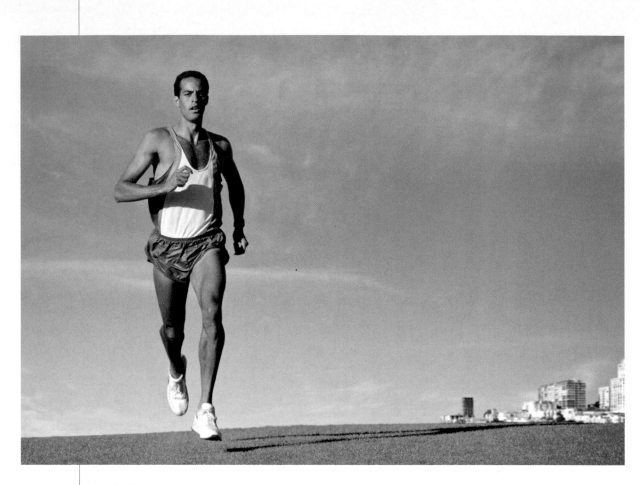

## Weak Core

**The effect:** a forward lean. "Keep your center of mass on a level plane, or you'll weaken progressively during the run," says Holdeman.

**The fix:** Not crunches; you want abdominal stabilization exercises, which involve all your core muscles. Try the bridge. Your body should form a straight line from head to

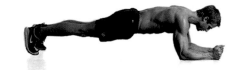

heels, as shown; don't let your back sag. Contract your abs and hold this position for 20 to 60 seconds, breathing steadily. Then relax.

# Revolutionize Your Leg Workout

## This is the best exercise you're not doing

### BY ALWYN COSGROVE, CSCS

As a trainer, I've witnessed some amazing things in the gym, most of which involved 300-pound powerlifters moving weight equal to that of a small SUV. (There was also the adult-film star I trained who had an orgasm every time she did hanging leg raises, but that's another story.)

The most impressive feat I've ever seen, though, came courtesy of a 160-pound guy named Steve Cotter. Steve's a martial artist, and one day he did a dozen single-leg squats while holding an 88-pound kettlebell in each hand. If that doesn't sound particularly jaw-dropping, try doing one—without any weights.

And therein lies an important point: Despite the plethora of gym equipment available, some of the greatest exercises remain the ones you can do with just your body weight—for instance, the single-arm pullup and the handstand pushup. Or the lower-body version, the best movement to build leg strength and improve athletic performance: the full-range, rock-bottom, single-leg squat.

So, while you may not be the strongest guy in the gym, you can still turn heads by banging out a set of single-leg squats. And the attention is just a side benefit. Master this one exercise, and you'll see gains in strength, speed, and balance. You'll squat more weight, jump higher, and discover athletic ability you never had before. The best part: You can do it all without setting foot in a gym.

## Test Your Best

To determine your training plan, do as many single-leg squats as you can. If you aren't able to perform at least two repetitions flawlessly, note the spot during your descent at which you can't control your speed of movement. This is your "breaking point"—and you'll need to know it to complete the routine. Once you've finished the test, proceed to the workout here that most closely matches your maximum effort.

**SINGLE-LEG SQUAT**

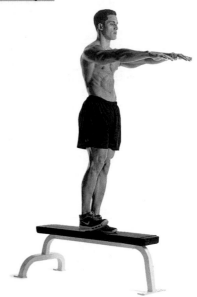

**Stand on a bench or box that's about knee height. Hold your arms in front of you and flex your right ankle so your toes are higher than your heel.**

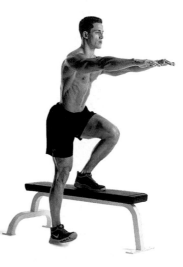

**Keeping your torso as upright as possible, bend your left knee and slowly lower your body until your right heel lightly touches the floor. Pause for 1 second, then push yourself up. That's one repetition.**

## Your Best Effort: Zero to One Reps

**The problem:** Individually, your legs aren't strong enough to support your body weight through the entire range of motion.

**The fix:** a two-pronged attack using "negatives" and "partials," both of which help you challenge your weak spots and lower your breaking point. Do this workout once every 4 days until you can perform at least two single-leg squats with perfect form.

### Your 4-Week Plan

| WEEK | SETS | REPS | REST |
|------|------|------|------|
| 1 | 8 | 50% of best effort | 60 seconds |
| 2 | 8 | 50% of best effort | 45 seconds |
| 3 | 8 | 50% of best effort | 30 seconds |
| 4 | 8 | 50% of best effort | 15 seconds |

## Step 1

**NEGATIVE SQUAT**

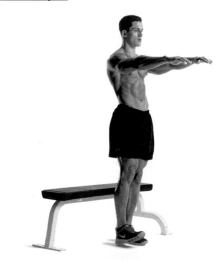

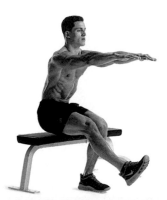

Stand on your left leg, facing away from a bench.

Holding your arms and your right leg in the air in front of you, slowly lower your body until your butt is slightly higher than your breaking point. (Ideally, this should take 5 to 7 seconds.) Sit, then stand up using both legs. That's one repetition. Do six reps with your left leg, then six more with your right. Complete a set. Rest for 2 to 3 minutes, then move on to step 2.

## Step 2

**PARTIAL SQUAT**

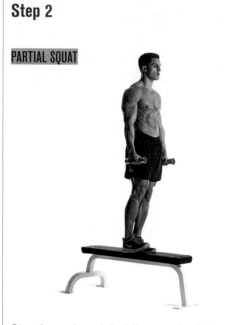

Stand on a bench holding a pair of 5-pound dumbbells.

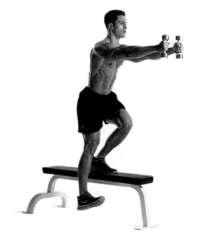

As you perform a single-leg squat, simultaneously lift the dumbbells in front of you to shoulder height. (This helps counterbalance your body, making the movement easier.) Again, lower your body until you're just above your breaking point, then pause for 2 seconds before pushing yourself back up. Do 10 repetitions with each leg, pausing for 10 seconds instead of 2 on the last rep with each.

## Your Best Effort: Two to Five Reps

**The problem:** Because you can't adjust the weight you're using, as you can with free weights, your muscles give out quickly, and that limits the total number of repetitions you can perform, a key factor in increasing strength.

**The fix:** a technique called escalating density training, or EDT. Popularized by Charles Staley, author of *Muscle Logic*, this method helps you slow the onset of fatigue, so you can complete more total repetitions than usual. Instead of doing as many reps as you can in each set, you'll do more sets of fewer repetitions. In addition, you'll further increase the challenge to your legs by adding two other single-leg exercises: the Bulgarian split squat and the high stepup.

## Step 1: Determine Your Starting Point

Take the number of single-leg squats you can complete with perfect form and divide it by two. That's how many repetitions you'll do each set. (If your best effort is three, round down to one.) Perform the 4-week EDT routine at right once every 4 days, doing the number of sets indicated and resting after each for the prescribed amount of time.

# Step 3

## BULGARIAN SPLIT SQUAT

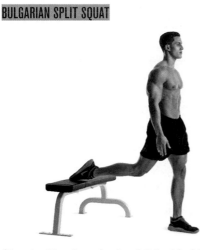

Stand with a bench about 2 feet behind you and place the instep of your right foot on the bench.

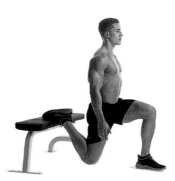

Keeping your torso upright, lower your body until your left thigh is parallel to the floor. Your left lower leg should remain perpendicular to the floor. Pause, then push yourself back to the starting position as quickly as you can. Do 12 to 15 repetitions, then repeat, this time with your left foot resting on the bench and your right foot in front. After you've worked both legs, immediately (without resting) complete step 3.

## HIGH STEPUP

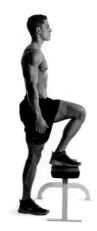

Stand facing a bench or step that's about knee height. Lift your left foot and place it firmly on the bench.

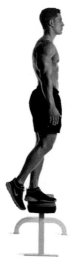

Push down with your left heel, and push your body upward until your left leg is straight and your right foot hangs off the bench. Lower yourself back down. That's one rep. Do 12 to 15, then do the same number of reps with your right leg.

### Your Best Effort: Six to Nine Reps

**The problem:** You have poor endurance.

**The fix:** training your muscles to resist fatigue. Perform the following routine once every 4 days for 5 weeks.

## Step 1

Do as many single-leg squats as you can, then rest for 60 seconds.

## Step 2

Repeat until you've completed twice the number of reps you achieved in your first set.

So, if you do seven reps in your first set, you'll do as many sets as needed to complete 14 reps. For each subsequent workout, this will be your repetition goal.

## Step 3

Each workout, try to reach your repetition goal in fewer sets. For instance, if you need five sets in your first workout, aim for your goal in four sets in your next session. After 5 weeks, repeat the entire process. In order to keep improving, do the exercise while holding dumbbells at your sides.

# Build Stamina

**BY MIKE MEJIA, CSCS**

The Tabata Protocol is not an action flick. It's a Japanese training technique, using basic body-weight exercises, that's been shown to improve aerobic and anaerobic fitness by as much as 28 percent in 6 weeks. Perform the first exercise below for 20 seconds, rest for 10 seconds, and repeat, continuing this back-and-forth sequence for 4 minutes. Rest for 60 to 90 seconds, then follow the same procedure with the other two exercises. Do this workout 3 days a week, with a day's rest between sessions.

**Chinup:** Hang from a chinup bar with an underhand grip (palms facing you), your elbows slightly bent.

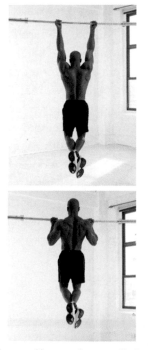

Pull yourself up until your collarbones almost touch the bar. Pause, then lower yourself to the starting position.

**Prisoner squat:** Stand with your feet slightly wider than shoulder-width apart and lace your fingers behind your head.

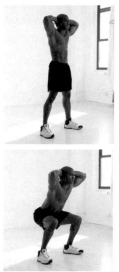

Keeping your elbows back, bend at the hips and knees to lower your body until your thighs are parallel to the floor. Press back up to the starting position and repeat. (If the basic prisoner squat is too easy for you, try this: At the bottom of the move, explode upward so your feet come off the floor a few inches. Land softly and sink into your next repetition.)

**Pushup:** Assume the classic pushup position, with your weight on your hands and the balls of your feet. Space your hands just wider than shoulder-width apart.

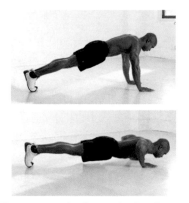

Keeping your back straight, bend your elbows to lower yourself to the floor. When your chest is just off the floor, push yourself back up to the starting position.

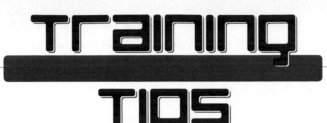

# Training Tips

**Are muscle and cardio mutually exclusive?**

Absolutely not. Ever seen a swimmer's back? Cycling, swimming, and running are great muscle builders and can act as a whole-body workout program if you cross-train. The trick is to maintain an anabolic, or muscle-building, state by having enough fuel to prevent sacrificing muscle for fuel. Eating enough calories before, during, and after exercise will help prevent this. Bonus: Including stairs in your running program and hills in your cycling routes is like adding weight.

**How should I approach hills— attack or downshift?**

That depends on your run. If you're out for a short one, attack. If you're going long, downshift to avoid generating excess lactic acid, which could come back to haunt you. Hill repeats are a great way to build strength and endurance, so training by attacking hills pays big dividends.

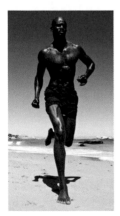

**How should I breathe when I run?**

Anything that hypnotizes you into a steady pace is worth trying—there's no one right way.

**I often suffer from terrible chafing when I run. Help!**

Chub rub ain't pretty. Try running in tights instead of shorts. They compress your skin and take the friction better than flesh on flesh. Or try BodyGlide Anti-Friction Skin Formula (www.bodyglide.com). It's a roll-on that isn't greasy and stays on no matter how much you sweat. There's also a powder that works, called Squeaky Cheeks. Don't try to fix the problem by modifying your stride. An unnatural gait can lead to injury.

**Is there any benefit to running backward?**

Whatever flips your switch, I guess. So-called retro running can be great for the joints, heart, lungs, and muscles. Research at the University of Oregon over the past 25 years shows that, compared with regular running, motoring in reverse works the lungs more efficiently, burns more calories, and allows the bones to absorb shock more effectively. And it helps patients recover from sprained ankles, pulled hamstrings, shin splints, groin injuries, and recently repaired knee joints. If you try it, watch out for curbs. You might want to practice on an elliptical trainer or treadmill.

**Which offers a better prerace boost—solid foods or liquids?**

Liquids are good for replacing water and electrolytes, and solid food provides sustained energy. But gels are best for a boost because they're easily digested and send fuel quickly into the bloodstream. We like GU and Hammer Gel. Train with one before using it before a race. Gel can take a little getting used to.

**I drink a protein shake after I lift. What should I have after I do aerobic exercise?**

The same thing. Many people down a sports drink after they bike or row and call it a day, but sports drinks only replenish electrolytes and glucose, which your muscles use for energy. If you want your muscles to grow—regardless of whether you used them to squat 150 pounds or run 15 miles—feed them protein. Look for shakes that contain a two-to-one carbs-to-protein ratio. We like Muscle Milk Ready-to-Drink ($3.69 for 17 ounces, www.cytosport.com). The carbs will elevate your insulin levels, driving the amino acids into your hungry muscles. In a pinch, you can also grab some chocolate milk. A recent study at Indiana University found that its high carbohydrate and

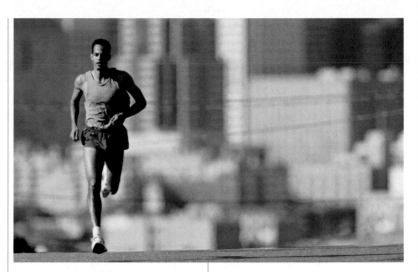

protein content is ideal for aiding muscle growth.

**Whenever I run, I have loose bowel movements. Is this weird?**

Nope. About 20 to 40 percent of runners suffer from "runner's trots." Symptoms include cramps, gas, or diarrhea during or after a strenuous run. The cause is unclear, but it probably has to do with all that bouncing, jarring, and sloshing. Running also boosts the hormones that move intestines, so it's a double whammy. See if diet changes help. You might want to avoid dairy 24 hours before racing. High-fiber foods can be problematic as well, so cut back on the bran flakes.

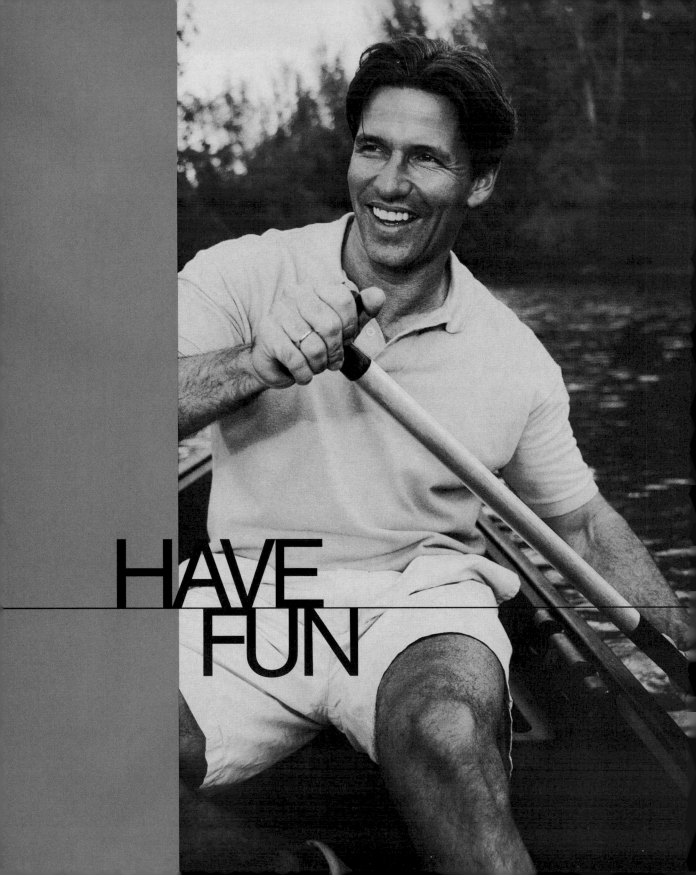

# HAVE FUN

## PART SIX

Open up the trunk of 72 percent of men's cars—or peer into the beds of their trucks—and you'll find sports equipment stowed there. No question, a lot of guys out there are actively pursuing the field of their dreams.

What's your passion? Whether it's skiing, skating, snowboarding, golf, bicycling, tennis, or basketball, you'll find something here for you. In this part of the book, dedicated to sports, you'll learn how to build a bigger, stronger, faster body, from one of the top trainers in college sports. Then, you'll build some muscle to shred the slopes this winter. In an effort to shrink your golf handicap, start working out like the pros with our workout. You'll unleash your golfing power and add 30 yards to your drive. Then, because nothing knocks a guy out of his sport faster than a bum knee, we also discuss how to get a handle on knee problems and get back in the game.

So without further ado, haul that sports gear out of your vehicle. Game on!

BY MYATT MURPHY

# Dominate Your Sport

One of the top trainers in college sports shows
you how to build a bigger, stronger, faster body

**J**ust like a protein shake, an effective sports workout depends on the right blend of ingredients. That's why this workout emphasizes four different types of exercises: explosive, knee-dominant, hip-dominant, and functional. Explosive movements improve your ability to generate power; knee-dominant exercises train your front thigh muscles; hip-dominant exercises strengthen your hamstrings, gluteal muscles, and lower back; and functional moves allow you to twist, turn, and balance. Together, they give you an edge.

"The athlete who can react explosively and move efficiently in all directions finishes first every time," says Robert dos Remedios, CSCS, director of speed, strength, and conditioning at College of the Canyons in Santa Clarita, California.

One of the many results of this workout is a more athletic physique. A combination of strength, stability, and flexibility is essential in order to excel in any sport, but most athletes fall short in at least one area. This plan improves all three, so you'll eliminate weaknesses in your game and your body.

The exercises in this workout, such as the woodchopper, jump squat, and barbell torque, mimic skills like swinging a racket and leaping for a rebound. The result: You'll develop power and strength that will transfer to your game. Also, because this plan mixes power training with core training, your body will be prepared for the demands of any athletic endeavor. Just as important, your workouts will stay exciting.

## The Workout

Follow the workout plan, alternating between Workouts A and B. Do three workouts a week and rest at least a day between sessions—so you might do Workout A on Monday, Workout B on Wednesday, and Workout A on Friday, then B, A, and B the following week. Perform each exercise for the specified number of sets and repetitions, and rest for 1 to 1½ minutes between sets.

## Benchmark of Success

### How do you measure up?

Professional and college coaches consider the vertical jump to be the single best way to gauge how well an athlete will perform. It measures two factors that are critical to performance: explosive lower-body power and the ability to generate force quickly. You'll need a wall you can mark on with chalk.

Stand with the wall at your side and the chalk in the hand next to the wall. Place your feet at whatever width feels comfortable. Dip down by bending your knees and hips, jump straight up as high as you can with your arm extended upward, and mark the wall at the top of your reach. Make three marks, resting a few seconds between jumps.

### Track Your Progress

Record your highest vertical jump in the chart below. Then follow the plan and retest yourself after 2 weeks and after 4 weeks.

Start (height in inches)_____

Week 2 (height in inches) _____

Finish (height in inches) _____

# WORKOUT A

## CLEAN PULL
(explosive exercise)

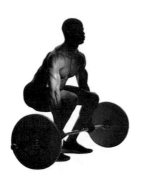

Load a barbell and roll it to your shins. Grab the bar with an overhand grip (palms facing you) and place your feet shoulder-width apart.

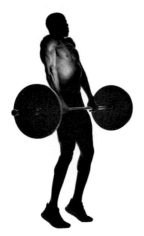

Keeping your back flat and arms straight, squeeze your glutes as you straighten your legs, rise onto your toes, and shrug your shoulders. Pause, then lower the bar to the floor.

**The plan:** Perform four sets of five repetitions in weeks 1 and 3. In weeks 2 and 4, do four sets, decreasing your repetitions and increasing the weight each set so that you do five reps in your first set, four in your second, three in your third, and two in your fourth.

## CURTSY LUNGE
(knee-dominant exercise)

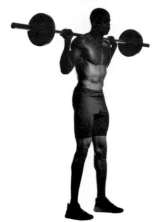

Stand with your feet shoulder-width apart and a barbell across the back of your shoulders.

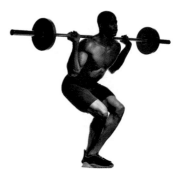

Keeping your hips facing forward, step back with your right foot and place it to the left of your left leg as you bend your knees, lowering your body. Push up to the starting position and repeat with your left leg back. That's one repetition.

**The plan:** Do three sets of 10 repetitions in weeks 1 and 3. In weeks 2 and 4, do four sets of five reps.

## GOOD MORNING
(hip-dominant exercise)

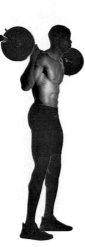

Stand with a light barbell across the back of your shoulders. Keep a slight bend in your knees and maintain a slight arch in your back throughout the move.

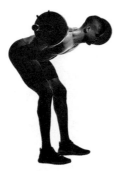

Push your butt back and bend forward at the hips until your chest is parallel to the floor. Contract your glutes, push your hips forward, and raise your torso to return to the starting position.

**The plan:** Perform three sets of 10 repetitions in weeks 1 and 3. In weeks 2 and 4, do four sets of five reps.

## WOODCHOPPER
(functional exercise)

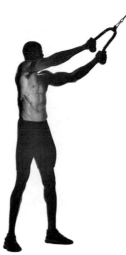

Attach a rope handle to a high-pulley cable. Stand with your left side toward the weight stack and your feet slightly more than shoulder-width apart. Grab the rope with both hands.

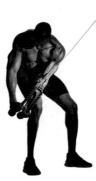

Keeping your arms straight, bend your knees as you pull the handle down and across your body until your hands reach the outside of your right lower leg. Reverse the motion and finish your reps before switching sides and repeating the move.

**The plan:** Do three sets of 10 repetitions in week 1, four sets of 10 reps in weeks 2 and 4, and five sets of five in week 3.

## WORKOUT B

### DUMBBELL JUMP SQUAT
(explosive exercise)

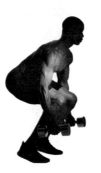

Stand with your feet slightly more than shoulder-width apart and hold a pair of light dumbbells at your sides. Lower your body until your thighs are parallel to the floor, then bend forward slightly at the hips so your shoulders move in front of your feet.

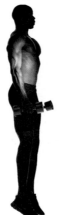

Push off the floor explosively to jump straight up as high as possible. Land with your knees soft and immediately sink down into your next squat.

**The plan:** Do four sets of five repetitions in weeks 1 and 3 and four sets of eight reps in weeks 2 and 4.

### FRONT SQUAT
(knee-dominant exercise)

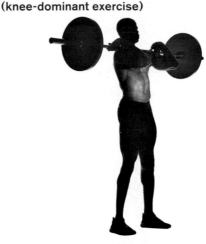

Stand with your feet shoulder-width apart and grab a bar with an overhand, shoulder-width grip. Bring your elbows forward so your palms face up, your upper arms are parallel to the floor, and the bar rests across the front of your shoulders.

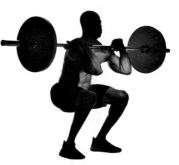

Keeping your elbows high, initiate the move by pushing your hips back. Lower your body until your thighs are parallel to the floor. Pause, then press yourself back up to a standing position.

**The plan:** In weeks 1 and 3, do four sets of five repetitions, and in weeks 2 and 4, do four sets of eight reps.

## SINGLE-LEG, SINGLE-ARM ROMANIAN DEADLIFT
(hip-dominant exercise)

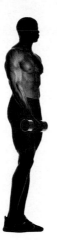

Stand holding a dumbbell in your right hand at arm's length in front of your right thigh. Lift your right foot slightly off the floor.

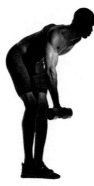

Keeping your knees slightly bent and your back flat, push your hips back to lower the weight toward the floor. Pause when your torso is as close to parallel to the floor as you can go without rounding your back, then push your hips forward to return to a standing position. Complete your repetitions on that leg, then switch sides and repeat.

**The plan:** Do four sets of five repetitions in weeks 1 and 3 and four sets of eight reps in weeks 2 and 4.

## BARBELL TORQUE
(functional exercise)

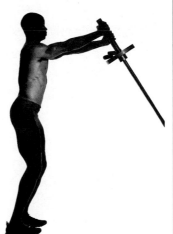

Load a barbell lightly on one end. Wrap the other end in a towel and place it in the corner of a room, wedged under a bench, or between the heels of a workout partner. Stand facing the loaded end (with the bar pointing toward you) and hold the bar in front of your face.

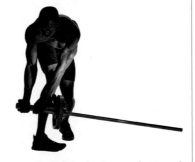

Keeping your arms straight, pivot your feet and torso as you bend at the knees to move the near end of the bar down and across your body toward the floor. Reverse the motion to lift the bar back up, then repeat to the opposite side. That's one repetition.

**The plan:** Perform four sets of 10 repetitions in weeks 1 and 3 and four sets of five reps in weeks 2 and 4.

BY DAVID SCHIPPER

# Shred the Slopes

Here's how to build some gold medal muscle

As a fitness tool, snow has never gotten its due. True, you can't pull it or pump it—you can only groom it. And consider the company it keeps: ski bums. No wonder it gets a bum rap.

In other words, snow is easy to underestimate, which is why gym memberships in this country rise as outdoor temperatures fall. But we're asking you to give the white stuff another look—specifically, to consider the total-body fitness benefits of five popular winter sports.

To help our hard-core sell—indeed, all of these sports solidify the midsection—we recruited five of the most ripped athletes in America. Each represented the United States at the 2006 Winter Olympic Games in Turin, Italy. More important, each proves you don't have to climb mountains to build big muscle. You can take the lift.

Your winter workout starts now.

## Downhill Skiing

**Burns:** 648 calories per hour
**Primarily builds:** cardiovascular fitness
**Also builds:** gluteals, quadriceps, hamstrings, calves

"Downhill skiing is one of the best outdoor sports for cardiovascular fitness," says Kevin Stone, MD, of the Stone Clinic in San Francisco. In fact, the higher the elevation and the thinner the air, the better your cardio workout. Daron Rahlves, the winningest downhill skier in U.S. history (who's been clocked at 92 mph), accelerates your on-slope workout.

**Arc, don't slide.** With shaped skis, you don't need to slide into a turn. "That's like throwing on the brakes," says Rahlves. Instead, lean forward ever so slightly on your inside foot and pull your outside ski back to initiate the turn, then arc through it smoothly.

**Look two turns ahead.** "The worst place to look is at your ski tips," says Rahlves. "You'll feel out of control, so you'll lose control." Instead, focus on where you want to go. You'll have more time to react to changing slope conditions.

**Stay grounded.** Big air will slow you down. "Keeping your skis on the ground," says Rahlves, "helps you link your turns smoothly and react quickly." Plus, you become a parachute when you're airborne.

**Tuck and roll.** Most intermediates tuck incorrectly, spreading their elbows like a bird's wings, creating drag. Bring those elbows in—way in. They should be in front of your knees, says Rahlves, with your poles parallel to the ground behind you. Likewise, bring your upper body down to parallel as well.

**HARD**TRUTH
Percentage of men who incorporate explosive training into their workouts:
**9**

## Cross-Country Skiing

**Burns:** 756 calories per hour
**Primarily builds:** gluteals, quadriceps, hamstrings
**Also builds:** cardiovascular fitness, latissimus dorsi, biceps, triceps, abdominals

Waddling across snow meadows on sticks may lack the thrill of the downhill, but it's a

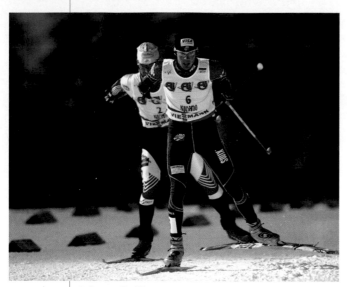

**Johnny Spillane**

monster total-body workout, cardio included. Johnny Spillane, the first American to win a World Championship in a Nordic event, explains how to amp up the workout—and the fun.

**Lose the poles.** In cross-country skiing, poles are like crutches, allowing you to favor your stronger side. As a result, says Spillane, your workhorse leg is exhausted faster, while your other leg rides along like the Grinch's dog. Skiing without poles streamlines your form and builds your lower body. Once you're solid below the belt, go ahead and add poles, but make sure both arms are pushing simultaneously. If you have trouble syncing them, practice on an elliptical machine.

**Slow down to speed up.** Running like Fred Flintstone won't make you faster. The secret is gliding longer. "On each kick, raise your body up as far and for as long as you can," says Spillane, "so you can explode down onto your poles for more power."

**Think small.** Lightweight, stable racing boots shorten the learning curve for beginners and help more-experienced skiers reach the finish line faster. The key, says Spillane, is to buy boots that are a half size too small. "Fit the boot as you would a running shoe," he says, "relatively tight but still comfortable." Spillane's choice: Salomon's Carbon Pro Skiathlon ($350), which has been worn by the past five world champions.

## Mogul Skiing

**Burns:** 864 calories per hour

**Primarily builds:** hamstrings, quadriceps

**Also builds:** chest, abdominals, gluteals, hip flexors

There's no bigger thrill than taming a mountain of moguls; nor is there a better leg workout. "Your hamstrings, quads, glutes, and hip muscles all act as stabilizers," explains Jeff Guerra, PT, CSCS, of the Boulder Center for Sports Medicine. In other words, your lower body becomes

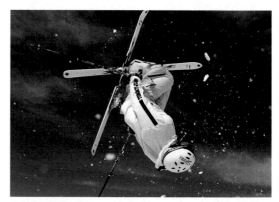

**Travis Cabral**

# Happy Landings!

Here are four ways to injury-proof your ski trip.

**Start 3 months before.** If you're out of shape, even just a little, you won't be long for the mountain, says Olympic skier Daron Rahlves. "I spend time at the gym 3 days a week strengthening my legs and core," he says, "and I spin and stretch for recovery." Rahlves recommends squats for coordination, single-leg hamstring curls for strength and balance, and interval training with sprints for explosive strength and aerobic endurance. He also suggests balancing gym time with tennis, soccer, surfing, mountain biking, or basketball. All are killer cardio workouts, and all develop the balance and agility necessary for skiing.

**Check your DIN.** Contrary to conventional winter wisdom, it's loose—not tight—bindings that blow out knees. Before you hit the slopes, swing by the ski shop and have a tech tweak the DIN setting. The more advanced the skier, the tighter the bindings should be. So when he asks your ability level, tell the truth—your knees depend on it.

**Drink like a fish.** Higher altitudes bring on dehydration more quickly, reducing endurance, causing fatigue, and lengthening recovery times. Drink water or a sports drink regularly while on the hill—don't wait until you're thirsty. Après-ski, "pound a glass of water after every beer," recommends Rahlves.

**Know how to fall.** "If you're sliding feet first down a hill, do what you can to swing around and go headfirst, and try to keep your legs up to avoid catching your skis in the snow," says Rahlves. "If you can't manage to keep your skis off the snow, at least keep your tips up and drag the tails."

---

stronger because preventing yourself from wiping out is yeoman's work. Travis Cabral, the youngest-ever freestyle-mogul World Cup champion, smooths your ride.

**Start strong.** If you don't have a strong upper and lower body, moguls will eat you alive. That's why Cabral box-jumps like a madman. The exercise mimics a mogul run, hitting the legs, abs, and chest. Set up a 12-inch-high box and perform a 30-second set of lateral jumps over it, aiming for one jump per second. Cabral does four sets using a 30-inch box, resting for 30 seconds after each set.

**See the future.** Surprise moguls will kill your rhythm and your knees. "Always look down the line," says Cabral, "never at the top of the mogul you're skiing over." Your eyes should be fixed at least three moguls ahead.

**Lean on your shins.** Absorb the rough terrain by keeping your body in a stacked position: knees bent, shoulders over your hips, hips over the balls of your feet—in other words, your body should be a bit more forward than it is in your stance on the downhill. If you're in the proper position, you'll feel pressure on your shins from the tongues of your boots.

## Speed Skating

**Burns:** 756 calories per hour

**Primarily builds:** gluteals, hip abductors, quadriceps

**Also builds:** biceps, triceps, abdominals

It's difficult to find a better total-body winter workout than speed skating. Of course, it's also difficult to find an ice rink that'll let you do it. But you'll want to train like a speed skater anyway—it builds coordination, balance, endurance, strength, and power at the same time. Derek Parra, who struck gold and silver in the 2002 Games and is the world record holder at 1500 meters, trains with these exercises.

**Build explosive power.** Stand with a bench about 12 inches behind you and rest the top of your right foot on it. Move your

left leg forward until your right leg is bent at 30 degrees. Now squat. Do three sets of 10 to 12 repetitions with each leg.

**Improve your balance.** "Speed skating is like doing a wall sit while balancing on two pencils moving at 30 miles per hour," says Parra. Build balance by standing with your left foot on the corner of a bench and your right foot hanging in the air next to it. Now squat, bringing your left thigh parallel to the floor. Reverse to a standing position, but don't let your knee lock. Do three sets of 10 to 12 reps with each leg.

**Increase lower-body strength.** Stand with both feet together and your hands on your hips. Step 3 feet forward with your right foot. Lower your body until the top of your right thigh is parallel to the floor. Your right knee should be over your toes. Pause, then forcefully push yourself up, taking a step forward with your left foot into the next lunge. Do 10 to 12, then turn around and repeat.

## Snowboarding

**Burns:** 545 calories per hour

**Primarily builds:** abdominals

**Also builds:** quadriceps, hamstrings, calves

Catch air, then abs. Because you have to rotate your upper body when you turn, snowboarding blasts your midsection like no other winter sport. The only thing standing between you and snowboard abs? The steep learning curve. World Champion snow-boarder Seth Wescott offers up three shortcuts.

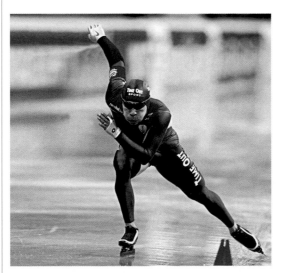

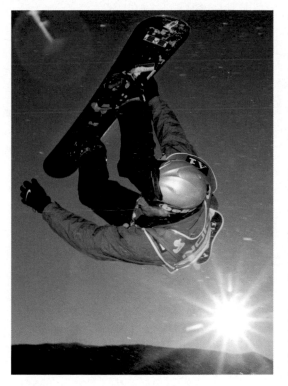

**Go fast to learn fast.** "Beginners take their lessons on terrain that's way too flat," says Wescott. "The slower you go, the easier it'll be for you to catch an edge and fall." His suggestion: Find an intermediate trail, and don't look back. See that first big turn ahead? Attack it, says Wescott. Commit yourself, and the board will do what it's designed to do: turn.

**Lower your stance.** "You want to use your knees and hips as shock absorbers," says Wescott. The lower you crouch, the more balanced you'll be through rough terrain. Plus, you won't fall as far. How low? Pretend you're doing a half squat in the gym, he advises.

**Fear fear.** When he's feeling faint-hearted, Wescott turns to bands like Green Day or the Killers. "In-your-face music will fire you up and make you go for it," he says. "If you worry about falling, you almost certainly will fall." His point: Keep the adrenaline flowing, and you'll be more alert and motivated and in an offensive position. Proactive tames the mountain; reactive gets airlifted to Boulder.

BY DAVID SCHIPPER

# Shrink Your Handicap

Want to add 30 yards to your drive? Start working out like the pros and unleash your golfing power

In high school, I worked at a driving range. When my buddy and I weren't retrieving balls (our job) or hitting balls (our pay), we'd hang out on the porch, watching customers hack their way through $8 buckets.

It was great comic relief: poor form, worse attitudes. And it was never more enjoyable than when big-muscle guys came over from the nearby Gold's Gym.

Ever watch a bodybuilder hit a golf ball? It's so ugly it's funny. "They can't put their joints in the right positions to access that strength," says Bill Hartman, PT, CSCS, an expert in golf-specific training based in Indianapolis. "That's why flexibility is so important." Without it, you're better off in a batting cage.

A golf swing is complicated, but there's one simple truth: Clubhead speed means distance. At the University of Pittsburgh's Sports Performance Complex, researchers found that a 5 percent increase in strength yields a 1.7 percent increase in clubhead speed. That's not much. On the other hand, they determined that improving your flexibility and body control can lead to a 14 percent increase in clubhead speed. That amounts to 20 or more yards on your drive.

Anyone who has met Charles Howell knows this. Howell, 26, is in his sixth year on the PGA Tour and is already one of its longest hitters, averaging 296 yards off the tee. And he's built like a 1-iron: 5'11", 155 pounds, 31" waist.

"It's easy to see why a John Daly or Tiger Woods is going to hit it long, but it's a little

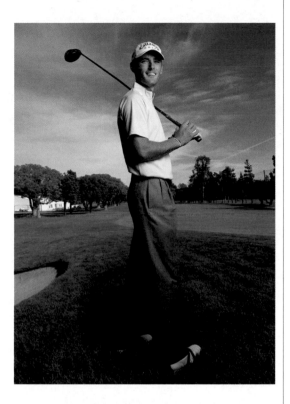

more difficult to see why a person like me would," says Howell, who doesn't work with Hartman but whose workouts are similar to those the trainer espouses.

The explanation is called transferable strength. In the gym, Howell activates muscle fibers in golf-specific positions. On the course, he turns on those fibers faster to produce greater force, says Hartman. "Weight lifting definitely goes into hitting it far, but the greater element is speed-and-flexibility training," Howell says.

Working with Hartman, we've created a workout with three goals: flexibility, power, and better swing mechanics. I followed Hartman's instructions for 1 month and increased my tee shots by 26 yards, peaking at 253 yards. Intrigued? Follow these steps.

## Flexibility

Increasing your range of motion ultimately means hitting the ball farther. "You'll elongate your shoulder turn during your backswing, which determines how much energy is transferred into the ball," says Howell. Perform one 20-repetition set of each of these three dynamic exercises.

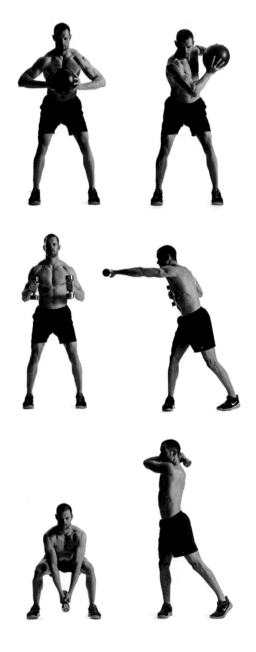

### GOLF TWIST

Stand in a golf-address position with your feet slightly more than shoulder-width apart, weight on the inside of each heel. Use both hands to hold a 5-pound medicine ball or dumbbell at the center of your chest, with your elbows extended out to your sides.

Keeping your head still and feet flat, bring the ball up and to the left, as in a backswing, until your right shoulder is underneath your chin. Return to the starting position and repeat to the right.

### GOLF PUNCH

Stand with your feet shoulder-width apart. In each hand, hold a 10-pound dumbbell in front of you with your elbows bent 90 degrees and your palms facing each other.

In one motion, pivot on your left foot as you turn your upper body to the right and throw a straight jab across your body with your left hand. As you punch, rotate your palm down. Return to the starting position and repeat the move to the opposite side.

### GOLF SQUAT

Stand holding a 10-pound dumbbell down in front of you with a hand-over-hand grip. Your feet should be more than shoulder-width apart. This is the starting position. Lower to a squat.

Rise, turning to the right while bending your elbows and raising the weight over your right shoulder. Your hips should face right, with your weight over your right foot and your left heel off the floor. Return to the starting position and repeat to the opposite side.

## Power

A golf club weighs about a pound, so superhuman strength isn't needed to swing it. Focus on "creating strength through the entire range of the golf swing," says Howell. "We all want to practice our strengths, not our weaknesses, but you need to target every area of your body when you work out for golf."

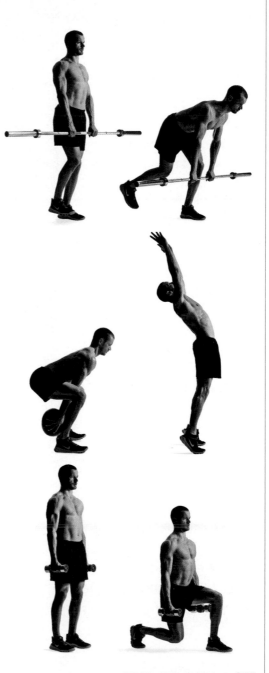

### SINGLE-LEG ROMANIAN DEADLIFT

Stand with your feet shoulder-width apart. Hold a barbell with your hands slightly more than shoulder-width apart. Move one foot slightly behind the other, holding it a few inches off the ground.

With your back flat and abs tight, slowly lower the bar toward your front foot. As you bend forward, allow your free leg to float behind you for balance. Once the barbell reaches midshin level, push through your grounded heel to return to the upright position, and repeat on the opposite leg. Perform two to four sets of eight reps.

### BACKWARD OVERHEAD THROW

Stand with your feet shoulder-width apart. Hold a moderately heavy (8- to 10-pound) medicine ball with both hands at arm's length down in front of you. Squat quickly, reaching back between your legs with the ball.

Reverse direction, exploding upward into a maximum-effort jump as you throw the ball above and behind you for maximum height and distance. Perform three sets of six reps, resting for 60 seconds after each set.

### FORWARD LUNGE

Stand with your feet hip-width apart, holding 10-pound dumbbells at your sides.

Stride forward with your left leg, so your left thigh ends up parallel to the floor with your left knee directly over your toes. Push back up to the starting position and repeat with the opposite leg. Perform two to four sets of eight reps.

## Five short-game stroke savers

Plenty of LPGA golfers can outdrive a typical male weekend player. But we can learn more about golf from watching them around the green, where strokes are saved and bets are won. Listen to LPGA hotshot Natalie Gulbis.

### Pitching and Chipping

**Lighten your grip.** Less hand tension means more clubhead speed and spin. "Don't be afraid to give it a little power, because the ball will check up," says Gulbis. "You won't produce any spin if you don't accelerate."

**Stick with a favorite.** Use the wedge you're most confident with, then adjust the distance "by gripping the club either high or low," says Gulbis. The lower you hold it, the less distance you'll go on the shot. "It's all about being comfortable," says Gulbis.

**Keep your hands ahead of the ball.** Press your hands forward before the stroke and "make sure to maintain that angle through impact," she says. Result: no more skulling or chunking.

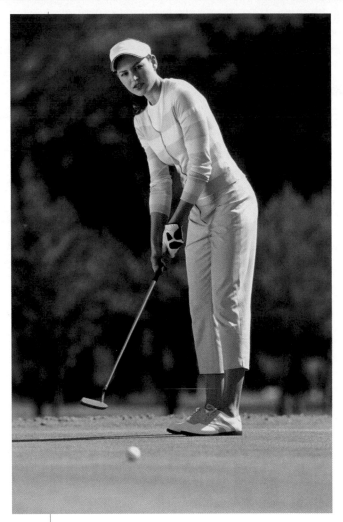

### Putting

**Open your stance.** By slightly facing the hole, "you'll be able to see the putting line better by using both eyes," says Gulbis. "I seem to gather more confidence by looking at the hole square." On the greens, confidence equals success.

**Try a 10-finger grip.** Wrist action ruins putting strokes. Gulbis limits it by separating her hands on the grip. "It allows me to use my shoulders more, taking the hands out of the stroke altogether," she says. This leads to a repeatable, consistent stroke.

## Mechanics

The last phase of the workout will help you keep your body under control as the club explodes through the hitting area. "These exercises are so specific that the benefit to your golf game will be huge," says Hartman.

## Stretch Your Game to the Max

Golfers are lousy stretchers, though it's a sport that "will challenge their flexibility and requires high levels of speed and strength," says Bill Hartman, PT, CSCS, an expert in golf training. "It's no wonder the injury rate is so high." Go to www.menshealth.com/flex for video demonstrations of five dynamic stretches that can stimulate your nervous system to produce power.

### DUMBBELL ROW WITH ROTATION

Stand with your feet shoulder-width apart and hold a 10-pound dumbbell in each hand. Bend forward at the waist, flex your knees, and let the dumbbells hang in front of your thighs, palms facing each other. Pull your right arm toward your rib cage while rotating your torso as far as you can to the right.

Pause, then lower your right arm while pulling up your left arm and rotating left. Perform two to four sets of eight reps.

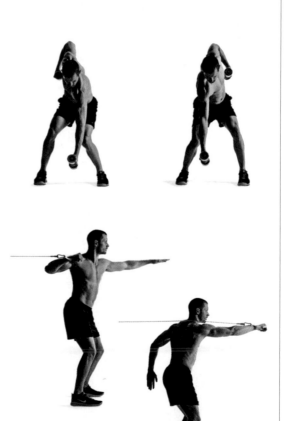

### STANDING CABLE PUSH

At a cable station, grab the high-pulley cable with your right hand. Face away from the weights with your feet at shoulder width and your right hand in front of your shoulder. Straighten your left arm and use it for balance.

Keeping your hips square, "punch" the handle forward until your right arm is fully extended. Return slowly to the starting position and punch eight times. Repeat on the other side. Perform two to four sets on each side.

## Standing Half Moon

This stretch is designed to wake up stubborn shoulder blades, improving flexibility and reducing the risk of injury.

Start by slowly raising your hands in a smooth arc, arms straight and palms facing forward.

As your hands ascend, shrug your shoulders to your ears. This movement causes your shoulder blades to move out and up. Finish by lowering your arms, pinching your shoulder blades in and down. To make it harder, hold a 2-pound dumbbell in each hand. Do two sets of 8 to 12 repetitions.

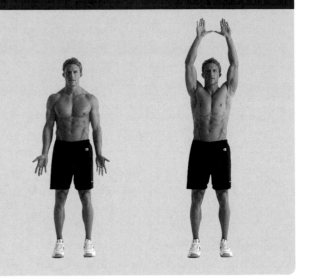

### MEDICINE-BALL LOWER-TRUNK ROTATION

Lie on your back with your knees bent and your feet in the air. Place a 5-pound medicine ball between your knees, holding it there so it doesn't drop. Keep your shoulders flat on the floor and your arms straight out to the sides with your palms up.

Rotate your lower body till your left leg touches the floor on your left side. Hold for 5 seconds, then rotate your legs to the center, maintaining the same leg position throughout. Complete 10 to 20 repetitions to the left side, then the same number to the right.

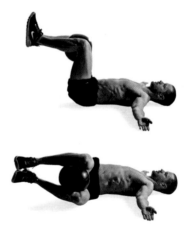

BY SARA WELLS

# Don't Be Knee-dy

Nothing knocks you out of the game faster than
a faulty knee. Here's how to get a handle on the problem
and get back in the swing of things

For a joint that's given us countless marriage proposals, bedside prayers, and jump shots at the buzzer, the knee turns out to be a fairly inferior piece of equipment. Knees are the Bobby Brown and Whitney Houston of the human anatomy: They're under a lot of pressure—each step loads your knees with many times your body weight—and "they're inherently unstable," says Ronald P. Grelsamer, MD, an orthopedic surgeon and associate professor at Mount Sinai Medical School in New York City. "Take away all of the ligaments and tendons, and [knees] just fall apart."

Which explains why more than 6 million men limped to the doctor in 2003 (the most recent year for which data are available). In fact, knee trouble ranks second only to back pain when it comes to the number of office visits related to musculoskeletal pain. And when you get up close and personal with the knee's construction, it's easy to see why: "It's like a bowling ball resting on a table that is entirely dependent on a series of very tight ropes—ligaments—to hold it in place," says Dr. Grelsamer. "If one rope is too tight or too loose, the knee can't function properly."

Fortunately, most knee injuries don't require surgery; in fact, most don't even require medical attention. "With self-care, a little rest, some icing, and some anti-inflammatories, most people do quite well on their own," says Brian Halpern, MD, a sports-medicine physician at the Hospital for Special Surgery in New York City and author of *The Knee Crisis Handbook*. Most doctors agree: Unless you've suffered a major trauma and your knee swells up like an overripe cantaloupe, you should try treating your aches and pains yourself before calling your doctor.

The RICE method—rest, ice, compression, and elevation—is the first step for almost all knee injuries. Wrap a bag of frozen peas or an ice pack in a towel, get off your dogs, and place the cold compress on your knee for about 20 minutes.

If you don't have swelling, skip the

## Inside View

The knee is dependent on tendons and ligaments to hold it together. If one is too tight or too loose, it can't function properly.

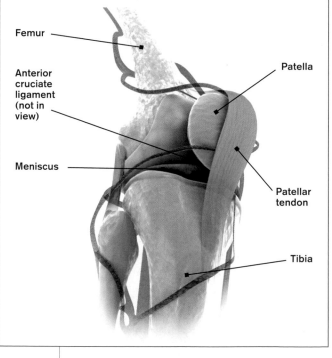

Femur

Anterior cruciate ligament (not in view)

Meniscus

Patella

Patellar tendon

Tibia

# On Mended Knee

## Five exercises to help you stay pain free, no matter how many miles you log

Most of us take our knees for granted. They bend perfectly through thousands of steps every day, carrying us effortlessly from one destination to another. But all it takes is one wrong step, one ill-fated twist, and suddenly we're clutching crutches and wondering how such an essential joint could do us so wrong. Rarely, however, is the joint itself to blame; most knee injuries occur because of an imbalance in the muscles surrounding it—weak quads, hamstrings, or calves, for example.

"By increasing your quad strength and working on balance and flexibility, you can cut your risk of injury dramatically," explains Terry Malone, PT, EdD, director of physical therapy at the University of Kentucky. Here are five exercises to help keep the spring in your step.

### Leg Press

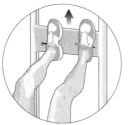

**Using a leg-press machine will help strengthen your quadriceps. The exercise places the same amount of stress on the knee that running does but in a more controlled manner. Work your legs together or separately—it doesn't matter. But aim for two sets of 10 to 12 repetitions, increasing the weight gradually as you grow stronger.**

### Single-Leg Stance

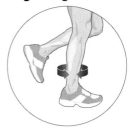

**Stand on one knee for 30 seconds to a minute, increasing the time as you get better at holding the pose without falling. This will strengthen the muscles and ligaments around your knee as they work to stabilize the joint. You can also do these while rotating slowly to your left and right. Do two repetitions on each leg two or three times a day.**

### Heel Raises

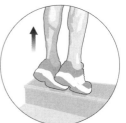

**Stand with both heels hanging off the back of a stair. Rise on your toes and hold; return to the starting position. This will strengthen and stretch your calf muscles. Do two repetitions on each leg two or three times a day.**

### Calf Stretch

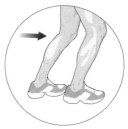

**Place one foot in front of the other and bend your knees. You should feel the stretch in the back of your lower legs. Do three repetitions, holding the stretch for 15 to 20 seconds. (Walk or jog for 5 to 10 minutes before stretching to warm up.)**

### Hamstring Stretch

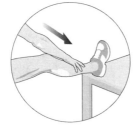

**Place one foot on a waist-high stationary object like a chair and slowly lean forward, reaching down the shin of the extended leg until you feel a stretch in the hamstring. Keep your back straight to avoid injury. Do three repetitions for each leg, holding the stretch for 15 to 20 seconds.**

compression and elevation parts, which involve wrapping the knee snugly with an elastic bandage and propping it up with pillows. Many physicians recommend their patients take an over-the-counter oral anti-inflammation medication such as Aleve or Motrin (for pain with swelling) or a pain-killer like Tylenol (for pain). Your next step, however, depends on your symptoms.

**Symptom:** pain under the kneecap or at the front of the knee. It generally hurts to go up and down stairs or to kneel or squat. It also tends to hurt if you've been sitting too long.

**Diagnosis:** patellofemoral pain syndrome. This is a fancy name for a multitude of problems that cause pain around the kneecap, including the early wear of carti-lage (the degeneration of the lining under the kneecap) or arthritis. It's often attributed to an alignment issue—your kneecap is higher than it should be or sits to the outside or inside of your thigh, where your muscles aren't as strong. Pain can also be from either flatfeet or ill-fitting shoes.

**Treatment:** Ice the sore spot for 20 minutes every couple of hours, and take anti-inflammatories. Limit or stop the aggravating activity, whether it's running, playing basketball, or using the stairclimber. Also stop doing squats or lunges until the pain subsides. "This type of pain is often caused by a muscle imbalance, so you want to work on

strengthening your quadriceps [front thigh muscle]," says Halpern, who recommends "quad sets" to correct the problem. Sit with your legs extended in front of you, your back straight, and your hands on the floor behind you for support. Place a rolled towel under the knee you're working on. Push the back of your knee into the towel, keeping your heel pressed against the floor. Hold for 10 seconds, release, and repeat. Do two sets of 15 repetitions. If you're not feeling better within a week, schedule an appointment with your doctor; physical therapy might be in order.

**Symptom:** pain just below the kneecap. If it's severe enough, you might feel the pain all the time, but generally it hurts during or after playing sports such as basketball.

**Diagnosis:** patellar tendinitis. Also known as jumper's knee, this is an overuse injury to the tendon that connects your patella, or kneecap, to your tibial tubercle, the bump on your lower-leg bone. It's usually caused by sports that involve jumping, such as basket-ball and volleyball, but runners can get it, too. "That part of the knee sees a lot of stress," says Grelsamer. "Anytime you lift your leg [walking, jumping, raising it in the air], all of the weight of your leg goes to that point. The entire lower leg is held up by that one tendon."

**Treatment:** Rest your knee; the tendon needs time to heal. "You really need to avoid the offending activity," says Dr. Grelsamer. "Otherwise, it's like having your foot on the gas and the brake at the same time." Treat it with ice and anti-inflammatories. Wearing a knee brace might also help because it takes tension off the tendon.

While the injury is healing, switch to exercises that won't irritate the tendon, such as swimming or very-light-resistance cycling, says Terry Malone, PT, EdD, director of physical therapy at the University of Kentucky. You should also work on strengthening your quadriceps. Malone suggests this exercise: On a leg–press machine, push out with both legs (again, using light resistance). Then take your right leg off and slowly bring the weight back down with just your left leg. Switch legs. Do two sets of 10 to 12 repetitions three times a week.

**Symptom:** pain, tenderness, or stiffness on the outside of the knee. Often you feel the pain only while exercising.

**Diagnosis:** iliotibial band syndrome Not. It's not actually a knee injury but an overuse injury to the ligament that runs down the outside of the thigh from the hip to the shin. As the band nears the knee, it narrows, and rubbing can occur between the band and the bone; this causes the ligament to become irritated and inflamed. It's most common in runners and usually triggered by a tightness or weakness in the ligament itself or by running on a sloped surface such as a beach or paved road.

**Treatment:** Cut back on mileage, take anti-inflammatories 1 to 2 hours before you run, and stretch and ice when you return. It's also important to avoid hills, sloped surfaces, and anything else that ups the risk of twisting your knee. Also, check your shoes. "The position of your foot has an effect on your knee, so if you're very flat–footed or have very high arches, you need running shoes that accommodate that," says Dr. Grelsamer. Worn-out shoes may also alter your gait and injure your knee.

**Symptom:** a pop, followed by intense pain, swelling, and a feeling of instability. Your knee may also buckle and give way. Chances are you won't be able to continue whatever it was that you were doing.

**Diagnosis:** sprained or torn ligament. There are four ligaments in the knee—two run alongside the knee joint, while the other two crisscross inside the joint holding it in place. (Ligaments are the ropelike tissues that connect the femur, or thighbone, to the tibia, or lower-leg bone.) The two most commonly injured are the medial collateral ligament (MCL) and the anterior cruciate ligament (ACL).

**Treatment:** Assuming you haven't injured your ACL, you'll probably do fine with a little rehab for the MCL, which usually involves icing the knee and doing exercises to regain strength and stability in the muscles surrounding the joint. Many people can start walking and jogging within a month.

If you've torn your ACL, however, more aggressive treatment might be in order. "Once it's torn, the ACL doesn't tighten and heal the way the other ligaments do," says Edward Laskowski, MD, codirector of the Mayo Clinic Sports Medicine Center.

**HARD TRUTH**

Percentage of men who've suffered a hamstring pull:

**29**

# PEAK
## performance

## Find your groove

Professional athletes are illusionists. What may look like raw power is often practiced restraint. The lesson: Pace, not force, is what can make the difference. Tips on setting your internal metronome:

### BICYCLING

**THE GOAL:** a pedal cadence around 100 revolutions per minute

**THE TIP:** "Think about lifting your knees higher," says Andy Applegate, a USA Cycling–certified coach.

**THE DRILL:** "Find the cadence right before you start to bounce off the saddle," he says. Start with three 1-minute intervals, resting 1 to 2 minutes. "Your legs will learn to spin fast while your body stays still, so you'll feel fine at greater speeds," Applegate says.

### TENNIS

**THE GOAL:** a smoother stroke

**THE TIP:** "Wait until the racket is about to make contact with the ball, then accelerate through it," says Andy Jackson, head coach of the men's tennis team at the University of Florida. You'll nail the sweet spot, generating power and spin.

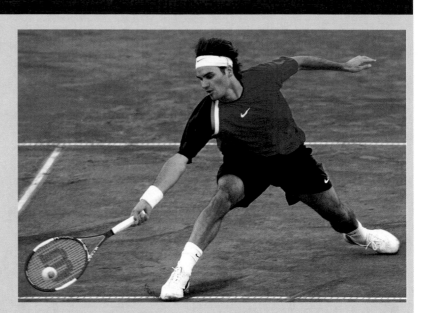

**THE DRILL:** Instead of hitting the ball, act "as if you were catching it with the racket," says Jackson.

### RUNNING

**THE GOAL:** a right foot strike of about 90 times per minute

**THE TIP:** Think quick, not fast. Shorter strides are more efficient.

**THE DRILL:** Run on a gradual downhill, says Jonas Holderman, a distance running coach at the University of Memphis. You'll take that muscle memory to flat ground. "Stay light on your feet, and focus on moving your legs," says Holderman.

### SWIMMING

**THE GOAL:** 30 strokes per 50 meters

**THE TIP:** Glide better, says Kevin Koskella, a coach at www.triswim-coach.com and the author of *The Complete Guide to Triathlon Swimming*. Make sure you always have one arm in front to break the water.

**THE DRILL:** Play golf. Count strokes as you do a six-lap stint. Aim to lower your score every week.

"There will be a risk of knee instability, especially with high-demand sports that really challenge that ligament, such as basketball, volleyball, and soccer." If you want to continue playing high-impact sports, you'll likely benefit from arthroscopic ligament reconstruction, says Dr. Laskowski. Afterward, it will take about

6 to 9 months to get back to aggressive activities.

If you do opt for surgery, don't rush into it. "We like to have people coming in for the surgery looking like they don't need it," says Dr. Laskowski. "Studies have shown that if you do the surgery too early, when the joint doesn't have much motion and there's a lot of swelling, there is an increased risk of joint stiffness, and the rehab afterward is tougher."

**Symptom:** a twinge or a tearing sensation in the knee. Serious pain and swelling may not show up until the next morning, at which point your knee may be very stiff. If a fragment of cartilage hinders motion, your knee may feel locked.

**Diagnosis:** torn meniscus. The meniscus is the cartilage or cushioning tissue that separates the thighbone (femur) and the larger lower-leg bone (tibia). Often, a torn meniscus accompanies an ACL tear.

**Treatment:** If you don't have a locked knee from a piece of cartilage caught in the joint (which keeps it from bending) or an associated injury like an ACL tear, you may do very well with physical therapy alone. "It's generally better to leave cartilage in the knee, even if it's torn, than to have no cartilage in the knee. If a person isn't in pain during activities, surgery may not be necessary," says Dr. Laskowski. "Some studies have shown that if you remove even a portion of the cartilage, arthritic changes occur within a few years in the affected region."

If you have a locked knee, caused by a tear known as a bucket handle tear, then you may need surgery to trim the cartilage. With arthroscopic surgery, you might be back on your feet within a few days.

BY JOHN BRANT

# Catch Your Breath

Every day, millions of men cycle, play tennis, shoot hoops, and run to improve their health and fitness. Are some of them speeding toward an early grave?

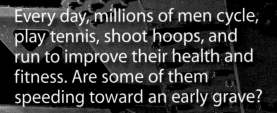

Five times a week for the past 5 years, I have been unwittingly but systematically poisoning myself.

Each lunch hour, I run for 30 minutes on a wood-chip trail in a leafy park in my hometown of Portland, Oregon. But there's a catch to my moderate, seemingly harmless routine: To reach the park, I must first jog nearly a mile along a busy thoroughfare named Fremont Avenue. Until recently, the screech of city buses and the reek of diesel trucks always felt like a small price to pay for the pleasures waiting on the trail.

Here's what I didn't know: With every deep draught of oxygen, I also gulp down alarming quantities of ozone, carbon monoxide, microscopic particulate matter, sulfur dioxide, nitrogen dioxide, lead, and a witch's brew of other pollutants. By conducting part of my workout at midday along a congested street, I am reducing my lung function, constricting my air passages, courting chest pain, increasing my chances of developing asthma, unleashing free radicals to catalyze carcinogens in my bloodstream, and activating cellular processes that might lead to a heart attack.

"When I see people running or bicycling along a busy street in the middle of the day, I want to tackle them and scream at them to stop," says Rachel Langford, coordinator of the Clean Air Project for the American Lung Association (ALA) in Oregon. "At some intersections, we ought to post 'No Exercise Allowed' signs."

It may be hard to imagine that vigorous outdoor exercise—generally trumpeted as an all-purpose antidote to disease and a retardant to mortality—could actually help bad air hurt you. But the explanation is simple: When you're running, cycling, playing tennis, or shooting hoops, you breathe in more of it. A lot more.

A sedentary person inhales approximately 15,000 liters of air per day, or 6 to 10 liters per minute. During heavy aerobic exercise, however, you draw in 60 to 150 liters per minute, delivering oxygen throughout 600 to 900 square feet of surface area in the lungs.

"That means the exerciser breathes in 10 to 15 times more pollution than the sedentary person, and he's sucking it deeper into his lungs," says Rob McConnell, MD, a researcher in the department of preventive medicine at the University of Southern California medical school. "In fact, just by stepping out the door, you could be exposed to five times the ozone you'd inhale if you stayed inside. So if you're outdoors and exercising—well, do the math."

The numbers grow more harrowing because you breathe primarily through your mouth during exercise. At the same time that I'm pulling vast clouds of bad air deep

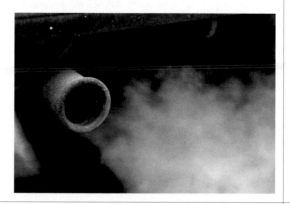

# Metrogrades: Ranking America's Cities

## Towns that breathe easy

Unlike with a trash-choked stream, it can be difficult to eyeball dirty air. If there isn't heavy smog or a horrid smell, the danger is invisible. So we analyzed 100 cities' daily Air Quality Index (AQI)—a chemical snapshot of ground-level ozone, particle pollution, carbon monoxide, sulfur dioxide, and nitrogen dioxide—and looked at how often the EPA

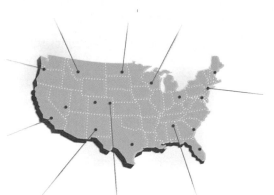

rated the AQI "good" or "bad" in '05. Then we evaluated the Texas Transportation Institute's Travel Time Index, a measure of traffic congestion and, by extension, traffic pollution. (Since diesel exhaust is a particularly noxious offender, we also gave credit to cities that had purchased hybrid-electric buses as of July 2005.) Finally, because the best gauge of a city's air quality is the lungs of the people who live there, we tracked asthma rates from the Centers for Disease Control and Prevention Behavioral Risk Factor Surveillance System. What should you do if your city has an unhealthy atmosphere? You have two choices: Suck it up, or air your concerns.

| | | |
|---|---|---|
| 1. Honolulu, HI | | A+ |
| 2. Fargo, ND | | A+ |
| 3. Lincoln, NE | | A |
| 4. Corpus Christi, TX | | A |
| 5. Fremont, CA | | A− |

into my lungs during my noon run, I'm also bypassing my body's remarkably effective air-filtering system: the nasal passages. (Mucus traps particulates, and then tiny, waving, hairlike structures called cilia push the old mucus up and out of the body.) The triple whammy of breathing fast, deeply, and through the mouth makes my daily run—and perhaps your regular workout—an ozone/particulate/carbon monoxide orgy.

Eventually, our bodies defend themselves against air pollution by breathing less. Air passages tighten, and breathing becomes labored. Our exercising bodies are ensnared in an intractable dilemma: While working furiously to process more air to feed oxygen-hungry muscles, they simultaneously strive to protect us from that air. Our pulmonary and cardiovascular systems strain like air conditioners in an extended heat wave and eventually, inevitably, break down. Early symptoms often include wheezing, coughing, scratchy throat, headache, chest pains, and watery eyes. Other, longer-term effects are considerably more dire.

In Scotland, for instance, researchers studied 30 healthy men cycling on exercise bikes while exposed to diluted diesel

| # | City | Grade | # | City | Grade | # | City | Grade | # | City | Grade |
|---|------|-------|---|------|-------|---|------|-------|---|------|-------|
| 6. | Cheyenne, WY | A– | 29. | Columbia, SC | B | 53. | Lexington, KY | C+ | 77. | Las Vegas, NV | D+ |
| 7. | Lubbock, TX | A– | 30. | Charleston, WV | B | 54. | Nashville, TN | C+ | 78. | Riverside, CA | D |
| 8. | Denver, CO | A– | 31. | Jacksonville, FL | B– | 55. | Fort Wayne, IN | C | 79. | Houston, TX | D |
| 9. | Anchorage, AK | B+ | 32. | Cleveland, OH | B– | 56. | Rochester, NY | C | 80. | St. Louis, MO | D |
| 10. | Colorado Springs, CO | B+ | 33. | Buffalo, NY | B– | 57. | Little Rock, AR | C | 81. | Providence, RI | D |
| 11. | Orlando, FL | B+ | 34. | Tampa, FL | B– | 58. | Austin, TX | C | 82. | Baltimore, MD | D |
| 12. | Richmond, VA | B+ | 35. | Burlington, VT | B– | 59. | Yonkers, NY | C | 83. | Fort Worth, TX | D– |
| 13. | Aurora, CO | B+ | 36. | San Jose, CA | B– | 60. | Seattle, WA | C | 84. | Columbus, OH | D– |
| 14. | Portland, OR | B+ | 37. | Wichita, KS | B– | 61. | Durham, NC | C | 85. | Louisville, KY | D– |
| 15. | Miami, FL | B+ | 38. | Raleigh, NC | B– | 62. | San Diego, CA | C | 86. | Albuquerque, NM | D– |
| 16. | Minneapolis, MN | B+ | 39. | Spokane, WA | B– | 63. | Kansas City, MO | C | 87. | Cincinnati, OH | D– |
| 17. | Anaheim, CA | B+ | 40. | Greensboro, NC | B– | 64. | Hartford, CT | C | 88. | Birmingham, AL | D– |
| 18. | Sioux Falls, SD | B+ | 41. | Tulsa, OK | B– | 65. | Norfolk, VA | C | 89. | Charlotte, NC | D– |
| 19. | Madison, WI | B+ | 42. | Des Moines, IA | C+ | 66. | Dallas, TX | C | 90. | Fresno, CA | F |
| 20. | Boise, ID | B+ | 43. | Baton Rouge, LA | C+ | 67. | Philadelphia, PA | C– | 91. | Atlanta, GA | F |
| 21. | Billings, MT | B+ | 44. | Manchester, NH | C+ | 68. | Modesto, CA | C– | 92. | Grand Rapids, MI | F |
| 22. | Jersey City, NJ | B+ | 45. | New York, NY | C+ | 69. | Salt Lake City, UT | C– | 93. | Arlington, TX | F |
| 23. | Tucson, AZ | B+ | 46. | St. Petersburg, FL | C+ | 70. | Toledo, OH | C– | 94. | Milwaukee, WI | F |
| 24. | Omaha, NE | B+ | 47. | San Francisco, CA | C+ | 71. | Boston, MA | D+ | 95. | Wilmington, DE | F |
| 25. | Jackson, MS | B | 48. | Oklahoma City, OK | C+ | 72. | Indianapolis, IN | D+ | 96. | Sacramento, CA | F |
| 26. | Bangor, ME | B | 49. | St. Paul, MN | C+ | 73. | Memphis, TN | D+ | 97. | Bakersfield, CA | F |
| 27. | Montgomery, AL | B | 50. | Washington, DC | C+ | 74. | Phoenix, AZ | D+ | 98. | Pittsburgh, PA | F |
| 28. | Oakland, CA | B | 51. | El Paso, TX | C+ | 75. | Newark, NJ | D+ | 99. | Chicago, IL | F |
|  |  |  | 52. | San Antonio, TX | C+ | 76. | Los Angeles, CA | D+ | 100. | Detroit, MI | F |

exhaust. After 1 hour's exposure to the fumes, the cyclists developed constricted blood vessels and showed a reduction in tPA, an enzyme that breaks down blood clots in the heart. In another study, 17 competitive cyclists were exposed to varying levels of ozone while exercising; their endurance decreased by approximately 30 percent, and their lung function, by 22 percent.

Research conducted in Finland shows an even clearer connection between dirty air and heart-attack risk. Every 2 weeks over a 6-month period, scientists monitored 45 volunteers as they exercised in simulated dirty-air conditions. Results linked both fine-particle pollution (the effluvia issuing out of smokestacks) and ultrafine-particle pollution (the invisible emissions from motor vehicles) with a threefold increase in the risk of ischemia, a potentially lethal shortage of oxygen reaching the heart muscle.

Perhaps most disturbing is how airborne toxins can harm us without triggering symptoms. In Southern California, for instance, researchers examined 107 fatal-accident victims, ranging in age from 14 to 25. Before their deaths, none reported breathing problems. Yet autopsies revealed that 86 of the deceased—80 percent—had chronic lung disease. The message to cardio devotees: Easy breathing can confer a false sense of security. "Healthy, active people tend to underestimate the harmful effects of polluted air because they don't wheeze or experience chest pain," says Henry Gong Jr., MD, an air-pollution researcher at USC. "Feeling invulnerable, they continue to exercise, putting themselves at greater risk."

**HARD** TRUTH
**Number of men who played organized basketball as kids:**
*3 in 4*

I wanted to know the kind and quantity of pollutants I was inhaling and thereby gain a rough sense of what my lungs might look like after years of unintentional abuse. My investigations took me from academic experts like Dr. McConnell to officials at the ALA, and finally, to a state DEQ air-monitoring station in my neighborhood in Portland. The station is overseen by Holly Stewart, a biologist and air-quality specialist.

A vigorous woman in her mid-forties who used to fight forest fires, Stewart takes me around the station, which lies less than a mile from the street where I run. She shows me the pumps and filters and computer monitors packed inside the 12- by 12-foot shed. She then leads me up a ladder to the flat roof, where there are more measuring devices. It's an abnormally sunny autumn day in western Oregon, with a cool breeze washing over the playground adjacent to the station and the steady din of traffic rising

from the I-5 freeway about a half mile to the west.

"Things are looking pretty good today," Stewart says, checking the nephelometer, a device that measures ozone levels. "And with that wind picking up from the east, we should stay well within the AQI [Air Quality Index] limits for the next several days."

Today's favorable air-pollution readings are characteristic of Portland, which made headlines in 2004 when results showed that the city's ozone-pollution level had decreased over the past decade, despite sharp rises in population, traffic, and economic growth. But over that same period, there was also an increase in Oregon's statewide incidence of asthma. The asthma spike is particularly pronounced among young people, who, with their high rates of physical activity, mimic the characteristics of healthy adult athletes.

The explanation for this might lie in two cutting-edge areas of inquiry: the study of pollutants other than the Big Six (ozone, carbon monoxide, nitrogen dioxide, sulfur dioxide, particulate matter, and lead) and analysis of air-pollution microclimates—i.e., localized areas in which the air is significantly dirtier than in regions as a whole. Among the former, diesel particulates—the black waste issuing primarily from trucks, buses, locomotives, and other large conveyances—are emerging as particularly worrisome.

"One of the dangers with diesel particulates is that they absorb other pollutants and

## The NBA Workout

In a recent study, Marquette University researchers surveyed 20 NBA strength-and-conditioning coaches and found that they all use plyometric training—explosive power movements—with their athletes. To improve your game, try any of these plyometric moves two or three times a week, courtesy of Aaron Nelson, CSCS, head athletic trainer for the Phoenix Suns. Do two sets of 5 to 10 repetitions, resting for 60 seconds between sets.

### Front Box Jump

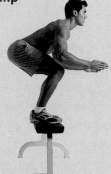

Stand facing a bench or a sturdy box (use one 12 inches high to start, and work your way up to taller boxes). Jump onto it with both feet, landing softly with your knees slightly bent. Step down and repeat.

### Side Box Jump

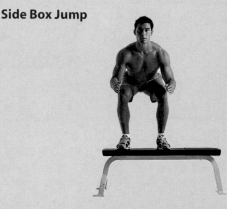

This time stand with the box or bench at your left side so you jump onto it laterally. Land softly, step down, and repeat. Perform the second set with the box at your right.

### Medicine-Ball Chest Pass

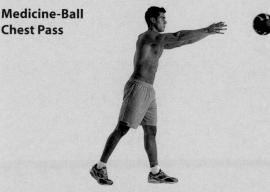

Stand facing a wall or a workout partner, and hold a medicine ball with both hands at your chest. With your feet staggered, forcefully toss the ball forward. Catch the rebound or return pass and repeat.

### Box Jump with Medicine-Ball Pass

Same as the front box jump, but hold a medicine ball in front of your chest. After you land on the box or bench and stabilize yourself, deliver a chest pass to a partner or against a wall.

# Be Seen, Not Hurt

## The best and brightest gear for exercising on a dark roadway

Early morning and early evening are the best times to run or cycle if you want to avoid inhaling tailpipe—and the worst times to avoid eating bumper. A third of all fatal pedestrian accidents occur from 6 a.m. to 9 a.m. and from 6 p.m. to 9 p.m., according to the Insurance Institute for Highway Safety. To help raise your visibility, we tested reflective and glow-in-the-dark gear and chose five shining examples. (We left out shoes, since buying a pair just because they're reflective could save your life but kill your feet.) Distances are those at which the wearer was visible to a driver on a dark street under realistic conditions.

**GoLite Fire Fly jacket** (shown above) Visibility factor: 1,150 feet

A pair of AA batteries powers the 69 inches of

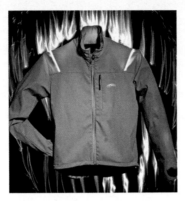

flashing LED piping stitched into this windproof and water-resistant shell. You'll be a beacon in the black. $250.

**Nathan Reflective LED gloves** Visibility factor: 900 feet

Slip them on, then tap the back of each hand to activate wide, flashing LEDs. Gloves that glow are a must for runners, since your hands are pumping at roughly eye level for drivers. $35. www.nathansports.com

**New Balance Seamless Reflective Night Vision socks** Visibility factor: 280 feet

These are one of your best defenses against becoming roadkill. The thousands of miniature glass beads that line

the cuffs will turn your ankles into hazard lights. $11.

**Brooks NightLight running hat** Visibility factor: 985 feet

You shouldn't get hit, because you'll be impossible to miss. Not only does this hat provide 360 degrees of visibility, but there's a flashing LED light on the back to ensure that you don't get rear-ended. $24. www.brooksrunning.com

**CamelBak SlipStream hydration pack** Visibility factor: 655 feet

Red and yellow reflective panels cover this 50-ounce hydration pack. These two hues raise by 20 percent the max distance at which you can be spotted, compared with other colors. $40.

**IllumiNite Alta Trac pants** Visibility factor: 360 feet

Pants with reflective stripes aren't new, but these may be the brightest. A third of their surface area is covered with reflective material. $60. www.illuminite.com

—Seth Porges

interact with them inside the body," says Fred Berman, PhD, director of the toxicology information center at Oregon Health & Science University. "They might prove to be closely linked to a variety of cancers. We're just beginning to understand the threat."

Since diesel particulates have only recently been identified as a health hazard, the EPA has yet to mandate caps on their levels. Instead, the agency issues voluntary "benchmarks." Thus, while a city like Portland can proudly point to a significant reduction in ozone, a rise in the level of diesel particulates may be canceling out the potential benefits, especially for outdoor exercisers.

"And the fact is that many things run on diesel now," Berman points out. "Trucks, locomotives—most things that move people and goods. Ironically, the conveyances doing the most to fight overall pollution—buses and recycling trucks—use diesel. Those are the vehicles spewing out the black stuff."

At the same time diesel particulates are mounting a growing hazard, scientists are recognizing that air pollutants can be meaningfully measured only on a localized basis. A neighborhood downwind from a freeway or pulp mill, for instance, might have dramatically dirtier air than someplace upwind. Yet, if the downwind area is factored in with more favorably positioned neighborhoods, the overall measurements might indicate that the city has healthy air.

"Where do we tend to build our schools and colleges?" asks Dr. McConnell. "Next to busy streets and intersections, due to convenience and the fact that land close to traffic is usually cheaper. When people run on the track at those schools or play tennis or swim laps in the outdoor pool, they are breathing much dirtier air than what's listed in the newspaper."

Despite the darkening diesel cloud, spiking asthma rates, and proliferation of scary studies, all the experts assure me that, on balance, I've been doing myself more good than harm with my daily run. "By all means, keep running," Dr. Gong says, "but for goodness' sake, stop running along that busy street. If you run just a block away, your risk will be significantly lower."

Dr. Gong also suggests exercising early in the day, when diesel particulates, ozone, and other air pollutants are at their lowest levels,

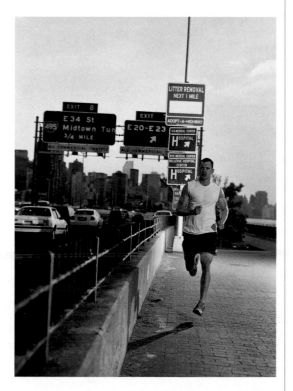

## Cycle Right

Flat roads are inviting, but you benefit the most from a cycling workout if you vary the terrain. According to a study in the *Journal of Sports Sciences*, the exertion required in a 3-mile hill climb equals 24 miles on the flats. And half a mile of off-road biking equals a mile on the road. Make sure you prepare your quads, glutes, and hamstrings for the added burn. In the gym, try these exercises from Robert dos Remedios, CSCS, director of speed, strength, and conditioning at the College of the Canyons in Santa Clarita, California.

### Split Squat

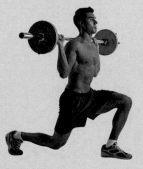

Hold a barbell across the back of your shoulders. Place your right foot back. Keeping your torso upright, lower your body until your left thigh is parallel to the floor. Pause, then push yourself back up. Perform three or four sets of 8 to 10 repetitions on each leg.

### Swiss-Ball Leg Curl

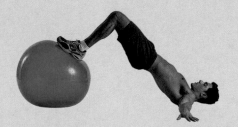

Start with your upper back and shoulders on the floor, arms to the sides, and calves on a Swiss ball. Raise your hips and pull the ball until your feet are flat against it. Pause, then push it away until your legs are straight. Do 5 to 10 repetitions.

### Drop Lunge

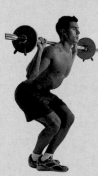

Holding a barbell across your shoulders, step back with your right foot and place it outside your left foot. Bend your knees, lowering your body a few inches. Push back up to the starting position and repeat with your other leg. Do 8 to 10 repetitions with each leg.

### Jump Landing

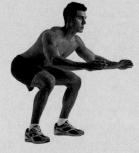

Stand with your feet at shoulder width on a semisoft surface, like a rubber mat. Jump straight up and land on the front two-thirds of your feet, with your heels just off the floor, knees bent, shoulders slightly forward, and butt and hips back. Do five jumps.

or after nightfall, when traffic abates. Ozone forms when sunlight reacts with automobile and industrial emissions, so it accumulates to significant levels by about 11 a.m. and peaks around 3 p.m. (After sunset, ozone can no longer form, so the concentration decreases.) By the same token, ozone levels are significantly higher during the sunnier months. Some experts, especially in notoriously smoggy cities such as Los Angeles and Houston, recommend tailoring training cycles to the season.

Other commonsense mitigating tactics include standing in front of the line of traffic at stoplights and busy intersections, as well as skipping your outdoor workout if the AQI exceeds 70. (Go to www.airnow.gov and click on "Local Air Quality Conditions and Forecasts.") Consuming fruits and vegetables high in vitamin C, such as peaches and red peppers, stimulates production of glutathione, a liver enzyme that helps prevent free-radical damage in the lungs. And just a few places down the antioxidant alphabet is vitamin E, which can also help repel radicals.

The most effective and logical response to air pollution, of course, is to drive less, consume less, and thereby reduce what you are, directly and indirectly, pumping into your city's atmosphere. No one is greener in this regard than bicycle commuters—and no one, ironically, breathes more traffic exhaust.

"I'm aware of the 'superpolluters' when I'm riding," says Scott Bricker, policy director for the Oregon Bicycle Transportation Alliance, an advocacy group. "When I ride behind one, I go into this thin, shallow style of nose breathing. That gets me through the worst of it. At least I like to believe it does."

Back at the air-quality station in Portland, the wind shifts, and the freeway din grows louder. Stewart opens the top of a PM10

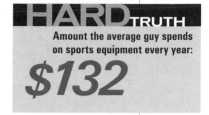

particulate sampler, a device that measures diesel particulates, and extracts a filter clogged with black soot. She explains that this grime has accumulated over just a 48-hour period. I recall all the miles I have logged along Fremont Avenue.

"Actually, this doesn't look so bad," Stewart says. She points to my black jacket. "Some cold days, when people have their fireplaces going, or during temperature inversions in the summer, it shows up darker than your jacket."

She replaces the filter, her expression thoughtful. "Besides, when you're talking about air pollution and exercise, it's often what you can't see that gets you."

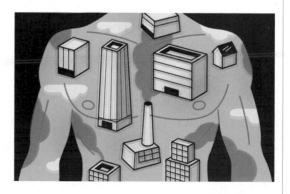

## Major League Muscle

Report to spring training—and get ripped by summer. In a recent study published in the *Journal of Strength and Conditioning Research,* Marquette University researchers surveyed 21 MLB strength coaches and found that these are their five essential exercises (in order of importance) for building muscle. Include them in your starting lineup.

### Squat

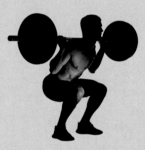

Stand holding a bar across the back of your shoulders. Keeping your back straight, lower your body as if sitting back in a chair, until your thighs are parallel to the floor. Pause, then press yourself back up.

### Lunge

Stand holding a pair of dumbbells, arms at your sides. Step forward with your right foot and lower your body until your front thigh is parallel to the floor. Push back up and repeat with your other foot.

### Lat Pulldown (Or Pullup)

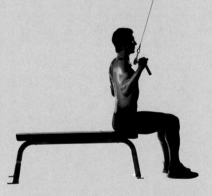

Sit at a lat-pulldown station and grab the bar overhead with your palms facing forward. Keeping your back straight, pull the bar to the top of your chest. Pause, then let the bar rise back above your head.

### Dumbbell Row

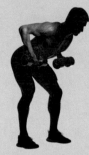

Stand holding a pair of dumbbells in front of your thighs. Bend forward at the waist until your torso is almost parallel to the floor. Pull the weights to the bottom of your rib cage, then slowly lower them.

### External Rotation

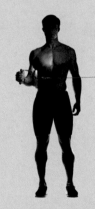

Place a towel under your right armpit and stand with a cable station at your left. Grab the handle with your right hand and rotate your arm to 2 o'clock, then return it. Repeat with your left hand.

# Get Big This Season

**T**his workout is specially designed to help your sports performance. Perform these five exercises, and your workout will take flight.

"These exercises help you handle more weight," says Jon Crosby, CSCS. Perform three sets of the lunge, resting 30 seconds between sets. Then do the Swiss-ball press and the Swiss-ball Y as a superset—that is, back-to-back, without rest—and do the chinup and leg curl as another superset. Rest 30 seconds after supersets. Do three sets of each pair.

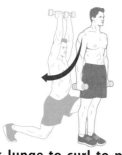

**Back lunge to curl to press:** Stand holding dumbbells at arm's length, palms facing your thighs. Step back with one leg and bend at the knees until your front thigh is parallel to the floor. Now do a curl and an overhead press, keeping your palms facing in. Lower the weights and step back up to the starting position. Repeat, this time stepping back with your other leg. Do six reps with each leg.

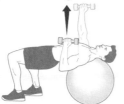

**Swiss-ball single-arm dumbbell press:** Grab a dumbbell with your right hand and lie on a Swiss ball so your head, shoulders, and upper back are in contact with the ball. Hold the weight at your shoulder, palm facing in. Squeeze your glutes and raise your hips so your body is straight from knees to ears. This is the starting position. Press the weight up, then lower it. Do eight reps, then switch to your left hand and repeat.

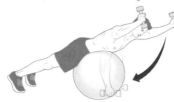

**Swiss-ball Y:** Holding a light dumbbell in each hand, lie facedown on a Swiss ball with your belly and pelvis on the ball, your toes on the floor, and your heels against a wall. Keep your palms in. With your legs straight and your core tight, raise your arms forward and out 45 degrees until they're in line with your torso. Lower the weights slowly and repeat for a total of 10 to 12 reps.

**Negative chinup:** Grab a chinup bar with an underhand grip (palms toward you), your hands about shoulder-width apart. Pull yourself up until the bar is below your chin, then slowly lower yourself for a count of four, until your arms are straight. Aim for four to six reps.

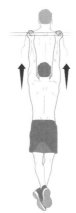

**Swiss-ball leg curl:** Lie on the floor with your calves on a Swiss ball and your arms at your sides. Squeeze your glutes to raise your hips off the floor so your body is in a straight line from your shoulders to your ankles. Pause for a second, then bend your legs to roll the ball toward your butt. Straighten your legs to roll the ball back out away from you, then lower your body to the floor. Do 10 to 12 reps.

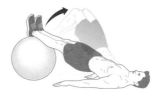

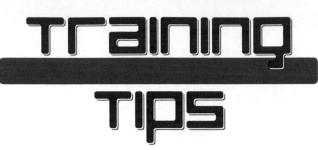

# Training Tips

**Trainers at my gym talk about working the "posterior chain." What is it?**

The posterior chain is a brawny team of muscles that includes those in your lower back, your glutes, your hamstrings, and your calf muscles. They're among the most powerful, yet most men ignore them because they can't see them in the mirror. Don't be one of those guys. Strengthening the posterior chain will help just about every part of your game, whether you want to jump higher, run faster, or change directions quicker. While these muscles can be addressed individually with isolation lifts, I suggest you focus on compound exercises like squats, deadlifts, back extensions, and jumps that promote intermuscular teamwork. Incorporate three sets of each exercise into your weekly routine, and see if you don't notice a difference.

**My stomach feels sore. Could it be a sports hernia like the one that sidelined Donovan McNabb?**

All hernias involve a breach in the abdominal wall. But sports hernias, which are common in twisting-and-turning sports such as football, ice hockey, and soccer, are harder to detect because they occur in the inguinal crease, alongside the lower abdomen, and seldom feature a protruding mass. They typically begin with a slow, dull ache and can include groin and testicle pain. Changing direction quickly, bending, and sneezing can all make the pain worse. Surgery is common, so prevention is the best medicine here. Strengthen the pelvic muscles, especially the hip flexors, to shore up your defenses.

**How can I throw farther?**

Try the cable wood chop in explosive fashion. Training your body to rotate more explosively through your core can add distance and velocity to your throw. You'll also protect your shoulder from injury, says Mike Gough, CSCS.

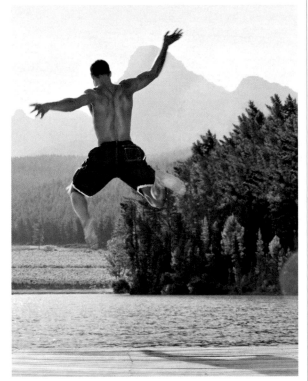

**Working the muscles of your backside will put more spring in your step.**

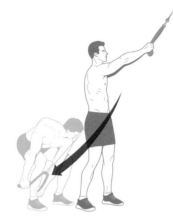

A cable wood chop, performed explosively, can help you throw the deep ball.

Attach a rope handle to a high-pulley cable. Stand with your left side toward the stack and your feet slightly more than shoulder-width apart. Grab the rope with both hands. Keeping your arms straight and your abs tight, bend your knees as you forcefully pull the handle down and across your body toward your right lower leg. Reverse the motion and finish your reps before switching sides. Do two or three sets of five to seven repetitions.

**Cycling makes my hips feel tight and inflexible. How can I keep them loose?**

Cycling causes your pelvis to tilt forward, pulling your glutes out of alignment and forcing you to rely too much on your hamstrings, quadriceps, and lower back. Since your hips act as a brace for your lower back, your back compensates by flexing, extending, and rotating. Release your tight hip flexors and retrain your glutes by performing these lower-body exercises twice a week. For each move, do 10 reps per side.

Active hip-flexor stretch (side-lying): Lie on your left side with your heels near your butt and your knees at waist level. Place your left hand on your left knee. Grab your right ankle, flex your foot toward your knee, then rotate your right leg downward. Pause, return, and repeat for 10 reps. Switch sides.

Back lunge (with side bend): From a standing position, step back with your left foot and bend your knees 90 degrees. At the same time, reach overhead with your left hand and bend your torso to your right. Then push back up.

Glute bridge (single leg): Lie on your back, knees bent 90 degrees and feet on the floor. Lift one leg off the floor and straighten it. Squeeze your glutes to lift your hips. Lower them.

**How can I boost my vertical leap?**

Your quads and hamstrings are your primary thrusters. But it's equally important to awaken and strengthen assisting muscles—your calves, the muscles around your hips, your glutes. Here's one exercise to get you started. It boosts mobility and improves your ability to generate power.

Forward lunge (forearm to instep): This exercise loosens tight hip flexors and ankles and powers up your calves. It boosts mobility and improves your ability to generate power.

Take a large step forward with your left leg into the lunge

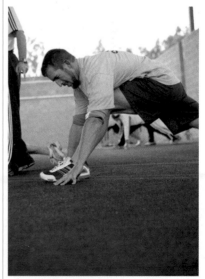

**Go low to fly high.**

position. Bend down and place your left elbow against the instep of your left foot while keeping your right knee off the floor. Pause, then place your left hand outside your left foot and your right hand on the floor for balance. Now push your hips toward the ceiling and lift the toes of your left foot toward your shin. Finally, stand up and stride into the next lunge.

## How can I hop without the hurt?

We tested two conventional ways of keeping your ankles safe: Fifteen men wore either athletic tape or a lace-up ankle brace on two separate occasions and played hoops for 15 minutes. A certified athletic trainer taped the men's ankles, but the tape still loosened as they played. The verdict: The men jumped, moved, and felt better wearing the brace.

If you've injured an ankle in the past, brace yourself before you take to the courts. In the weight room, strengthen your calves with calf raises to protect your ankles, and try the NBA workout on page 331.

## Ice baths look so cold–there must be a reason football players always use them. Right?

The cold dunk isn't bunk: Cryotherapy can ease inflammation and pain after high-intensity exercise. A 2004 study even showed that cold-water immersion after a high-intensity session helped cyclists bounce back better the next day.

Taking the plunge might be worth it if you're in training camp, but I'd suggest light exercise the next day to improve bloodflow to sore body parts. Sore legs? Try an easy jog, or hop on an exercise bike. If your upper body aches, work out the sore muscles with about 20 percent of the amount you can lift one time, performing

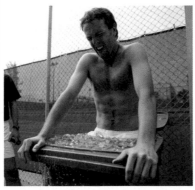

**A site for sore thighs.**

two sets of 20 repetitions. Researchers at the University of Massachusetts found that a similar method significantly reduced markers of muscle damage.

## Does it matter what color the lens is on my ski goggles?

Sure does. Stay away from blue. Research shows that it increases your risk of developing age-related macular degeneration, meaning you could go blind. Blue light triggers the release of harmful free radicals in the retina, says Janet Sparrow, PhD, a professor of ophthalmic science at Columbia University medical center. Go for yellow or amber, which filters out blue light best, she says. Amber lenses are also best for seeing the shadows of moguls in fog. Other tints skiers swear by: rose for low light and dark green in bright light. Mirror coatings are okay but won't block glare.

# Credits

**Cover Photograph**
© Beth Bischoff

**Interior Photographs**
© AP Photo/Fabian Bimmer: page 324
© AP Photo/Matthew S. Gunby: page 140
© AP Photo/Scott Martin: page 137
© AP Photo/Sergey Ponomarev: page 310
© Banana Stock: pages 141 (middle top), 144 (right), 200
© Ben Baker: page 45
© Big Cheese Photo: page 75
© Beth Bischoff: pages 3, 60, 62, 63, 64, 65, 84, 101, 102, 103, 104, 105, 106, 138, 139, 144 (left), 154, 164, 166, 167, 168, 174, 175, 180, 181, 183, 186, 187, 190, 191, 193, 194, 195, 197, 204, 205, 206, 207, 208, 209, 212, 213, 214, 215, 216, 217, 219, 220, 221, 224, 228, 229, 230, 231, 232, 233, 234, 235, 237, 238, 239, 240, 241, 244, 245, 246, 247, 248, 249, 250, 252, 253, 254, 255, 256, 257, 258 (right), 261 (left), 284 (exercises), 286, 287 (bottom left), 288 (bottom), 289, 290, 291, 292, 293, 295, 302, 303, 304, 305, 314, 315, 317, 318, 331, 334, 336
© Blend Images: page 74
© Bob Carey: page 159
© Jamie Chard: page 287 (top)
© Lynda Churilla: page 143 (right)
© Corbis: page 146
© Bettmann/Corbis: page 107
© Pier Nicola D'Amico: pages 86, 88, 89, 91, 92, 93, 95, 96, 98, 99
© Michael Darter: pages 110, 113, 116
© Digital Vision: pages 14, 56, 145, 273, 284 (soccer player), 287 (bottom right), 297, 338
© Gallo Images: page 296
© Morgan Mazzoni/Stone/Getty Images: page 281
© Agence Zoom/Getty Images Sport: page 308 (left)
© Tom Hauck/Getty Images Sport: page 127 (far left)
© Doug Pensinger/Getty Images Sport: page 134
© Clive Rose/Getty Images Sport: page 340
© Jeff Topping/Getty Images Sport: page 129
© Patrik Giardino: 264, 266, 268, 271, 272, 285
© Mark Hanauer: pages 312, 313
© Terry Heffernan: pages 54, 59
© Image Source: page 259
© Ingram Publishing: page 280
© Brian Klutch: page 260
© Robert Landau: pages 50, 51, 52, 53

Courtesy of © Alexander Ruesche?EPA/Landov: page 327
© Henry Leutwyler: page 80
© Steven Lippman: pages 100, 117, 118, 119, 120, 122, 123
© Benjamin Lowy: pages 124, 127 (top, Andreu Swasey, bottom), 130, 131
© Scott McDermott: page 189
© Jens Mortensen: page 283
© Sean Murphy: pages 136, 339 (right)
© Photodisc: pages 76 (left), 77 (left), 258 (left), 319
© Photographer's Choice: page 288 (top)
© Carrie Prophett: page 83
© Purestock: page 78
© Tom Rafalovich: page 222 (left)
© Reuters/Alexandra Beier: page 311
© Jennifer Rocholl: pages 170, 172, 173
© Rodale Images: pages 43, 69, 332
© John Hamel/Rodale Images: pages 76 (right), 142
© Mitch Mandel/Rodale Images: pages 5, 7, 21, 22, 23, 24, 25, 26, 28, 29, 30, 31, 32, 33, 34, 35, 36, 37, 38, 39, 40, 143 (left), 199, 202, 300
© Margaret Skrovanek/Rodale Images: page 141 (left, middle bottom)
© Embry Rucker: page 121
© Gregg Segal: page 108
© Jonathan Selkowitz: pages 306, 308 (right)
© Piotr Sikora: pages 177, 210, 226, 242
Courtesy of © Space Cycle: page 149
© Justin Steele: page 326, 333
© Stockbyte: pages x, 2, 77 (right), 141 (right), 262, 298, 316
© ThinkStock: page 10
© Tim Turner: pages 66, 71
© Al Messerschmidt/wireimage.com: page 127 (Reggie Wayne)
© James Worrell: pages 44, 47, 48

**Interior Illustrations**
© Samuel Velasco/5W Infographic: page 58
© Harry Campbell: page 328, 335
© Digital Vision: page 198
© 3D4Medical.com/Getty Images: page 320
© Kurt Ketchum: pages 9, 12
© Mika Grondahl/Lumi Inc. Illustration: page 321
© Josh McKible/McKibillo: pages 161, 162
© Kagan McLeod: pages 73, 151, 152, 156, 157, 222 (right), 223, 261 (right), 337, 339 (left)
© Ben Hasler/NB Illustration: page 275
© Rodale Images: page 128

# Index

Boldface page references indicate photographs. <u>Underscored</u> references indicate boxed text.